ANESTHESIOLOGY AND PAIN MANAGEMENT

DEVELOPMENTS IN
CRITICAL CARE MEDICINE AND ANESTHESIOLOGY

Volume 29

The titles published in this series are listed at the end of this volume.

ANESTHESIOLOGY AND PAIN MANAGEMENT

edited by

T.H. STANLEY AND M.A. ASHBURN

Department of Anesthesiology,
The University of Utah Medical School,
Salt Lake City, Utah, U.S.A.

SPRINGER-SCIENCE+BUSINESS MEDIA, B.V.

Library of Congress Cataloging-in-Publication Data

Anesthesiology and pain management / edited by T.H. Stanley and M.A. Ashburn.
p. cm. -- (Developments in critical care, medicine, and anesthesiology ; v. 29)
"Presentations of the 39th Annual Postgraduate Course in Anesthesiology which took place at the Cliff Conference Center in Snowbird, Utah, February 18-22, 1994"--Pref.
ISBN 978-0-7923-2662-5 ISBN 978-94-011-0816-4 (eBook)
DOI 10.1007/978-94-011-0816-4
1. Anesthesia--Congresses. 2. Pain--Congresses. 3. Analgesia--Congresses. I. Stanley, Theodore H. (Theodore Henry), 1940- II. Ashburn, M. A. (Michael A.) III. Postgraduate Course in Anesthesiology (39th : 1994 : Snowbird, Utah) IV. Series: Developments in critical care medicine and anaesthesiology ; 29.
[DNLM: 1. Pain--therapy--congresses. 2. Anesthetics--therapeutic use--congresses. 3. Analgesics--therapeutic use--congresses. 4. Palliative Treatment--congresses. W1 DE997VRL v.29 1994 / WL 704 A5791 1994]
RD78.4.A543 1994
617.9'6--dc20
DNLM/DLC
for Library of Congress 93-44398

ISBN 978-0-7923-2662-5

Printed on acid-free paper

TABLE OF CONTENTS

Preface

Theodore H. Stanley, M.D.

Anesthesiology and Pain Management contains the Refresher Course manuscripts of the presentations of the 39th Annual Postgraduate Course in Anesthesiology which took place at The Cliff Conference Center in Snowbird, Utah, February 18-22, 1994. The chapters reflect new data concepts within the general framework of "pain research and basic science," "clinical topics in pain management." The purposes of the textbook are to 1) act as a reference for the anesthesiologists attending the meeting, and 2) serve as a vehicle to bring many of the latest concepts in anesthesiology to others within a short time of the formal presentation. Each chapter is a brief but sharply focused glimpse of the interests in anesthesia expressed at the conference. This book and its chapters should not be considered complete treatises on the subjects addressed but rather attempts to summarize the most salient points. This textbook is the twelfth in a continuing series documenting the proceedings of the Postgraduate Course in Salt Lake City. We hope that this and the past and future volumes reflect the rapid and continuing evolution of anesthesiology in the late twentieth century.

LIST OF CONTRIBUTORS

Allan I. Basbaum, Ph.D.
Department of Anatomy, University of California, San Francisco, California, U.S.A.

Michael J. Cousins, M.B., B.S., M.D. (SYD), F.R.C.A., F.A.N.Z.C.A.
Department of Anaesthesia and Pain Management, University of Sydney, Royal North Shore Hospital , St. Leonards, NSW, Australia

Jørgen B. Dahl, M.D.
Department of Surgical Gastroenterology, Hvidovre University Hospital, Hvidovre , Denmark

Ronald Dubner, D.D.S., Ph.D.
Neurobiology and Anesthesiology Branch, National Institute of Dental Research, National Institutes of Health, Bethesda, Maryland, U.S.A.

Perry G. Fine, M.D.
Department of Anesthesiology, University of Utah School of Medicine, Salt Lake City, Utah, U.S.A.

Kathleen M. Foley, M.D.
Chief, Pain Service, Department of Neurology, Memorial Sloan-Kettering Cancer Center, New York City, New York, U.S.A.

Brian Fredman, M.B., B.Ch.
Department of Anesthesiology and Pain Management, The University of Texas Southwestern Medical Center at Dallas, Dallas, Texas, U.S.A.

Bradford D. Hare, M.D., Ph.D.
Department of Anesthesiology, University of Utah School of Medicine, Salt Lake City, Utah, U.S.A.

Girish P. Joshi, M.D., F.F.A.R.C.S.I.
Department of Anesthesiology and Pain Management, The University of Texas Southwestern Medical Center at Dallas, Dallas, Texas, U.S.A.

Henrik Kehlet, M.D., Ph.D.
Department of Surgical Gastroenterology, Hvidovre University Hospital, Hvidovre, Denmark

Donald H. Lambert, Ph.D., M.D.
Brigham and Women's Hospital, and Harvard Medical School, Boston, Massachusetts, U.S.A.

Laurence E. Mather, M.Sc., Ph.D., F.A.N.Z.C.A.
Department of Anaesthesia and Pain Management, University of Sydney, Royal North Shore Hospital , St. Leonards, NSW, Australia

Terence M. Murphy, M.D.
Department of Anesthesiology, University of Washington School of Medicine, Seattle, Washington, U.S.A.

L. Brian Ready, M.D.
Acute Pain Service, University of Washington School of Medicine, Seattle, Washington, U.S.A

P. J. Siddall, M.B., B.S., Ph.D. (SYD)
Department of Anaesthesia and Pain Management, University of Sydney, Royal North Shore Hospital, St. Leonards, NSW, Australia

Neil Smart, M.B., Ch.B., F.R.C.A.
Department of Anaesthesia and Pain Management, University of Sydney, Royal North Shore Hospital, St. Leonards, NSW, Australia

James B. Streisand, M.D.
Department of Anesthesiology, University of Utah School of Medicine, Salt Lake City, Utah, U.S.A.

Donald C. Tyler, M.D.
Department of Anesthesiology, Children's Hospital and Medical Center, Seattle, Washington, U.S.A.

Paul F. White, Ph.D., M.D.
Department of Anesthesiology and Pain Management, The University of Texas Southwestern Medical Center at Dallas, Dallas, Texas, U.S.A.

Deborah White, B.Sc., Ph.D.
Department of Anaesthesia and Pain Management, University of Sydney, Royal North Shore Hospital, St. Leonards, NSW, Australia

Alon P. Winnie, M.D.
Department of Anesthesiology and Critical Care, Cook County Hospital, Chicago, Illinois, U.S.A.

MECHANISMS OF SUBSTANCE P-MEDIATED NOCICEPTION AND OPIOID-MEDIATED ANTINOCICEPTION

A. I. Basbaum

INTRODUCTION

Since a detailed review of the organization of the primary afferent input to the dorsal horn has recently been published (1), the purpose of my discussion will be to highlight three areas in which considerable new information is available about pain processing and pain control mechanisms. Specifically, I will discuss some new perspectives on the problem of the processing of the afferent input at the level of the dorsal horn, mechanisms of opioid regulation of nociceptive processing and new studies of the factors that contribute to the development of opiate tolerance.

Primary Afferent Neurotransmitters

Anatomical studies have demonstrated that unmyelinated primary afferent fibers contain a variety of neuroactive substances. In general, there is coexistence of glutamate and a variety of neuropeptides (2). Glutamate is released by high intensity peripheral stimulation and probably mediates the fast depolarization of dorsal horn nociresponsive neurons. The receptors through which glutamate exerts its effects are, however, rather complicated (3,4). Two types of receptors predominate, a non-NMDA and a NMDA receptor. NMDA refers to N-methyl-D-aspartate, a compound that mimics the action of glutamate, but which is not the endogenous ligand. The non-NMDA receptor almost certainly mediates the short-term activation of second order neurons by small diameter primary afferent fibers. Under resting conditions, the NMDA receptor is plugged by magnesium ions. These, however, are removed

T. H. Stanley and M. A. Ashburn (eds.), Anesthesiology and Pain Management, 1–17.

when the cell is depolarized, resulting in additional action of primary afferent derived glutamate at the NMDA site. This results in an influx of Ca^{2+} into the cells, which in turn, results in many long term changes in the cell, many of which involve complex enzymatic changes and induction of various genes. Wind-up, the phenomenon whereby repetitive stimulation results in increasing discharges of the dorsal horn neuron, appears to be mediated by the NMDA receptor (5,6).

In addition to glutamate, which is localized in agranular vesicles, C fiber terminals contain a variety of neuroactive peptides, including Substance P, neurokinin A (NKA) and calcitonin gene-related peptide (CGRP). These peptides are located in dense core vesicles within the same terminal that stores glutamate. Electron microscopic immunogold studies, in fact, demonstrated that the same dense core vesicle contains several different peptides. There is considerable evidence that the peptides, in particular, Substance P, enhance the action of the released glutamate, thus contributing to long term changes in the dorsal horn neurons, changes that are particularly manifest when there is intense stimulation of nociceptive primary afferents, or when there is persistent injury (7).

Although the differential contribution of the different peptides is not clear, recent studies have provided some very interesting information concerning the targets of neuropeptides. The analysis requires a brief discussion of the receptors through which the primary afferent peptides interact. Substance P is a member of the tachykinin family, which includes NKA and NKB. These peptides interact with the neurokinin receptors, several of which have been identified. Substance P preferentially binds to the NK-1 receptor, NKA to the NK-2 receptor, and NKB (which is not found in primary afferents) to the NK-3 receptor (8).

Of great interest are studies which compare the distribution of Substance P immunoreactivity in the spinal cord and the distribution of its putative receptor, the NK-1 tachykinin receptor; these studies reveal considerable mismatch. Early studies used labelled SP to identify the distribution of the SP binding sites/receptors. More recently we have mapped the distribution of the NK-1 receptor using an antibody directed against the NK-1 receptor. This approach revealed several important aspects of the localization of this receptor. First, it is most heavily concentrated in lamina I of the dorsal horn, which, of course, contains high concentrations of SP. On the other hand, there was minimal receptor labelling in the substantia gelatinosa (SG), despite the fact that the SG also contains high concentrations of SP. Another important feature of the NK-1 labelling is that it was exclusively on cell bodies and dendrites. *Indeed the entire surface of the neuron was labelled, indicating that that entire neuron is a possible target of released SP.*

We also found several well labelled neurons in lamina III. Some of these contained dendrites that extended dorsally up to lamina I. These latter neurons were unexpected because neurons in lamina III receive large diameter primary afferent input and predominantly respond to non-noxious stimulation; if they receive an input from small diameter SP containing primary afferents, it is likely that these neurons would respond to noxious stimulation. Other SP-receptor laden neurons were found in the region of the central canal and in the intermediolateral cell column. They almost certainly contribute to the regulation of autonomic outflow.

Finding mismatch at the light microscopic level only provides a clue to what is happening at the level of the synapse. To address the peptide receptor mismatch at the EM level, we used a double label approach to co-localize the peptide and the receptor at the synaptic level. This study established that the receptor is indeed located over the entire surface of the neuron. Large patches of the neuron are covered with receptor; these are broken by small area of membrane that did not contain receptor. *Importantly, receptor patches were only occasionally apposed by synapses and only some of these were SP-immunoreactive.* The presence of the receptor in regions that did not contain synapses suggests that the receptor is targeted by peptide that diffuses from the site of release. If that is true, it would indicate that the co-released neurotransmitters can target different neurons.

With a view to addressing the distribution of released peptide, Duggan and colleagues have developed a very interesting technique. It involves coating glass microelectrodes with antibodies directed against the peptide of interest. The electrode is inserted into the spinal cord and then a particular stimulus is administered. If the peptide is released in the region of the electrode, it will bind to the antibody. To identify the site of binding, the electrode is dipped in a solution of labelled peptide. That region of the electrode which does not bind the labelled peptide identifies the site of release in the spinal cord. Using this approach, it was demonstrated that the release of SP is focused in the substantia gelatinosa, precisely where the C fiber terminals are concentrated and where immunocytochemistry reveals the greatest concentration of SP terminals (9). These results are, therefore, expected. Completely unexpected results, however, were revealed when these authors monitored the release of NKA, a peptide that is made on the same precursor as SP, coexists with SP in primary afferent terminals, and binds the NK-2 receptor. In contrast to the localized distribution of SP in the substantia gelatinosa, *NKA was found throughout the dorsal horn,* despite the fact that it clearly is located in primary afferents that terminate within the superficial dorsal horn, as does SP (10). The authors concluded that NKA is released and can then diffuse considerable distances to act on neurons that are not innervated by NKA containing synapses.

Since the mechanism of termination of action of peptides does not involve a reuptake system (as exists for monoamines), but rather involves enzymatic degradation, the authors hypothesized that NKA is not a substrate for the peptidase that normally degrades Substance P. To test the hypothesis, the following experiment was performed. They used a noxious stimulus in the presence of an enzyme inhibitor (11). Under these conditions, they found that the distribution of Substance P increased dramatically, indicating that regulation of the enzyme is a major factor in determining the distribution of released peptides. Interestingly, the other peptide which co-occurs with SP in the dense core vesicle, i.e., CGRP, has been shown to decrease activity of the enzyme. This indicates that a given primary afferent terminal can indirectly regulate the targets acted upon by the transmitters that are released from that terminal.

The possibility that a primary afferent peptide can diffuse large distances is, in fact, not surprising. Many earlier studies had used recovery from the spinal cord CSF to monitor the effects of stimulation (12). Since SP is most likely derived from terminals located in the superficial dorsal horn, the peptide must have diffused a considerable distance to reach the CSF. This indicates that under *physiological* conditions, i.e., not merely when an enzyme inhibitor is added, a primary afferent peptide can diffuse from its site of release.

Differential Contribution of Spinal Cord Nociresponsive Neurons to Pain Behavior

Although anatomical and electrophysiological studies have identified the location of neurons that receive small diameter primary afferent input and respond to noxious stimulation, these studies cannot identify whether any particular subpopulation of nociresponsive neurons is more critical to the generation of pain behavior. For example, nociresponsive neurons are located in laminae I and outer II of the superficial dorsal horn, in lamina V and in the ventral horn. The neurons in these different regions do not have identical receptive field properties. Thus, marginal neurons, many of which project to supraspinal targets (in particular, the parabrachial region of the dorsolateral pons), typically have very small receptive fields and many are nociceptive specific, i.e., respond exclusively to noxious stimulation. Neurons in lamina V typically have large receptive field sizes and respond to both non-noxious and noxious stimuli. Many of these belong to the class of wide dynamic range neurons; they project to several supraspinal targets, including the thalamus. Finally, the neurons in laminae VII and VIII of the ventral horn typically have much larger, often whole body, receptive fields with complicated inhibitory and excitatory components. These neurons have a diverse projection, including the reticular formation of the medulla, pons and midbrain, as well as the intralaminar nuclei of the thalamus. To determine the differential contribution of these different classes of nociresponsive neurons to pain behavior, it would be necessary to correlate the firing of single cells with pain behavior. A few studies have attempted this approach, however, the sample of cells is very small. In the primate trigeminal nucleus caudalis, the trigeminal homologue of the spinal cord dorsal horn, evidence suggests that the firing of neurons in the region of lamina V, rather than lamina I, correlates best with pain behavior (13).

Our laboratory has used a different approach to monitor the activity of neurons and to correlate their activity with pain behavior. Specifically, it has been demonstrated that the c-fos proto-oncogene, the cellular homologue of a viral oncogene, is induced in neurons that are active. By staining for the protein product of this gene, it is possible to identify large populations of active neurons (14,15). The spinal cord has proven to be a particularly useful place to use this technique because the basal levels of expression of the gene are quite low. Indeed, basal expression is largely confined to the nucleus proprius, laminae III and IV, which is consistent with the fact that neurons in these regions respond to non-noxious stimuli, that, of course, predominate in the awake freely-moving rat. A great advantage of the fos technique is that the studies can be performed in awake animals so that the behavior of the animals (e.g., pain score) can be evaluated and correlated with the pattern of fos expression.

The procedure is to stimulate a rat with a noxious stimulus (we typically use hindpaw injection of formalin) and then monitor the rat's behavior for one hour. The rat is then anesthetized and perfused with aldehydes so that the spinal cord can be immunostained with antibodies directed against the fos protein. The fos protein is located in the nucleus, where it presumably acts to regulate transcription of many, as yet undefined, gene populations (16). Our first studies demonstrated that different noxious stimuli evoke distinct patterns of fos expression in the lumbar spinal cord. The most dense staining is in the superficial laminae, I and II. Many labelled cells are also found in the region of the neck of the dorsal horn, lamina V, and in more ventral regions, laminae VII and VIII. These results are, of course, consistent with the electrophysiological studies which identified single neurons and provided confirmation of the utility of the fos approach to identifying populations of active neurons. Importantly, in other studies we demonstrated that the numbers of fos-immunoreactive neurons correlates very highly with the pain score obtained in the formalin test, a test that purportedly best models tonic/persistent pain characteristic of clinical pain states (17).

Mechanisms of Opioid Analgesia

Having revealed these patterns of noxious stimulus evoked c-fos expression, we next evaluated the effects of analgesic doses of opioids, administered either systemically, intracerebroventricularly or intrathecally. Before addressing these results, I will very briefly review information on the analgesic action of opioids. Opioids (which includes exogenous opiate analgesics, e.g., morphine and the endogenous opioids)exert their analgesic effect through interactions with opioid receptors located at several sites in the central nervous system. After systemic injection, it has been hypothesized that opioids bind to receptors in the midbrain periaqueductal gray, which activates a descending inhibitory control system that blocks the firing of nociresponsive neurons in the spinal cord (18). In part, this inhibition is mediated via connections with serotonergic and noradrenergic cell groups in the brainstem.

Opioids, of course, also act directly at the level of the spinal cord (19). Two major targets have been implicated. First, opioid receptors are located on dorsal horn neurons, providing a basis for an opioid-mediated postsynaptic inhibition of the firing of these neurons (20) There is also a high concentration of opioid receptors on the terminals of small diameter primary afferent fibers (20). Although there is considerable evidence that opioids presynaptically block the release of neurotransmitters (e.g., substance P) from these afferents (12,21,22), the differential contribution of pre- and postsynaptic opioid inhibition to spinal analgesia has not been determined.

In addition, to the supraspinal and spinal sites of opioid action, there is recent experimental and clinical evidence that opioids can exert an analgesic action in the periphery, presumably via an action on the peripheral terminals of small diameter afferents. Opioid receptors are synthesized in the cell bodies of small diameter afferents and then are transported both centrally and peripherally. Several laboratories demonstrated that injection of small amounts of morphine into the periphery can produce analgesia under conditions of inflammation (23-25). Equivalent doses of morphine are without effect when administered into the brain.

Of particular interest is the observation that the peripheral analgesic action of opioids is *only* demonstrable under conditions of inflammation or after tissue is sensitized, for example, with prostaglandins (24). Stein and colleagues hypothesize that under conditions of inflammation there is an up-regulation of opioid receptor synthesis by the cell bodies of small diameter afferents which are then transported to the periphery (26), where they can be acted upon by local injection of morphine to produce analgesia. The most interesting question is whether there is an endogenous opioid ligand that acts upon these receptors under conditions of inflammation. Immunohistochemical studies provide evidence that a variety of inflammatory and immunocompetent cells synthesize endorphins (27,28). Since these cells are attracted to a site of injury, it is likely that they provide the endogenous ligand that normally operates to reduce analgesia. Consistent with this hypothesis, the authors reported that naloxone decreased thresholds in the inflamed paw (below that already produced by the inflammation). This was presumed to have resulted from an antagonism of a hypoalgesia produced by a local action of the opioids released from inflammatory cells.

Following this experimental evidence, the authors evaluated the effect of intraarticular morphine in postarthroscopy patients and reported a significant and prolonged analgesic effect (29). The effect of morphine was not only equivalent to, but significantly outlasted, the analgesia produced by intraarticular bupivacaine. There was also a significantly reduced use of postoperative pain medication in the morphine group. The very long post-injection effect (up to 24 hours), was presumed to reflect the inability of the morphine to escape the joint space.

These results are intriguing and raise interesting questions as to the extent to which the analgesia produced by systemic injection of morphine involves a peripheral as well as a central mechanism. It should be emphasized, however, that another group has not found that intraarticular morphine is more efficacious than bupivacaine, under apparently similar conditions (30). Time will tell whether this is an important approach for the management of postoperative pain and what other conditions may be treatable with this approach.

Opioid Regulation of Noxious Stimulus-evoked C-fos Expression

After systemic injection, we found a dose-dependent inhibition of fos expression (31). On the other hand, we found that it was possible to produce complete inhibition of pain behavior in the formalin test, without eliminating the expression of fos in the cord. The densest residual staining was found in the superficial dorsal horn, where up to 50% of the cells continued to express the protein, despite the fact that the animal was behaviorally analgesic. Very similar results were found after intraventricular injection of either morphine or the mu-selective opioid ligand, DAMGO (17). The best correlation between pain behavior and the expression of the fos protein was in lamina V and the ventral horn. As a result, we concluded that activity in these latter regions is particularly important, and possibly necessary, for the expression of pain behavior. In contrast, activity in the more superficial laminae, which may contribute to activity that is generated in neurons located more ventrally, did not have to be completely eliminated.

This hypothesis assumes that there is transmission of nociceptive information to the brain arising in lamina I, even when the rat is analgesic. Another hypothesis as to the residual activity has, however, been proposed. Specifically, it is possible that the residual labelling only occurred in interneurons of the superficial dorsal horn. That is, if all the activity in the *projection* neurons of lamina I were blocked, then the brain would not be *aware* of the persistent activity in the cord, and absence of pain behavior would be expected. To test this hypothesis the following experiment was performed. We injected rats with a retrograde tracer in the parabrachial region, a major target of neurons in lamina I. One week later, the rats received an injection of formalin, however, it was performed after injection of a large, analgesic dose of morphine. To determine whether residual labelling exists in projection neurons, we stained tissue for *both* the fos protein and for the retrograde tracer. Although we found that there was an almost 50% inhibition of fos expression in the superficial laminae (consistent with our previous studies) we found that the percentage of double-labelled projection neurons was *not* changed in the morphine-treated animals. These results indicate that under conditions of morphine analgesia, there is persistent activity in a population of lamina I neurons that project to the parabrachial region. We do not know the physiological significance of this persistent activity. It could represent a population of nociresponsive neurons that is specifically concerned with the activation of descending controls, i.e., this may represent part of the afferent limb of a negative feedback mechanism that results in the attenuation of pain when there is persistent noxious input. Injection of opiates, of course, would further contribute to antinociception. It makes sense, however, that a system which is designed to regulate nociception not, itself, be blocked by opiates (which presumably means that it is not regulated by endogenous opioids).

A different hypothesis is that the output from these "opiate-resistant" neurons in the marginal zone provides nociceptive information to the brain that does not access those systems which generate a perception of pain and related behavior. It is of interest in this regard that the parabrachial neurons are not part of the traditional spinothalamic/ spinoreticular pathway. Rather the parabrachial region projects to the amygdala, a major component of the limbic system (32,33). Conceivably, this pathway provides nociceptive information to the circuitry that engages emotional behavior, but that it is only manifested if there is concomitant transmission of information over the somatic pathways to thalamus and reticular formation.

Regardless of the functional consequences of persistent activation of neurons in the superficial dorsal horn, these data emphasize the value of monitoring fos expression to identify the populations of neurons that are involved in the transmission of nociceptive messages. Our present studies are focusing on the differential regulation that is produced by opioid ligands selective for the mu, delta and kappa receptors. In preliminary studies, we found that kappa agonists administered supraspinally produce behavioral analgesia, but have little effect on the expression of fos at the level of the spinal cord. This result indicates that kappa agonists may exert their effects predominantly via activation of supraspinal antinociceptive controls. These are clearly very distinct from those that are activated by mu selective agonists; these significantly influence the expression of fos in spinal cord neurons.

A New Perspective on the Mechanism of Opiate Tolerance

Although there is controversy as to the extent to which patients become tolerant with continuous use of opiates for the relief of pain, there are sufficient reports indicating that it is a significant concern. Recent studies have provided new insights into the mechanisms through which tolerance develops and have introduced potential approaches to overcoming or preventing its development. The latter studies are based on the premise that tolerance develops differently at the different opioid receptor subtypes. Thus, if tolerance develops at the mu receptor through repeated use of a mu selective agonist, it is possible to reestablish analgesia by introducing an opioid that acts at a different receptor, for example, the delta receptor. Other studies have emphasized the value of using more efficacious ligands for the receptor that has become tolerant. That approach is based on the assumption that a more efficacious ligand (e.g., sufentanil *vs.* morphine) needs fewer receptors in order to exert a maximal effect. If only a fraction of the available receptors were made tolerant with continued used of morphine, it may still be possible to induce analgesia with the "spare" receptors. Sufentanil is a very efficacious mu agonist that can generate analgesia in an animal that is tolerant to morphine, presumably because there are sufficient receptors available (34).

There are several hypotheses concerning the mechanisms through which tolerance develops. An early idea was that there is a downregulation of the number of receptors for a particular opiate. That hypothesis has not been substantiated. It is possible to demonstrate behavioral and biochemical tolerance well before there is a downregulation of the receptor. The more accepted assumption is that there is a loss or decrease of the coupling between the receptor and the second messenger systems (typically G-protein coupled systems) through which the opiate ligand exerts its downstream effects. The opiate receptor is linked to an inhibitory G protein (Gi), the action of which leads either to a decrease in the level of cyclic AMP, and/or an increase in potassium conductance, which mediates the hyperpolarization of neurons (35).

Although this hypothesis is attractive and appears to account for much of the tolerance phenomenology, there are some observations that are at odds with this formulation. Specifically, in an opiate tolerant animal, it is possible to precipitate an abstinence syndrome, i.e., withdrawal, by injection of an opiate antagonist, naloxone or naltrexone. *These latter drugs never elicit the syndrome in an opiate naive animal,* i.e., they have no intrinsic activity; all that they can do is antagonize the effect of an opiate. If this is true, it follows that under conditions of tolerance, i.e., when the effect of the opiate (e.g., behavioral analgesia) can no longer be demonstrated, *the opiate must still be operating.* How else could an antagonist produce an effect that involves displacement of the opiate ligand, unless the opiate ligand was still functional? Apparently, the opiate is operating, but there is a compensatory response to the continued presence of the opiate that is induced in the neurons upon which the opiate acts. Indeed the opiate is not only working, but it is preventing the development of withdrawal!

With this hypothesis in mind, we began a series of studies to evaluate whether we could identify aspects of the compensatory response. Which populations of neurons are affected? In these studies we plotted the distribution of neurons that expressed the fos protein in response to noxious stimulation under conditions of opiate tolerance. We also evaluated the patterns of fos expression produced by naltrexone, i.e., during withdrawal. Our results provided a new insight into the nature of the nervous response to the continued presence of opiate.

As in the studies described above, we evaluated fos expression in the formalin test. To begin these studies it was necessary to determine the extent to which a rat becomes tolerant in the formalin test. Indeed, Abbott and colleagues (36) previously reported that tolerance does not develop in the formalin test. They suggested that this test, which is a tonic pain test, is more comparable to clinical pain states, many of which appear not to be become tolerant to opiates. Our results, in fact, demonstrated that tolerance to morphine does develop in the formalin test. We used a tolerance-inducing paradigm that involved daily implantation of a morphine pellet. On the sixth day the rats were injected with formalin into the hindpaw and the behavior monitored. We found that there was not only a normal response to the formalin, i.e., tolerance had developed, but that an injection of 10 mg/kg morphine (which would normally block the response to formalin) on the sixth day of pellet implantation was without effect. We conclude that in this test there is indeed a strong development of tolerance.

One hour after the formalin was injected, the rats were perfused for immunocytochemistry for the fos protein. Although the overall pattern of staining was comparable to that seen when formalin was injected into control rats, we found that there was significant increase in the number of labelled cells. This was not only true on the side of the cord ipsilateral to the noxious stimulus, but there was also an increase on the contralateral side. Of particular interest was that in some rats the densest staining in the superficial dorsal horn contralateral to the formalin injection was in the topographically identical region, i.e., the medial two-thirds of laminae

I and II. This result indicates that there is probably cross talk between the two halves of the cord, in topographically identical regions. This almost certainly occurs through local connections, rather than via supraspinal links, which would probably result in a loss of the topography. In addition to the increased contralateral staining, we found a significant increase in the rostrocaudal spread of neurons that expressed the fos protein. We believe that the enhanced fos staining is indicative of a latent sensitization of spinal cord neurons when they are rendered tolerant to morphine. We consider that the sensitization is latent because it was only manifested when a noxious stimulus was presented. These results suggest that the failure of the opiate may not be due to its loss of efficacy, but rather to the fact that the compensatory response that counteracts the effect of the opiate results in an enhanced nociceptive message (which may, in fact, result in greater pain produced by the same noxious stimulus).

When we evaluated the pattern of fos expression in rats in which we precipitated withdrawal with naltrexone, we found further evidence for a latent central sensitization. More importantly, we found suggestive evidence as to where these changes occur. When tolerance was precipitated in awake rats, we found a significant increase in fos expression in neurons of laminae I, III, and IV. There was also considerable increase in staining in neurons around the central canal and in the region of the parasympathetic preganglionic neurons of the sacral spinal cord. Interestingly, the substantia gelatinosa, the neurons of which express fos in the presence of a noxious stimulus, did not "light up" during withdrawal. To determine to what extent the behavior associated with withdrawal contributed to the pattern of staining in the withdrawing rat, we repeated these studies under conditions in which withdrawal was precipitated under halothane anesthesia. This not only eliminated the behavior, but also significantly reduced the staining in laminae III and IV, indicating that neurons in these regions probably expressed the fos protein secondary to the movement and afferent drive associated with the hyperactivity of withdrawal.

On the other hand, the staining in lamina I, which was present at all levels of the spinal cord, persisted in the animals that withdrew under anesthesia. These data suggest that the latent sensitization that is characteristic of the tolerant state is focused in marginal neurons of the superficial dorsal horn. Interestingly, these same neurons have been shown to contribute to central sensitization following injury or C-fiber stimulation (37). For example, a noxious stimulus results in long term changes in these cells, such that subsequent inputs evoke a greater response. After sensitization has occurred, the receptive fields of marginal neurons are enlarged and they begin to respond to stimuli of much lower, often innocuous, intensities. These data suggest that sensitization that results from noxious stimulation and latent sensitization, that we believe occurs during opiate tolerance, have many features in common.

In this regard, it is of particular interest that the pharmacology of sensitization is comparable to that which has recently been implicated in the development of tolerance and dependence. Specifically, it has been reported that treatment with an NMDA antagonist not only reduces central sensitization but reduces the development of tolerance to morphine (38). Moreover, blocking the NMDA receptor completely prevented the withdrawal syndrome produced by injection of the opiate antagonist in morphine tolerant rats. We are presently evaluating whether MK-801, a non-competitive NMDA antagonist, blocks the expression of fos in lamina I neurons during withdrawal. If our hypothesis is confirmed, it will provide important evidence that the locus of changes that contribute to the development of tolerance is indeed in the dorsal horn. More importantly, it will offer new suggestions to mitigating the problem of tolerance. Interestingly, since tolerance to opiates (in the clinical setting) would usually occur under conditions in which there is persistent injury/pain, the development of central sensitization would be exacerbated and possibly occur more rapidly. Hopefully, these new approaches to understanding the changes that occur in the spinal cord under conditions of tolerance and persistent injury may lead to better methods for their prevention.

REFERENCES

1. Levine JD, Fields HL, Basbaum AI: Peptides and the primary afferent nociceptor. J Neurosci 13:2273-2286, 1993
2. De Biasi S, Rustioni A: Glutamate and substance P coexist in primary afferent terminals in the superficial laminae of spinal cord. Proc Natl Acad Sci U S A 85:7820-7824, 1988

3. Lodge D, Johnson KM: Noncompetitive excitatory amino acid receptor antagonists. Trends Pharmacol Sci 11:81-86, 1990
4. Zeman S, Lodge D: Pharmacological characterization of non-NMDA subtypes of glutamate receptor in the neonatal rat hemisected spinal cord in vitro. Br J Pharmacol 106:367-372, 1992
5. Woolf CJ, Thompson SW: The induction and maintenance of central sensitization is dependent on N-methyl-D-aspartic acid receptor activation. Implications for the treatment of post-injury pain hypersensitivity states. Pain 44:293-299, 1991
6. Dickenson AH: A cure for wind up: NMDA receptor antagonists as potential analgesics. Trends Pharmacol Sci 11:307-309, 1990
7. Dougherty PM, Willis WD: Enhancement of spinothalamic neuron responses to chemical and mechanical stimuli following combined micro-iontophoretic application of N-methyl-D-aspartic acid and substance P. Pain 47:85-93, 1991
8. Yashpal K, Dam TV, Quirion R: Effects of dorsal rhizotomy on neurokinin receptor sub-types in the rat spinal cord: A quantitative autoradiographic study. Brain Res 552:240-247, 1991
9. Duggan AW, Hendry IA, Morton CR, et al: Cutaneous stimuli releasing immunoreactive substance P in the dorsal horn of the cat. Brain Res 451:261-273, 1988
10. Duggan AW, Hope PJ, Jarrott B, et al: Release, spread and persistence of immunoreactive neurokinin A in the dorsal horn of the cat following noxious cutaneous stimulation. Studies with antibody microprobes. Neuroscience 35:195-202, 1990
11. Duggan AW, Schaible HG, Hope PJ, Lang CW: Effect of peptidase inhibition on the pattern of intraspinally released immunoreactive substance P detected with antibody microprobes. Brain Res 579:261-269, 1992
12. Yaksh TL, Jessell TM, Gamse R, et al: Intrathecal morphine inhibits substance P release from mammalian spinal cord in vivo. Nature 286:155-157, 1980
13. Dubner R, Kenshalo DR Jr, Maixner W, et al: The correlation of monkey medullary dorsal horn neuronal activity and the perceived intensity of noxious heat stimuli. J Neurophysiol 62:450-457, 1989
14. Basbaum AI, Presley R, Menétrey D, et al: Somatic, articular, and visceral noxious stimulus-evoked expression of c-fos in the spinal cord of the rat: Differential patterns of activity and modulation of analgesic agents, Processing of Sensory Information in the Superficial Dorsal Horn of the Spinal Cord. Edited by Cervero F, Bennett GJ, Headley PM. New York, Plenum Press, 1989, pp. 365-382
15. Menétrey D, Gannon A, Levine JD, Basbaum AI: Expression of c-fos protein in interneurons and projection neurons of the rat spinal cord in response to noxious somatic, articular, and visceral stimulation. J Comp Neurol 285:177-195, 1989

16. Morgan JI, Curran T: Stimulus-transcription coupling in neurons: Role of cellular immediate-early genes. Trends Neurosci 12:459-462, 1989
17. Gogas KR, Presley RW, Levine JD, Basbaum AI: The antinociceptive action of supraspinal opioids results from an increase in descending inhibitory control: Correlation of nociceptive behavior and c-fos expression. Neuroscience 42:617-628, 1991
18. Basbaum AI, Fields HL: Endogenous pain control systems: Brainstem spinal pathways and endorphin circuitry. Ann Rev Neurosci 7:309-338, 1984
19. Yaksh TL, Rudy TA: Analgesia mediated by a direct spinal action of narcotics. Science 192:1357-1358, 1976
20. Besse D, Lombard MC, Zajac JM, et al: Pre- and postsynaptic distribution of mu, delta and kappa opioid receptors in the superficial layers of the cervical dorsal horn of the rat spinal cord. Brain Res 521:15-22, 1990
21. Jessell TM, Iversen LL: Opiate analgesics inhibit substance P release from rat trigeminal nucleus. Nature (Lond) 268:549-551, 1977
22. Suarez-Roca H, Maixner W: Morphine produces a multiphasic effect on the release of substance P from rat trigeminal nucleus slices by activating different opioid receptor subtypes. Brain Res 579:195-203, 1992
23. Ferreira SH, Nakamura M: II. Prostaglandin hyperalgesia: the peripheral analgesic activity of morphine, enkephalins and opioid antagonists. Prostaglandins 18:191-200, 1979
24. Levine JD, Taiwo YO: Involvement of the mu-opiate receptor in peripheral analgesia. Neuroscience 32:571-575, 1989
25. Stein C, Millan MJ, Yassouridis A, Herz A: Antinociceptive effects of μ- and k-agonists in inflammation are enhanced by a peripheral opioid receptor-specific mechanism. Eur J Pharmacol 155:225-264, 1988
26. Hassan AH, Ableitner A, Stein C, Herz A: Inflammation of the rat paw enhances axonal transport of opioid receptors in the sciatic nerve and increases their density in the inflamed tissue. Neuroscience 55:185-195, 1993
27. Przewlocki R, Hassan AH, Lason W, et al: Gene expression and localization of opioid peptides in immune cells of inflamed tissue: Functional role in antinociception. Neuroscience 48:491-500, 1992
28. Stein C, Hassan AH, Przewlocki R, et al: Opioids from immunocytes interact with receptors on sensory nerves to inhibit nociception in inflammation. Proc Natl Acad Sci U S A 87:5935-5939, 1990
29. Stein C, Comisel K, Haimerl E, et al: Analgesic effect of intraarticular morphine after arthroscopic knee surgery. New Engl J Med 325:1123-1126, 1991
30. Raja SN, Dickstein RE, Johnson CA: Comparison of postoperative analgesic effects of intraarticular bupivacaine and morphine

following arthroscopic knee surgery. Anesthesiology 77:1143-1147, 1992

31. Presley RW, Menétrey D, Levine JD, Basbaum AI: Systemic morphine suppresses noxious stimulus-evoked Fos protein-like immunoreactivity in the rat spinal cord. J Neurosci 10:323-335, 1990
32. Bernard JF, Peschanski M, Besson JM: A possible spino (trigemino)-ponto-amygdaloid pathway for pain. Neurosci Lett 100:83-88, 1989
33. Bernard JF, Alden M, Besson JM: The organization of the efferent projections from the pontine parabrachial area to the amygdaloid complex: A Phaseolus vulgaris leucoagglutinin (PHA-L) study in the rat. J Comp Neurol 329:201-229, 1993
34. Yaksh TL: Tolerance: Factors involved in changes in the dose-effect relationship with chronic drug exposure, Towards a New Pharmacotherapy of Pain. Edited by Basbaum AI, Besson J-M. Chisester, John Wiley & Sons, 1991, pp. 157-179
35. Cox BM: Molecular and cellular mechanisms in opioid tolerance, John Wiley & Sons. Edited by Basbaum AI, Besson J-M. Chisester, Towards a New Pharmacotherapy of Pain, 1991, pp. 137-156
36. Abbott FV, Franklin KB, Ludwick RJ, Melzack R: Apparent lack of tolerance in the formalin test suggests different mechanisms for morphine analgesia in different types of pain. Pharm Biochem Behav 15:637-640, 1981
37. Cook AJ, Woolf CJ, Wall PD: Prolonged C-fibre mediated facilitation of the flexion reflex in the rat is not due to changes in afferent terminal or motoneurone excitability. Neurosci Lett 70:91-96, 1986
38. Trujillo KA, Akil H: Inhibition of morphine tolerance and dependence by the NMDA receptor antagonist MK-801. Science 251:85-87, 1991

ACKNOWLEDGEMENT

This work was supported by grants from the NIH: NIDA08377, NS14627 and NS21445. Parts of this manuscript were reproduced with permission from the International Association for the Study of Pain.

SPINAL CORD NEURONAL PLASTICITY: MECHANISMS OF PERSISTENT PAIN FOLLOWING TISSUE DAMAGE AND NERVE INJURY[1]

R. Dubner

SUMMARY

Injury to peripheral tissues following trauma or surgery results in hyperalgesia that is characterized by increased sensitivity to painful stimuli. Often innocuous stimuli are perceived as painful. Similarly, nerve injury produced by trauma or metabolic disease can give rise to hyperalgesia. Until recently, it was thought that the increase in pain was due to changes at the site of injury. It is now becoming clear that the increase in pain also involves altered processing and hyperexcitability in the central nervous system. Animal models of hyperalgesia produced by inflammation or nerve injury have been developed. The injection of an inflammatory agent into the rat's hindpaw produces an increase in the spinal cord dorsal horn levels of the opioid peptide, dynorphin, and an increase in messenger RNA that codes for the dynorphin precursor protein. The change in dynorphin gene expression parallels the development and time course of the hyperalgesia produced by the inflammatory agent. Hyperalgesia can also be produced by placing loose ligatures around the sciatic nerve of the rat. Similar to changes seen in inflammation models, there is a large increase in dynorphin gene expression that parallels the development of hyperalgesia in this nerve injury model. Changes in the response properties of spinal dorsal horn neurons accompany the hyperalgesia produced by injury. After inflammation, dorsal horn neurons exhibit increased excitability. There is

---

[1]Excerpted from Dubner R: Spinal cord neuronal plasticity: Mechanisms of persistent pain following tissue damage and nerve injury, New Trends In Referred Pain And Hyperalgesia. Edited by Vecchiet and Lindblom U. Amsterdam, Elsevier (in press).

T. H. Stanley and M. A. Ashburn (eds.), Anesthesiology and Pain Management, 19–34.

often an enlargement of receptive fields as well as increased responsiveness to stimulation. The enlargement of receptive fields leads to a greater overlap between receptive fields so that more neurons are activated by a stimulus than the number activated in the absence of receptive field expansion. The increase in neural activity may be perceived as more intense pain. Spinal administration of dynorphin results in expansion of receptive fields and increased responsiveness of some dorsal horn neurons. This increase in excitability involves activation of neurons at N-methyl-D-aspartate (NMDA) receptor sites by excitatory amino acids such as glutamate and aspartate. The release of excitatory amino acids and their effects on dorsal horn neurons are enhanced by neuropeptides such as dynorphin, substance P (SP), and calcitonin gene-related peptide (CGRP). The expanded receptive fields and hyperexcitability can be blocked or reduced by the administration of NMDA antagonists. The hyperalgesia following tissue or nerve injury can also be blocked or reduced by NMDA antagonists. A model has been proposed wherein dynorphin, SP and CGRP enhance excitability at NMDA receptor sites, leading first to dorsal horn hyperexcitability, and then to excessive depolarization and excitotoxicity. Small, inhibitory local circuit neurons would be most affected by the excitotoxicity leading to a loss of inhibitory mechanisms. The combined effects of depolarization and loss of inhibition contribute to the expansion of receptive fields and hyperexcitability, and lead to an increase in pain. These findings have important therapeutic implications because the pain of tissue and nerve damage can now be attacked at the site of injury where it is initiated and at central nervous system sites where it is maintained. New treatment strategies for controlling persistent pain following injury have developed based on these new research advances.

Injury to peripheral tissues following trauma, infection or surgery produces inflammation, hyperalgesia, and spontaneous pain. The hyperalgesia is characterized by increased sensitivity to noxious or painful stimuli. Often innocuous stimuli such as a light touch are perceived as painful. In a similar fashion, nerve injury produced by trauma or metabolic disease can give rise to hyperalgesia and spontaneous pain. The mechanisms underlying these clinical pain states are incompletely understood. Until recently, it was thought that the increase in pain was due to changes taking place at the site of injury. It is now clear that the increase in pain following tissue or nerve injury also involves altered processing and hyperexcitability in the central nervous system.

Tissue damage results in an increased sensitivity of receptors, called nociceptors, at the site of injury. The two most common types of peripheral nociceptors are myelinated mechanothermal nociceptors and unmyelinated polymodal nociceptors. They both appear to contribute to the hyperalgesia following injury to the skin [see Dubner (1) for review]. After tissue injury, they exhibit spontaneous activity, lowered thresholds, and increased responsiveness to noxious stimuli. This increased nociceptor activity leads to hyperexcitability and altered neuronal processing in the spinal cord and brain that contribute to the hyperalgesia and spontaneous pain. Similarly, nerve damage also can lead to increased activity at the site of injury. When a nerve is damaged, axons begin to sprout from the discontinuity and form a neuroma. The nerve sprouts emit spontaneous discharges and are responsive to mechanical, thermal and chemical stimulation. Spontaneous nerve activity also originates from the cell bodies of damaged nerves located in the dorsal root ganglia. The increase in nerve activity arising from neuromas and the dorsal root ganglia results in hyperexcitability and altered processing in the central nervous system contributing to the hyperalgesia and spontaneous pain. Thus, both tissue and nerve injury lead to prolonged changes in the nervous system. The prolonged changes are similar to those associated with increased nerve activity during development and learning (2). These nerve activity-dependent changes following injury involve the major classes of chemical mediators participating in pain transmission including neuropeptides and excitatory amino acids (3). In this chapter I, will review some of the neurochemical changes that occur at the molecular level following tissue and nerve injury and that contribute to the resulting prolonged increases in pain. In addition, I will describe some new pain treatment strategies that have been proposed based on this new knowledge.

Animal models of hyperalgesia produced by inflammation or nerve injury have recently been developed. The injection of an inflammatory agent into the rat's hindpaw produces redness, swelling and hyperalgesia limited to the injected paw. Other than showing guarding behavior of the limb, the animals exhibit normal behaviors such as grooming and socialization with littermates and they maintain their body weight. Inflammation produced in one limb as described above results in the increased expression of various genes in those dorsal root ganglia and in those spinal cord dorsal horn segments that receive signals from the site of tissue injury. Neuropeptides in the nervous system are coded by specific genes in the cell nucleus (Figure 1). These genes transcribe messenger RNA which is then released into the cytoplasm and translated into precursor molecules (proteins) that contain active neuropeptide sequences. These proteins are then enzymatically cleaved to yield the active peptide products. This includes opioid peptides such as dynorphin, and other neuropeptides such as substance P (SP), calcitonin gene-related peptide (CGRP), and vasoactive intestinal peptide (VIP).

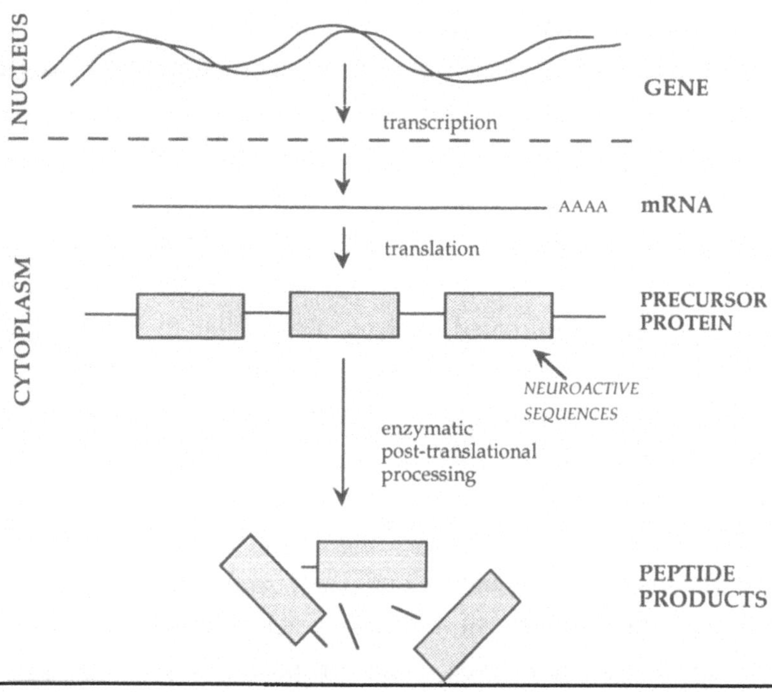

Figure 1. Gene transcription in the nervous system. See text for details.

Inflammation of the hindpaw in the rat produces an increase in the level of the opioid peptide, dynorphin, in the spinal dorsal horn (4-6). The unilateral inflammation also produces an increase in messenger RNA that codes for the dynorphin precursor protein (6). The increase in dynorphin message is present as early as four hours with a peak 8-fold increase occurring between 2 and 5 days and returning to control levels by 10 to 14 days. The change in dynorphin gene expression parallels the development and time course of behavioral hyperalgesia produced by the inflammatory agents. The increase in dynorphin peptide content occurs later; it is apparent by two days and a 3-fold increase can be detected by 4 days after the induction of inflammation (5-7). The changes in dynorphin gene expression and dynorphin peptide levels are segmentally-specific and only occur in that part of the spinal cord receiving input from the inflamed paw. The dorsal horn of the contralateral, non-injected side appears the same as in normal animals and thus serves as an appropriate control.

Using molecular and histochemical methods, the neurons showing an increase in dynorphin gene message can be localized autoradiographically in tissue sections of the spinal cord (8). There is approximately a 3-fold increase in the number of labeled cells on the experimental as compared to the control side. The increase in labeling is concentrated in the medial part of the superficial laminae of the dorsal horn and the neck of the dorsal horn, areas that receive innervation from the inflamed hindpaw. An increase in neuronal labeling for dynorphin peptide is also observed ipsilateral to the site of inflammation in the same regions. These are the two regions of the dorsal horn that contain neurons involved in pain transmission. The dynorphin-containing neurons in the superficial laminae of the dorsal horn are both projection neurons and local circuit neurons (9). Dynorphin-containing neurons receive monosynaptic input from small myelinated and unmyelinated afferents (10), and high-frequency stimulation of unmyelinated nerve fibers has been shown to result in the release of dynorphin peptides into the superficial dorsal horn (11).

Hyperalgesia can also be produced in rats by placing loose ligatures around the sciatic nerve of the rat (12). The animals exhibit signs of nerve injury pain that closely mimic those seen in patients with reflex sympathetic dystrophy or causalgia. In all other respects, the animals appear healthy: there is minimal loss of body weight, grooming behavior is normal, and they socialize with their littermates. The hyperalgesia exhibited by these animals begins as early as day two and at this time a high percentage of myelinated nerve fibers exhibits conduction block through the site of injury (13). Spontaneous discharges appear mainly in myelinated nerve fibers at the same time and originate from the dorsal root ganglia (14). Similar to the changes seen in inflammation models, there is a large increase in dynorphin gene expression that peaks at 5 days, coincident with the peak of hyperalgesia seen in this nerve injury model (15). The increase in dynorphin peptide peaks at 10 days (16). The increases in dynorphin peptide are localized to the superficial laminae and the neck of the dorsal horn, those regions of the spinal dorsal horn that are involved in pain transmission.

Tissue and nerve injury also produce changes in the expression of other genes in the dorsal root ganglia. Inflammation induces increases in messenger RNA coding for the neuropeptides SP and CGRP (17,18). These neuropeptides increase in dorsal root ganglion cells after inflammation (19) and are then released into the spinal cord. The increase in messenger RNA is in response to the increased release and the need for further SP and CGRP synthesis. In contrast, nerve injury produces marked reductions in SP and CGRP immunoreactivity in the dorsal root ganglion (20). The functional significance of these changes in gene expression following nerve injury is not known.

Recently, a new class of genes called cellular immediate-early genes have been discovered and appear to regulate gene expression by coding for proteins that bind to DNA in the promotor region of other target genes (21). These nuclear proteins are thought to regulate initial genetic events leading to prolonged functional changes in the nervous system. One such gene, c-fos, is the cellular homologue of the viral oncogene, v-fos, the transforming gene of mouse osteogenic sarcoma viruses. The expression of c-fos occurs within 30 minutes after injection of an inflammatory agent into the rat hindpaw (22). This increase precedes the increase in dynorphin gene expression (see above). There is a peak elevation at 2 hours, a decrease to one-half maximal levels by 4 hours, and nearly complete recovery to control levels by 8 hours after injection. An examination of the distribution of the protein product of c-fos, using immunocytochemistry, reveals that, following inflammation and partial nerve injury, the Fos protein is localized to neurons in the superficial laminae and the neck of the spinal dorsal horn, the same sites exhibiting increases in dynorphin message (23,24). Recent studies (24) have demonstrated that over 80% of these neurons in the superficial laminae and neck of the dorsal horn showing increases in dynorphin gene expression following inflammation also exhibit Fos protein in their nuclei. These findings suggest that Fos proteins may bind to the promotor region of the dynorphin gene and regulate its transcription.

These findings are consistent with the idea that signals from peripheral nerve fibers, including neuropeptide release, activate cellular messages (second messengers) in dorsal horn neurons. These second messengers appear to regulate the transcription of various genes. The protein products of immediate-early genes such as c-fos appear to be transcription factors that regulate the expression of target genes induced by neuronal activity associated with injury as well as learning and memory. Fos protein is thought to bind cooperatively with Jun protein, the product of another immediate-early gene, at a DNA binding site (the AP-1 element) in the promotor region of various genes. Recently, an AP-1 like binding site in the promotor region of the rat dynorphin gene has been shown to bind Fos and Jun and to induce dynorphin gene transcription (25). However, there is evidence that other nuclear proteins also bind to the dynorphin promotor and induce transcription (26).

What is the functional significance of the increased expression of dynorphin peptide in the dorsal horn following tissue or nerve injury? The answer may come from studies of the inflammation-induced changes in the response properties of dorsal horn neurons involved in pain transmission. Inflammatory agents or repeated tissue injury leads to the expansion of receptive fields of spinal dorsal horn neurons (27-30). Following inflammation, many lamina I projection neurons exhibit an enlargement of their receptive fields (2.4 times larger on the average) and many have discontinuous fields responding to noxious stimulation (Figure 2) (29). There also is a significant increase in the number of cells exhibiting spontaneous activity as compared to control animals (87% to 24%). Other studies, in addition, have reported decreased thresholds of dorsal horn neurons to mechanical stimulation following inflammation and injury (28,30). When the response properties of lamina I neurons are studied between 4 and 8.5 hours after CFA administration, changes in receptive field size parallel the time course of development of the

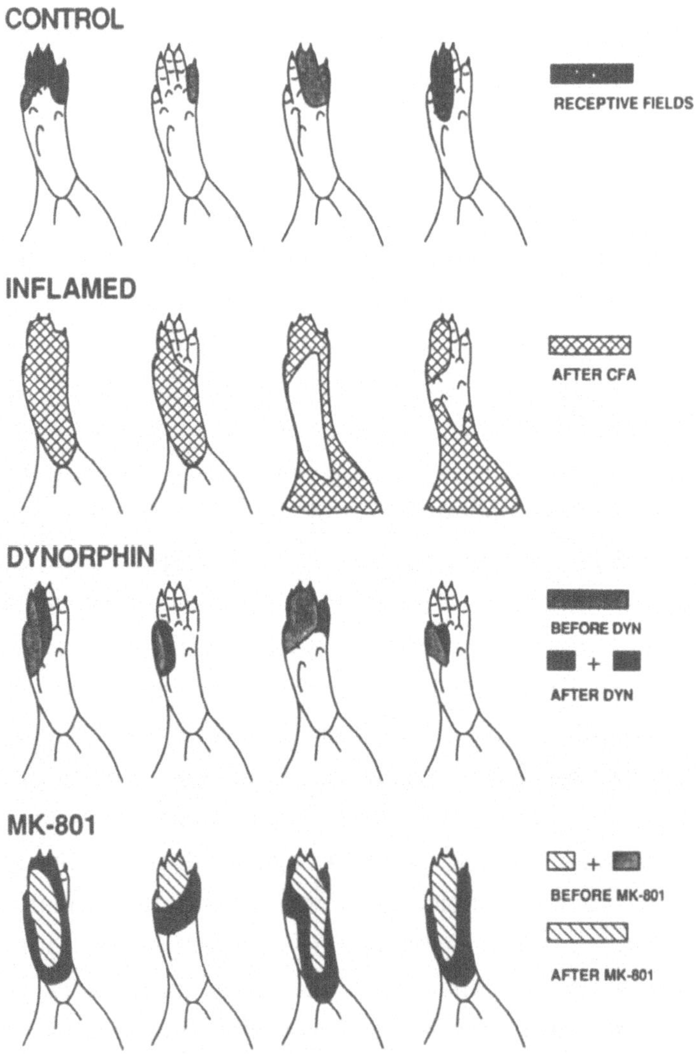

Figure 2. Changes in the receptive fields of superficial dorsal horn neurons produced by inflammation and drug manipulations. The first row illustrates examples of the small receptive fields found in control animals. The second row shows examples of enlarged receptive fields after inflammation. The third row illustrates the small enlargement of the receptive fields in control animals following the application of dynorphin peptide to the surface of the spinal cord. The fourth row illustrates that MK-801 applied to the surface of the spinal cord of rats with unilateral inflammation produces a reduction in receptive field size, but the receptive fields are still larger than those found in control animals. The findings suggest that the very large receptive fields found in rats with inflamed paws are a result of multiple

behavioral hyperalgesia (29). Following the placement of loose ligatures around the sciatic nerve, there are changes in the responses of dorsal horn neurons that parallel the hyperalgesia produced in this model of neuropathic pain (31,32). The most profound changes are found 14 days after inducing the neuropathy, and include both an increase in spontaneous activity of the neurons and abnormally prolonged afterdischarges.

How does the expansion of the receptive fields of nociceptive neurons lead to hyperalgesia? One hypothesis (1) is that expanded receptive fields will result in greater overlap of the receptive fields of neurons and, therefore, will lead to a greater number of neurons activated by a stimulus than the number activated by the same stimulus applied in the absence of receptive field expansion. The increase in neuronal activity may ultimately be perceived as more intense pain.

It appears that both the observed changes in receptive field size of superficial dorsal horn neurons and the alterations in dynorphin gene expression are closely correlated with the development of behavioral hyperalgesia. To test whether dynorphin or related compounds acting at kappa-opioid receptor sites could induce changes in receptive field size, the effects of spinally-administered dynorphin or a kappa-opioid agonist, on superficial dorsal horn neurons in rats without inflammation, were examined (33). Dynorphin applied to the surface of the spinal cord induced an average 50% expansion of the receptive fields of 5 of 15 superficial dorsal horn neurons (Figure 2). A separate group of 8 of 23 cells exhibited an average expansion of their receptive fields of 30% after spinal administration of the active isomer of the kappa-opioid receptor agonist, U50,488H. After the administration of U50,488H, there also was either enhanced or suppressed responsiveness of neurons to mechanical and thermal stimuli. Approximately one-third of the cells exhibited enhanced responses to mechanical stimuli (most of them also had expanded receptive fields), whereas, a few exhibited a suppression of activity. Approximately one-third of the cells also demonstrated a facilitation of their heat-evoked response, but about one-half of these exhibited suppression of activity at higher doses. About one-third of the cells only exhibited suppression of the thermal response. These results suggest that dynorphin and kappa-opioid receptor agonists have dual effects in the spinal dorsal horn. They result in expanded receptive fields of some neurons often accompanied by increased sensitivity to mechanical and thermal stimuli; in other neurons there is a suppression of responsiveness to mechanical and thermal stimuli. Related studies have also reported facilitation or inhibition of dorsal horn neuronal activity after the administration of kappa opioid receptor agonists (34,35). The two types of responses may represent activation of two functionally different populations of neurons, or alternatively, the two responses may reflect interaction of the agonists at more than one receptor type. Recent data support the argument that kappa opioid receptor agonists have a role in the antinociceptive response to inflammatory pain (36). Other findings (35) suggest that dynorphin-induced potentiation and the subsequent loss of C-fiber reflexes involves excessive excitation and possible excitotoxicity mediated at N-methyl-D-aspartate receptor sites, ultimately leading to cell dysfunction (see below).

The increase in excitability of spinal cord dorsal horn neurons appears to involve excitation at receptor sites activated by excitatory amino acids. Rapid neurotransmitter excitatory events in nociceptive neurons are mediated by excitatory amino acids such as glutamate and aspartate that act at N-methyl-D-aspartate (NMDA) receptor sites [see Dubner and Ruda (3) for review]. The release of excitatory amino acids in the spinal dorsal horn is enhanced by neuropeptides such as SP and CGRP (37,38). SP and CGRP potentiate the dorsal root stimulation-evoked release of glutamate and aspartate from spinal cord in vitro preparations (39). SP has been found to enhance the responses of spinothalamic tract neurons in the monkey to NMDA and these responses are blocked by an NMDA antagonist (40). These effects may be important in increasing synaptic efficacy in the spinal cord and likely participate in the long-lasting hyperexcitability found following inflammation and hyperalgesia.

The expanded receptive fields of pain transmission neurons following inflammation can be blocked or reduced by the administration of NMDA antagonists, chemicals that block the excitatory effects at NMDA receptors (41) (Figure 2). These NMDA antagonists also significantly attenuate the hyperalgesia induced by inflammation and by partial nerve injury (41,42). It appears that altered processing and hyperexcitability in dorsal horn pain transmission neurons involves the release of excitatory amino acids and their action at NMDA receptor sites. These effects are modulated by various neuropeptides including dynorphin, SP and CGRP.

We have proposed a model that takes into account the increased nociceptive afferent fiber activity at the site of tissue or nerve injury leading to spinal cord dorsal horn hyperexcitability and behavioral hyperalgesia (1,3). It is counterintuitive to think of nerve injury producing increases in nociceptive afferent fiber activity since there is a loss of normal nerve fiber function after such injury. However, as mentioned above, nerve injury leads to ectopic spontaneous activity of peripheral nerve fibers arising from neuromas, from the dorsal root ganglia and from demyelinated zones. On the other hand, tissue injury results in a sensitization of peripheral nociceptors and increased spontaneous and evoked activity. Although the mechanisms of altered activity arising from the sites of tissue and nerve injury are different, they both produced an increased neuronal barrage reaching the central nervous system. The sequence of events is diagrammed in Figure 3. Increased neural activity from the site of injury will lead to increased depolarization or excitation by excitatory amino acids at NMDA receptor sites. This depolarization is facilitated by neuropeptide release (SP, CGRP and dynorphin). The result is an expansion of receptive fields and hyperexcitability leading to an increase in pain. This hyperexcitability, or increased depolarization, if excessive, can lead to a pathological state by promoting excitotoxicity, cell dysfunction, and a loss of inhibitory mechanisms. The effect is similar to the cell loss found in experimental epilepsy associated with the loss of inhibition and excessive excitatory amino acid transmission (43,44). Neurons most sensitive to this excitotoxicity are small local circuit neurons which likely are inhibitory. Small neurons in the superficial dorsal horn exhibit morphological changes suggestive of dysfunction following partial nerve injury (45). The combined effects of excessive excitation and loss of inhibition would further contribute to the expansion of receptive fields, hyperexcitability and increased pain.

These findings have led to the development of new treatment strategies for pain arising after tissue or nerve injury. One exciting advance is the use of preemptive local anesthesia for the treatment of postoperative pain (46,47). Local anesthetics are administered before

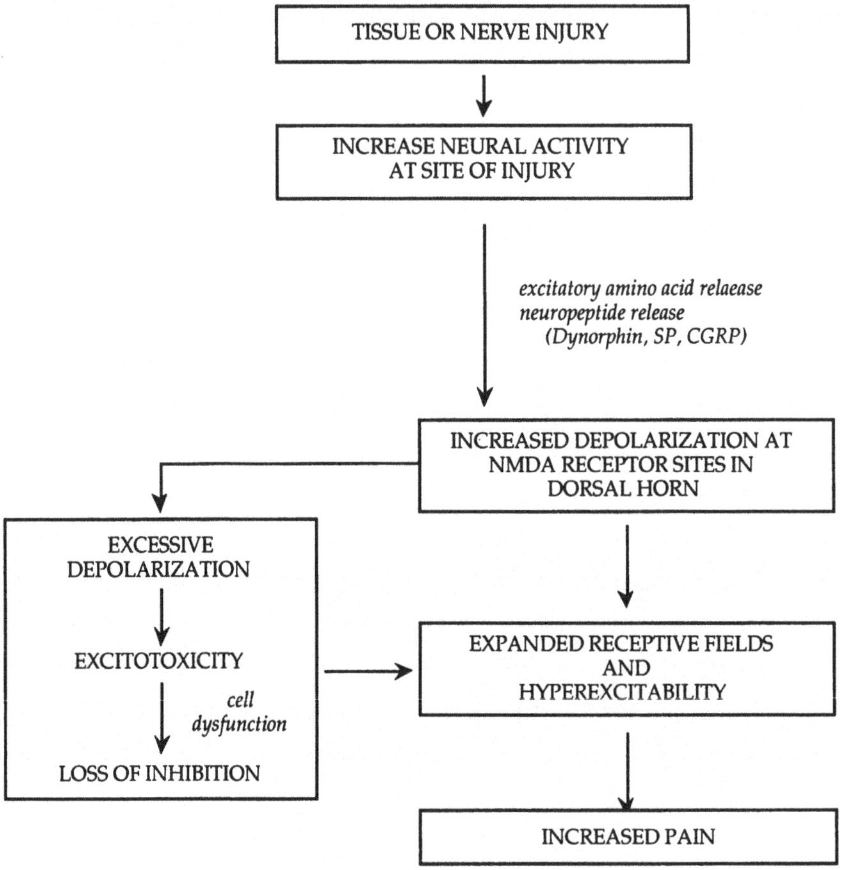

Figure 3. Sequence of events that may occur following peripheral tissue inflammation or peripheral nerve injury. See text for details.

surgery under general anesthesia in order to prevent or reduce the neural barrage from the site of tissue damage reaching the spinal cord. This should prevent the development of hyperexcitability in the spinal dorsal horn. The preoperative administration of aspirin-like drugs should have a similar though not as complete an effect. The attack on postoperative pain can also be directed at the spinal cord. Opioid drugs, or in the future, clinically acceptable NMDA antagonists (48), can reduce or eliminate the central hyperexcitability, resulting in a reduction in postoperative pain.

A similar approach can be used to reduce or eliminate the pain associated with nerve injury. Nerve activity originating from neuromas or dorsal root ganglia can be blocked by local anesthetics. It may be important in cases of nerve injury produced by trauma to administer local anesthetics as soon as possible and for the first few days after injury. Drugs that reduce central nervous system hyperexcitability such as anticonvulsants and NMDA antagonists should also be effective.

The findings presented here are important because they suggest that pain is not a passive symptom, but an aggressive symptom that produces central nervous system changes underlying the pathophysiology leading to persistent and increased pain. Such pain produces changes in behavior, often with resulting depression and maladaptive personal relationships. It also can produce changes in immune function and slowing of tissue repair (49). It is imperative to block or reduce this excessive neural activity, not only to improve patient comfort, but to prevent these harmful pathophysiological consequences.

REFERENCES

1. Dubner R: Neuronal plasticity and pain following peripheral tissue inflammation or nerve injury, Proceedings of the VIth World Congress on Pain. Amsterdam, Elsevier, 1991, pp. 263-276
2. Goelet P, Castellucci VF, Schacher S, Kandel ER: The long and short of long-term memory—a molecular framework. Nature 322:419-422, 1986
3. Dubner R, Ruda MA: Activity-dependent neuronal plasticity following tissue injury and inflammation. Trends Neurosci 15:96-103, 1992
4. Millan MJ, Millan MH, Czlonkowski A, et al: A model of chronic pain in the rat: Response of multiple opioid systems to adjuvant-induced arthritis. J Neurosci 6:899-906, 1986
5. Millan MJ, Czlonkowski A, Morris B, et al: Inflammation of the hind limb as a model of unilateral, localized pain: Influence on multiple opioid systems in the spinal cord of the rat. Pain 35:299-312, 1988
6. Iadarola MJ, Douglass J, Civelli O, Naranjo JR: Differential activation of spinal cord dynorphin and enkephalin neurons during hyperalgesia: Evidence using cDNA hybridization. Brain Res 455:205-212, 1988
7. Weihe E, Iadarola MJ, Nohr D, et al: Sustained expression and co-localization of proenkephalin and prodynorphin opioids and c-fos proteins in dorsal horn neurons revealed in arthritis rats, Proceedings of the International Narcotics Research Conference. Edited by Ree JMV, Mulder AH, Wiegant VM, Greidanus TBVW. Amsterdam, Excerpta Medica, 1990, pp. 92-94
8. Ruda MA, Iadarola MJ, Cohen LV, Young WS III: In situ hybridization histochemistry and immunocytochemistry reveal an increase in

spinal dynorphin biosynthesis in a rat model of peripheral inflammation and hyperalgesia. Proc Natl Acad Sci U S A 85:622-626, 1988
9. Nahin RL, Hylden JLK, Iadarola MJ, Dubner R: Peripheral inflammation is associated with increased dynorphin immunoreactivity in both projection and local circuit neurons in the superficial dorsal horn of the rat lumbar spinal cord. Neurosci Lett 96:247-252, 1989
10. Takahashi O, Traub RJ, Ruda MA: Demonstration of calcitonin gene-related peptide immunoreactive axons, contacting dynorphin A(1-8) immunoreactive spinal neurons in a rat model of peripheral inflammation and hyperalgesia. Brain Res 475:168-172, 1988
11. Hutchison WD, Morton CR, Terenius L: Dynorphin A: In vivo release in the spinal cord of the cat. Brain Res 532:299-306, 1990
12. Bennett GJ, Xie Y-K: A peripheral mononeuropathy in rat that produces disorders of pain sensation like those seen in man. Pain 33:87-107, 1988
13. Kajander KC, Bennett GJ: The onset of painful peripheral neuropathy in rat: A partial and differential deafferentation and spontaneous discharge in Aß and Aδ primary afferent neurons. J Neurophysiol 68:734-744, 1992
14. Kajander KC, Wakisaka S, Bennett GJ: Spontaneous discharge originates in the dorsal root ganglion at the onset of a painful peripheral neuropathy in the rat. Neurosci Lett 138:225-228, 1992
15. Draisci G, Kajander KC, Dubner R, et al: Up-regulation of opioid gene expression in spinal cord evoked by experimental nerve injuries and inflammation. Brain Res 560:186-192, 1991
16. Kajander KC, Sahara Y, Iadarola MJ, Bennett GJ: Dynorphin increases in the dorsal spinal cord in rats with a painful peripheral neuropathy. Peptides 11:719-728, 1990
17. Iadarola MJ, Draisci G: Elevation of spinal cord dynorphin mRNA compared to dorsal root ganglion peptide mRNAs during peripheral inflammation, The Arthritic Rat as a Model of Clinical Pain? Edited by Besson J-M, Guilbaud G. Amsterdam, Elsevier Science Publishers BV, 1988, pp. 173-183
18. Noguchi K, Morita Y, Kiyama H, et al: A noxious stimulus induces the preprotachykinin—A gene expression in the rat dorsal root ganglion: A quantative study using in situ hybridization histochemistry. Brain Res 464:31-35, 1988
19. Nahin RL, Byers MR: Local inflammation induces alterations of calcitonin gene-related peptide immunoreactivity within cutaneous primary afferents. Pain (Suppl) 5:S134, 1990
20. Bennett GJ, Kajander KC, Sahara Y, et al: Neurochemical and anatomical changes in the dorsal horn of rats with an experimental painful peripheral neuropathy, Processing of Sensory Information in the Superficial Dorsal Horn of the Spinal Cord. Edited by Cervero F, Bennett GJ, Headley PM. New York, Plenum Press, 1989, pp. 463-471

21. Morgan JI, Curran T: Stimulus-transcription coupling in neurons: Role of cellular immediate-early genes. Trends Neurosci 12:459-462, 1989
22. Draisci G, Iadarola MJ: Temporal analysis of increases in c-fos, preprodynorphin and preproenkephalin in mRNAs in rat spinal cord. Brain Res Mol Brain Res 6:31-37, 1989
23. Kajander KC, Wakisaka S, Draisci G, Iadarola MJ: Labeling of Fos protein increases in an experimental model of peripheral neuropathy in the rat. Soc for Neurosci Abs 16:1281, 1990
24. Noguchi K, Kowalski K, Traub R, et al: Colocalization of Dynorphin and fos proteins in spinal cord neurons following inflammation induced hyperalgesia. Brain Res Mol Brain Res 10:227-233, 1991
25. Naranjo JR, Mellström B, Achaval M, Sassone-Corsi P: Molecular pathways of pain: Fos/Jun-mediated activation of a noncanonical AP-1 site in the prodynorphin gene. Neuron 6:607-617, 1991
26. Iadarola MJ, Mojdehi G, Gu J, et al: A protein complex differing from the fos/jun complex binds at an AP-1 variant sequence in the dynorphin promoter and is induced in spinal cord by peripheral inflammation. Soc for Neurosci Abs 17:905, 1991
27. McMahon SB, Wall PD: Receptive fields of rat lamina I projection cells move to incorporate a nearby region of injury. Pain 19:235-247, 1984
28. Calvino B, Villanueva L, LeBars D: Dorsal horn (convergent) neurones in the intact anaesthetized arthritic rat. I. Segmental excitatory influences. Pain 28:81-98, 1987
29. Hylden JLK, Nahin RL, Traub RJ, Dubner R: Expansion of receptive fields of spinal lamina I projection neurons in the rats with unilateral adjuvant-induced inflammation: the contribution of dorsal horn mechanisms. Pain 37:229-243, 1989
30. Laird JMA, Cervero F: A comparative study of the changes in receptive-field properties of multireceptive and nocireceptive rat dorsal horn neurons following noxious mechanical stimulation. J Neurophysiol 62:854-863, 1989
31. Laird JMA, Bennett GJ: Responses of spinal dorsal horn neurons in rats with an experimental peripheral mononeuropathy. Soc for Neurosci Abs 17:537, 1991
32. Palecek J, Paleckova V, Dougherty PM, et al: Responses of spinothalamic tract cells to mechanical and thermal stimulation of skin in rats with experimental peripheral neuropathy. Soc for Neurosci Abs 17:437, 1991
33. Hylden JLK, Nahin RL, Traub RJ, Dubner R: Effects of spinal kappa-opioid receptor agonists on the responsiveness of nociceptive superficial dorsal horn neurons. Pain 44:187-193, 1991
34. Knox RJ, Dickenson AH: Effects of selective and non-selective kappa-opioid receptor agonists on cutaneous c-fibre-evoked responses of rat dorsal horn neurones. Brain Res 415:21-29, 1987

35. Caudle RM, Isaac L: Influence of dynorphin(1-13) on spinal reflexes in the rat. J Pharmacol Exp Ther 246:508-513, 1988
36. Millan MJ, Colpaert FC: Opioid systems in the response to inflammatory pain: Sustained blockade suggests role of κ- but not μ-opioid receptors in the modulation of nociception, behaviour and pathology. Neuroscience 42:541-553, 1991
37. Murase K, Ryu PD, Randic M: Excitatory and inhibitory amino acids and peptide-induced responses in acutely isolated rat spinal dorsal horn neurons. Neurosci Lett 103:56-63, 1989
38. Randic M, Hecimovic H, Ryu PD: Substance P modulates glutamate-induced currents in acutely isolated rat spinal dorsal horn neurones. Neurosci Lett 117:74-80, 1990
39. Kangrga I, Randic M: Tachykinins and calcitonin gene-related peptide enhance release of endogenous glutamate and aspartate from the rat spinal dorsal horn slice. J Neurosci 10:2026-2038, 1990
40. Dougherty PM, Willis WD: Enhancement of spinothalamic neuron responses to chemical and mechanical stimuli following combined micro-iontophoretic application of N-methyl-D-aspartic acid and substance P. Pain 47:85-93, 1991
41. Ren K, Hylden JLK, Williams GM, et al: The effects of a non-competitive NMDA receptor antagonist, MK-801, on behavioral hyperalgesia and dorsal horn neuronal activity in rats with unilateral inflammation. Pain 50:331-344, 1992
42. Yamamoto T, Yaksh TL: Spinal pharmacology of thermal hyperesthesia induced by constriction injury of sciatic nerve. Excitatory amino acid antagonists. Pain 49:121-128, 1992
43. Sloviter RS, Damiano BP: Sustained electrical stimulation of the perforant path duplicates kainate-induced electrophysiological effects and hippocampal damage in rats. Neurosci Lett 24:279-284, 1981
44. Sloviter RS: Decreased hippocampal inhibition and a selective loss of interneurons in experimental epilepsy. Science 235:73-76, 1987
45. Sugimoto T, Bennett GJ, Kajander KC: Transsynaptic degeneration in the superficial dorsal horn after sciatic nerve injury: Effects of a chronic constriction injury, transection, and strychnine. Pain 42:205-213, 1990
46. Wall PD: The prevention of postoperative pain (editorial). Pain 33:289-290, 1988
47. Tverskoy M, Cozacov C, Ayache M, et al: Postoperative pain after inguinal herniorrhaphy with different types of anesthesia. Anesth Analg 70:29-35, 1990
48. Dubner R: Pain and hyperalgesia following tissue injury: New mechanisms and new treatments. Pain 44:213-214, 1991
49. Liebeskind JC: Pain can kill (editorial). Pain 44:3-4, 1991

LOCAL ANESTHETIC PHARMACOLOGY

D. H. Lambert

STRUCTURE ACTIVITY RELATIONSHIPS

Local anesthetics are drugs used to produce anesthesia in circumscribed regions of the body by blocking nerve transmission. Most local anesthetics contain an aromatic group and an amine group separated by an intermediate chain (Table 1). The clinically useful local anesthetics fall into one of two chemical groups. Amino-esters (procaine, chloroprocaine and tetracaine) contain an ester link between the aromatic portion and the intermediate chain. Amino-amides (lidocaine, mepivacaine, prilocaine, ropivacaine, bupivacaine and etidocaine) have an amide link between the aromatic end and the intermediate chain. The ester and amide compounds differ in terms of their stability in solution, metabolism, and allergic potential. Amides are extremely stable in solution, while esters are unstable. The amino-esters are hydrolyzed in plasma by the enzyme pseudocholinesterase, whereas the amide compounds undergo enzymatic degradation in the liver and excretion in the urine. Para-aminobenzoic acid (PABA) is an amino-ester metabolite, which causes allergic reactions in some patients. The amino-amides are not metabolized to PABA and they rarely cause allergic reactions.

GENERAL CONSIDERATIONS

The clinically important properties of local anesthetics include potency, duration of action, speed of onset, and differential sensory/motor blockade. The clinical profile of the individual agents depends on their chemical structure, which determines their physico-chemical characteristics. The physico-chemical properties that influence anesthetic

T. H. Stanley and M. A. Ashburn (eds.), Anesthesiology and Pain Management, 35–64.

Table 1. Chemical structure of local anesthetics.

	Aromatic Group (Lipophilic)	Intermediate Chain	Amine Group (Hydrophilic)
ESTERS			
PROCAINE	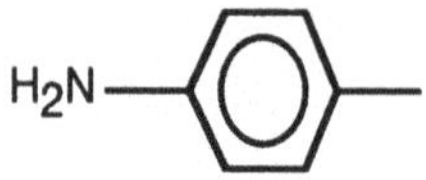	$—COOCH_2CH_2—$	$—N(C_2H_5)(C_2H_5)$
CHLOROPROCAINE	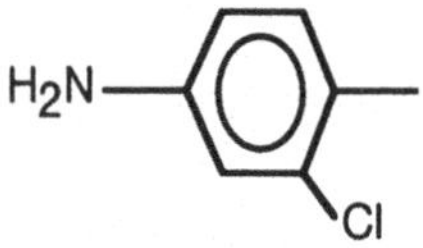	$—COOCH_2CH_2—$	$—N(C_2H_5)(C_2H_5)$
TETRACAINE	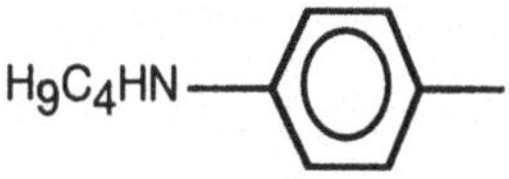	$—COOCH_2CH_2—$	$—N(CH_3)(CH_3)$
AMIDES			
PRILOCAINE	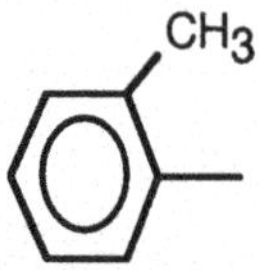	$— NHCOCH(CH_3) —$	$—N(H)(C_3H_7)$
LIDOCAINE	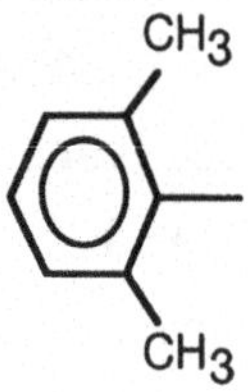	$—NHCOCH_2 —$	$—N(C_2H_5)(C_2H_5)$
MEPIVACAINE	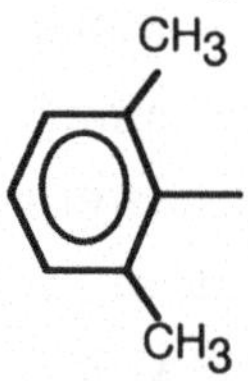	— NHCO —	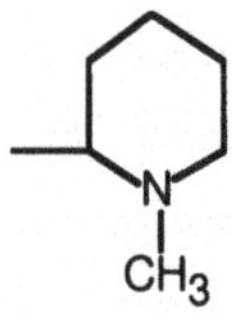
ROPIVACAINE	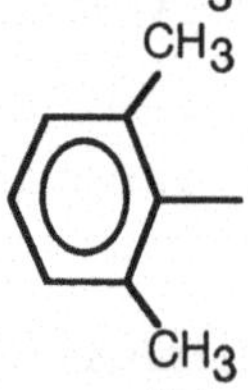	— NHCO —	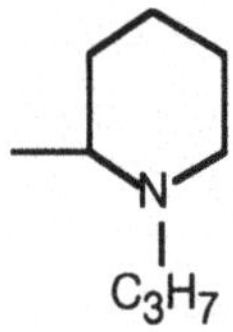
BUPIVACAINE	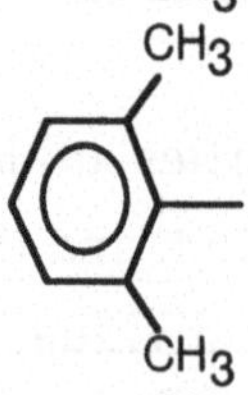	— NHCO —	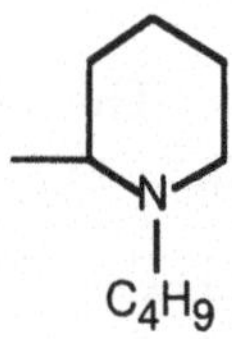
ETIDOCAINE	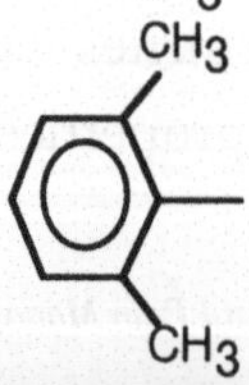	$— NHCOCH(C_2H_5) —$	$—N(C_2H_5)(C_3H_7)$

activity are lipid solubility (potency), protein binding (duration), and pK_a (onset). Minor changes in molecular structure have dramatic effects on these properties (Table 2).

Anesthetic Potency—Lipid Solubility

Lipid solubility is responsible for intrinsic anesthetic potency. The axolemma is a matrix of lipid (90%) and protein (10%). Thus, highly lipophilic chemical compounds penetrate the nerve membrane more easily, so fewer molecules are required for conduction blockade, resulting in enhanced potency. In vitro studies on isolated nerves show a correlation between the partition coefficient of local anesthetics and the minimum concentration (Cm) required for conduction blockade (1,2). For example, the weakest amino-amides, mepivacaine and prilocaine, are the least lipid soluble, while etidocaine is the most lipophilic and the most potent (Figure 1). There is a similar relationship between lipid solubility and the potency of the ester local anesthetics. Procaine is the least lipid soluble and the weakest agent while tetracaine is the most lipophilic and the most potent ester drug.

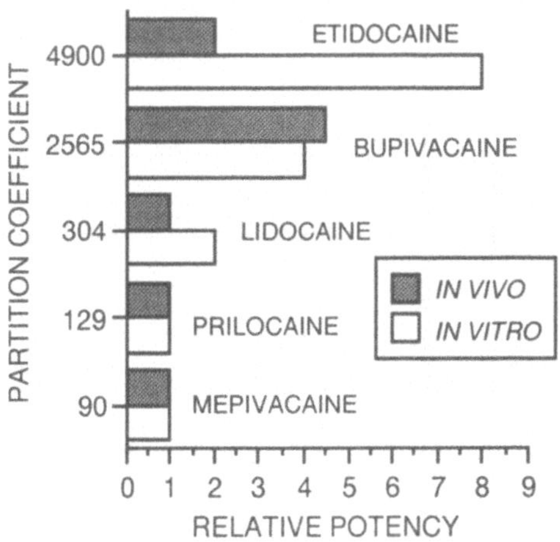

Figure 1. Relationship of lipid solubility (partition coefficient) to *in vitro* and *in vivo* anesthetic potency.

Factors other than lipid solubility also influence anesthetic potency. A comparison of the partition coefficients of the base form of esters and amides with their relative anesthetic potencies indicates that the amino-esters are more potent than the amino-amides. The amino-esters may

Table 2. Properties of local anesthetics.

	Physico-Chemical Properties				Pharmacological Properties		
Agent	**Molecular Weight† (base)**	**pK_a**	**Partition Coefficient (25 C°)**	**Percent Protein Binding**	**Onset**	**Relative Potency**	**Duration**
Esters							
Procaine	236	8.9	81	6	slow	1	short
Chloroproc.	271	8.7	720	---	fast	1	short
Tetracaine	264	8.5	3615	76	slow	8	long
Amides							
Prilocaine	220	7.9	129	55	fast	2	intermediate
Lidocaine	234	7.9	304	64	fast	2	intermediate
Mepivacaine	246	7.6	90	65	fast	2	intermediate
Ropivacaine	274	8.1	775	94	intermediate	6	long
Bupivacaine	288	8.1	2565	96	intermediate	8	long
Etidocaine	276	7.7	4900	94	fast	8	long

interact with a greater number of local anesthetic receptors and this may explain their inherently greater potency (3).

In vivo studies in man indicate that the correlation between lipid solubility and anesthetic potency is not as precise as in an isolated nerve (Figure 1). Lidocaine is approximately twice as potent as prilocaine and mepivacaine in an isolated nerve preparation, but in man there is little difference in potency between these agents. Similarly, etidocaine is more potent than bupivacaine in isolated nerve, while clinically etidocaine is less potent than bupivacaine. The difference between *in vitro* and *in vivo* results is believed related to the vasodilator or tissue distribution properties (diffusibility) of the various local anesthetics. For example, lidocaine causes more vasodilation than either mepivacaine or prilocaine. Thus, lidocaine is more rapidly absorbed making less available for neural blockade *in vivo*. The extremely high lipid solubility of etidocaine results in a greater uptake of this agent by adipose tissue (e.g., the epidural space). This results also in fewer etidocaine molecules available for neural blockade compared to the less lipid soluble drugs like bupivacaine.

Duration of Action—Protein Binding

The duration of local anesthesia is related to the ability of local anesthetics to bind protein. Local anesthetics are believed to combine with a protein receptor located within the sodium channel of the neurolemma. Chemical compounds with a high binding affinity for the receptor site remain in the channel longer and this prolongs the duration of conduction blockade. Most of this protein binding information comes from binding studies of local anesthetics to plasma proteins. It is assumed that there is a relationship between the plasma protein binding of local anesthetics and the degree of binding to membrane proteins.

In vitro studies demonstrate that poorly protein bound agents, like procaine, are rapidly washed out from isolated nerves whereas highly protein bound drugs like tetracaine, bupivacaine and etidocaine are removed very slowly. *In vivo* studies including clinical investigations in man confirm this relationship between local anesthetic protein binding and duration of action (4). For example, the duration of brachial plexus blockade is 30 to 60 minutes with procaine but 6 to 10 hours with bupivacaine (Figure 2).

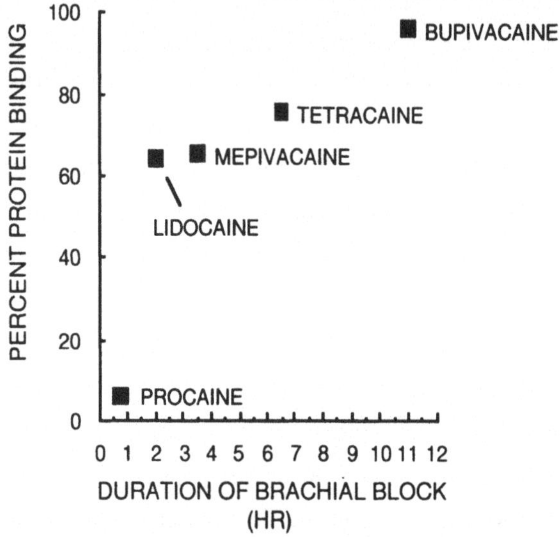

Figure 2. Relationship of protein binding of various local anesthetics to the duration of brachial plexus blockade.

In man, the duration of anesthesia is influenced also by the peripheral vascular effects of the local anesthetic agents. All local anesthetics, except cocaine, have a biphasic effect on vascular smooth muscle. At low concentrations, they cause vasoconstriction whereas at clinically used concentrations they cause vasodilation (5,6). Vasodilatation causes more rapid removal of drug from the injection site, decreasing the amount that enters the nerve. This, in turn, decreases the duration of anesthesia. However, the various drugs produce different degrees of vasodilation. For example, lidocaine is a more potent vasodilator than mepivacaine or prilocaine. Thus, while there is little difference in the duration of block between these agents in an isolated nerve, lidocaine's duration *in vivo* is shorter than that of mepivacaine or prilocaine. Adding a vasoconstrictor drug to these three local anesthetics results in a similar duration of action, because the vasoconstrictor blunts lidocaine's vasodilatation, while mepivacaine's and prilocaine's vasodilatation is meager to begin with.

Onset of Action -pK$_a$

The onset of block in isolated nerves is determined by the pK_a of the local anesthetic. The pK_a is defined as the pH at which the ionized and non-ionized forms of the local anesthetic are equal. Since the uncharged (non-ionized) ***base*** form of the local anesthetic is responsible for its diffusion across the nerve sheath and nerve membrane, the onset of action is directly related to the amount of ***base*** available (Figure 3). The percentage of local anesthetic drug, which is present in the base form when injected into tissue whose pH is 7.4, is inversely proportional to that agent's pK_a. For example, the pK_a of mepivacaine, lidocaine, prilocaine and etidocaine is approximately 7.7. When these agents are injected into tissue at a pH of 7.4, approximately 65% of these drugs is ionized and 35% is in the non-ionized base form. Likewise, tetracaine has a pK_a 8.6 and only 5% is present as non-ionized base at pH 7.4, and 95% is in the charged cationic form. The pK_a of bupivacaine is 8.1, which means that 15% of this agent is in the non-ionized base form at pH 7.4, and 85% is in the charged cationic form. Therefore, lidocaine, mepivacaine, prilocaine and etidocaine with low pK_a have a rapid onset, whereas procaine and tetracaine, with high pK_a, have a slow onset time (Figure 3). Bupivacaine is intermediate in terms of pK_a and onset of block.

The onset of blockade *in vivo* depends also on other miscellaneous factors. Onset time may be affected by diffusion through non-nervous connective tissue. For example, lidocaine and prilocaine have similar

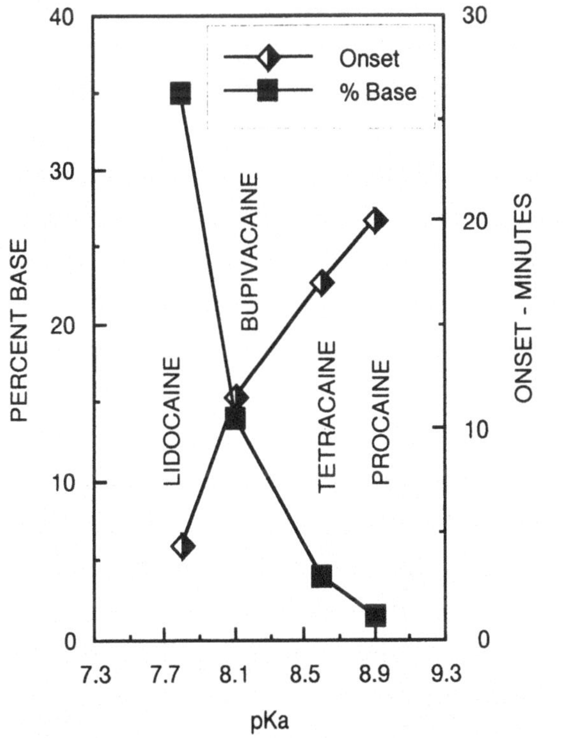

Figure 3. Relationship of onset of anesthesia of various local anesthetic agents to their pKa and percentage of drug in un-ionized (base) form.

p*K*a's and similar onset times in isolated nerve. However, *in vivo* prilocaine may be slower in onset than lidocaine. This difference may be related to lidocaine's ability to better diffuse through non-nervous tissue. More important, however, is the concentration of local anesthetic. For example, 0.25% bupivacaine has a slow onset of action. Increasing the concentration to 0.75% significantly decreases onset time. The rapid onset of chloroprocaine *in vivo* may be related in part to better diffusion through non-nervous tissue, but also to its high (3%) concentration. The pK_a of chloroprocaine is approximately 9 and its onset in isolated nerve is relatively slow (7). However, its low systemic toxicity allows it to be used in high concentrations. Therefore, its rapid onset time *in vivo* may be due to the large number of molecules injected around the nerves.

Differential Sensory/Motor Block

Another important clinical consideration is the ability of local anesthetics to differentially block sensory and motor fibers. The intrathecal administration of varying concentrations of procaine produces differential blockade of sensory, sympathetic and motor fibers. However, with spinal anesthesia, it is nearly impossible to produce sensory anesthesia sufficient for surgery without impairing motor function. Bupivacaine is relatively specific for sensory fibers and adequate sensory epidural analgesia, with little motor block can be achieved for surgical, obstetrical and acute and chronic pain therapy. Although they are both potent long acting anesthetic agents, bupivacaine and etidocaine provide an interesting contrast in terms of their differential sensory/motor blocking activity (Figure 4). Bupivacaine is widely used epidurally for both surgical and obstetrical procedures and for postoperative pain relief because of its ability to produce sensory analgesia with minimal motor blockade, particularly when used as a 0.25% or 0.5% solution. One of the primary reasons why this agent enjoys such popularity for continuous epidural blockade during labor is that the patient in labor can be pain free and still be able to move her legs. Increasing the concentration of bupivacaine to 0.75% increases the depth of both sensory and motor blockade while also shortening onset and prolonging duration (8). Etidocaine on the other hand shows little separation of sensory and motor

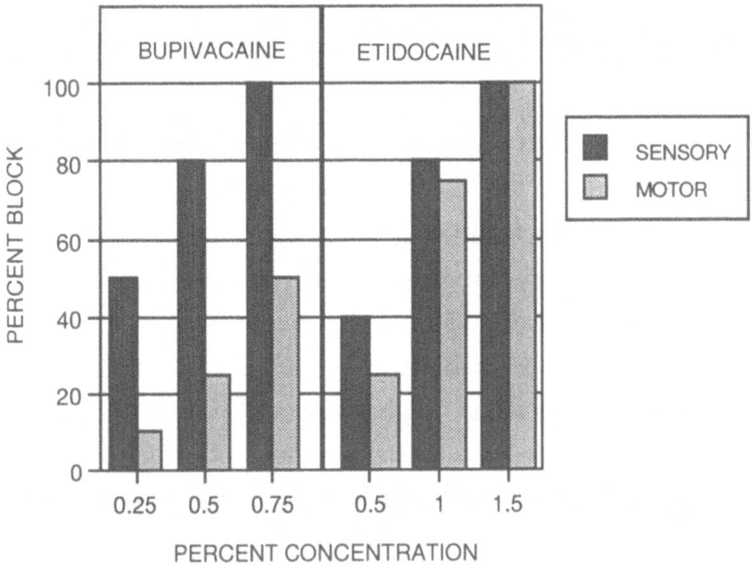

Figure 4. Comparative sensory and motor blockade of bupivacaine and etidocaine following epidural administration—relationship to dose.

blockade. In order to achieve adequate epidural sensory anesthesia with etidocaine, a concentration of 1.5% is usually required. At this concentration, etidocaine has an extremely rapid onset and prolonged duration of anesthesia. However, the sensory anesthesia is associated with profound motor blockade. Thus, etidocaine is a valuable agent for epidural blockade in operations where intense muscle relaxation is desirable. However, the marked motor blockade makes etidocaine unusable for obstetric analgesia and for postoperative pain relief.

The factors responsible for bupivacaine's differential sensory/motor separation are unknown. Studies on isolated nerves show that low concentrations of bupivacaine initially block unmyelinated C fibers followed by block of myelinated A fibers (9). On the other hand, etidocaine blocks both A and C fibers at approximately the same rate. Bupivacaine's slow blockade of A fibers is believed to be due to its relatively high p*K*a, such that fewer uncharged molecules are available to penetrate the diffusion barriers surrounding large A fibers. The lack of diffusion barriers around the small sensory C fibers allows sufficient bupivacaine molecules to reach the C fiber receptor sites to cause sensory anesthesia.

Thus, bupivacaine may possess the optimal pK_a and lipid solubility characteristics required for differential sensory/motor blockade.

In summary, the pharmacological activity of local anesthetic agents is related to their physico-chemical properties. However, the activity of these agents in vivo may be altered by factors unrelated to their physico-chemical properties. On the basis of anesthetic activity in man, the various agents may be classified as follows:

1. Agents of low anesthetic potency and short duration of action: procaine and chloroprocaine.
2. Agents of intermediate anesthetic potency and duration of action: lidocaine, mepivacaine and prilocaine.
3. Agents of high anesthetic potency and prolonged duration of action: ropivacaine, tetracaine, bupivacaine and etidocaine.

In terms of onset of action, chloroprocaine, lidocaine, mepivacaine, prilocaine and etidocaine are rapid, bupivacaine intermediate, while procaine and tetracaine are slow.

FACTORS INFLUENCING ANESTHETIC ACTIVITY

Although the inherent pharmacologic properties of the various local anesthetics determine their anesthetic profile, other factors influence the quality of regional anesthesia. These include:

1. The dosage of local administered.
2. The addition of a vasoconstrictor.
3. The site of administration.
4. Carbonation or pH adjustment.
5. Additives.
6. The mixing of local anesthetics.
7. Pregnancy.

Dosage of Local Anesthetic

The mass of drug administered influences the onset, depth and duration of anesthesia (Figure 5). As the dose of local anesthetic increases, the frequency of satisfactory anesthesia and the duration of anesthesia increase, while the onset of anesthesia decreases. The dosage of local

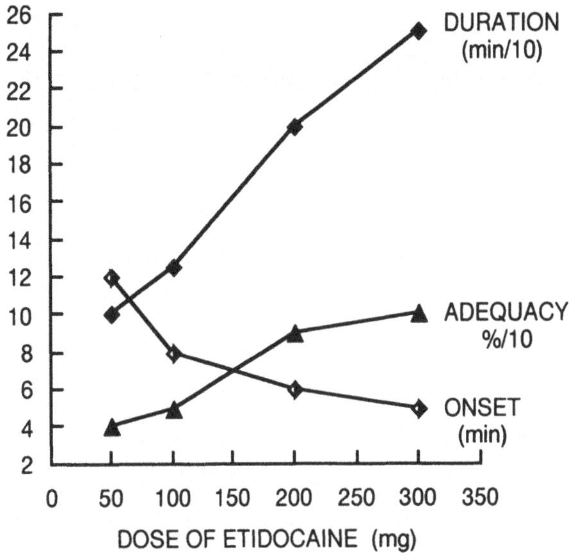

Figure 5. Effect of dose of epidural etidocaine on onset, frequency and duration of anesthesia. Note that the duration and adequacy are ÷ 10. Thus, a duration of 26 = 260 min and an adequacy of 10 = 100%.

anesthetic can be increased by administering either a larger volume or a more concentrated solution. However, in clinical practice dosage is usually increased by injecting a more concentrated solution. For example, increasing the concentration of epidurally administered bupivacaine from 0.125% to 0.5%, while maintaining the same volume (10 ml), results in decreased onset time, more frequent satisfactory analgesia, and increased duration of analgesia. Similarly, increasing the concentration of epidural bupivacaine from 0.5% to 0.75% so that the dosage increases from 100 mg to 150 mg produces more rapid onset, prolonged duration, greater frequency of satisfactory anesthesia, and enhanced depth of motor blockade (8). When prilocaine (600 mg) is given epidurally, either as 30 ml of a 2% solution or 20 ml of 3% there is no difference in onset, adequacy of analgesia, and duration of sensory and motor blockade. This indicates that dosage rather than volume or concentration is the primary determinant of local anesthetic activity. The volume of anesthetic solution may influence the spread of anesthesia. For example, epidural anesthesia with 30 ml of 1% lidocaine produces a level of anesthesia which is 4 dermatomes higher than that achieved with 10 ml of 3% lidocaine. Thus, except for the possible effect on the spread of anesthesia, the onset, depth, quality and duration of blockade are due to the mass of drug injected, that is, the product of volume times concentration.

Addition of Vasoconstrictor Agent

Epinephrine is frequently added to local anesthetic solutions to decrease vascular absorption of the drug. This allows more anesthetic molecules to reach the nerve membrane and improves the depth and duration of anesthesia. Epinephrine is usually added to local anesthetic solutions in a 1:200,000 dilution (5 μg/ml). This concentration of epinephrine produces optimal vasoconstriction when added to lidocaine for epidural or intercostal block. Norepinephrine and phenylephrine have also been added to local anesthetic solutions. Equipotent concentrations of epinephrine and phenylephrine prolong the duration of tetracaine spinal anesthesia to roughly the same extent (10) (Figure 6). When used to prolong spinal anesthesia, the dose of phenylephrine is 2 to 5 mg compared to 0.2 to 0.4 mg of epinephrine.

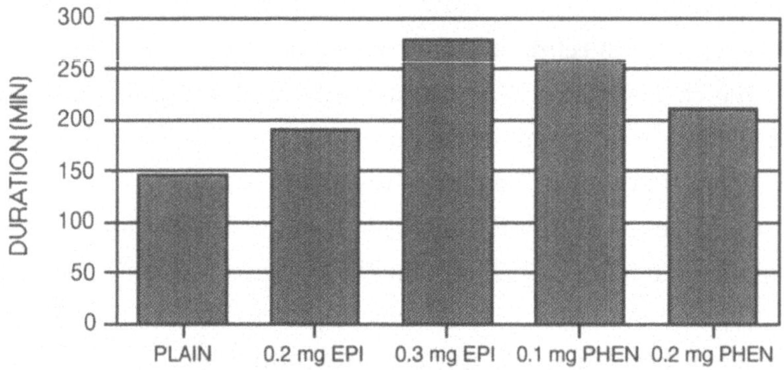

Figure 6. Effect of epinephrine and phenylephrine on the duration of spinal anesthesia produced by tetracaine. (Data from Ref. 10).

The ability of epinephrine to prolong the duration of anesthesia depends on the local anesthetic to which it is added and the site of injection. For example, the duration of infiltration anesthesia and peripheral nerve block is prolonged when epinephrine is added to any local anesthetic. Epinephrine increases also the duration of <u>epidural</u> anesthesia when added to procaine, mepivacaine and lidocaine but does not do so when administered with prilocaine, bupivacaine or etidocaine. The inability of epinephrine to prolong the duration of epidural prilocaine compared to lidocaine is believed to be due to the fact that prilocaine causes less vasodilation than lidocaine. The high lipid solubility of bupivacaine and etidocaine may account for the diminished effect of epinephrine when given epidurally with these drugs. These agents are sequestered by epidural fat and then slowly released. This overcomes any vasodilation effects of these drugs and contributes to their long duration of action. Nevertheless, epinephrine can prolong the action of epidural bupivacaine, but this is concentration dependent. For example, in epidural labor analgesia, the frequency and duration of adequate analgesia is improved when 1:200,000 epinephrine is added to 0.125% and 0.25% bupivacaine. However, adding epinephrine to 0.5% or 0.75% bupivacaine does not improve the adequacy or prolong the regression of epidural anesthesia in obstetrical or surgical patients. The profoundness but not the duration of motor blockade is enhanced when epinephrine is added to epidural solutions of bupivacaine or etidocaine. In spinal anesthesia, epinephrine significantly prolongs the duration of tetracaine (10). Two or four segment regression of lidocaine or bupivacaine spinal anesthesia is not prolonged by epinephrine. However, anesthesia in the lower thoracic and lumbosacral areas is prolonged. Thus, epinephrine added to spinal solutions of lidocaine (11) and bupivacaine (12) does not significantly prolong the duration of "effective surgical anesthesia" in the abdominal dermatomes but seems to extend duration in the lower limbs.

Site of Injection

Although local anesthetics are classified as agents of short, moderate or long duration with slow or rapid onset, these properties are affected by the type of anesthetic procedure performed. In general, the most rapid onset but the shortest duration occurs with intrathecal or subcutaneous injections, while the slowest onset and the longest durations are seen with brachial plexus blocks. For example, spinal bupivacaine has an onset of approximately five minutes and a duration of some 3 to 4 hours. However, when bupivacaine is used for brachial plexus blockade, the onset time is 20 to 30 minutes and the duration averages 6 to 10 hours. These differences in onset and duration are due in part to the anatomy of the injection site, the rate of vascular absorption, and the amount of drug used. In the case of spinal anesthesia, the absence of a sheath around the spinal nerves and the spinal cord, and the injection of the local anesthetic close to the target tissue is responsible for the rapid onset. On the other hand, the small amount of drug used for spinal anesthesia accounts for its short duration. In the case of brachial plexus blockade, the onset of anesthesia is slow because the local anesthetic is injected at some distance from the targeted nerves, and it must diffuse through various tissue barriers before reaching the nerves to be blocked. The long duration of brachial plexus blockade is probably due to decreased vascular absorption as well as the larger doses of drug routinely used for this anesthetic technique.

Carbonation and pH Adjustment of Local Anesthetics

One of the drawbacks of regional blocks is the slow onset of anesthesia due to diffusion barriers and the time required for the local anesthetic to reach the sodium channel inside the nerve. Diffusion depends on pKa and pH:

$$pH - pKa = \log [base/cation] \text{ (Henderson-Hesselbach equation),}$$

which determine the amount of ***base*** present. The higher the base concentration, the more rapid is the onset of anesthesia (Figure 3). Theoretically, there are three ways to quicken the onset of local anesthesia: 1) carbonation of the local anesthetic, 2) pH adjustment, and 3) "gassing" with CO_2.

Carbonation of Local Anesthetics. It must be appreciated that adding $NaHCO_3$ to a local anesthetic is *pH adjustment* and not *carbonation* of the local anesthetic. Because lidocaine base is poorly soluble, lidocaine solutions are prepared as an HCl salt to increase its solubility. On the other hand, carbonated salt solutions of lidocaine are prepared by bubbling CO_2 through a watery emulsion of lidocaine base in the cold. In this way, a carbonated salt solution of lidocaine is formed without addition of HCl. This solution has a pH of 6.5 (about the same as the plain hydrochloride solution). Unfortunately, carbonated local anesthetics are only commercially available in Canada and some other countries. The mechanism by which carbonation enhances conduction blockade is not precisely known, but several possibilities exist: 1) carbon dioxide may have a direct local anesthetic effect, 2) the increase in CO_2 inside the nerve decrease the pH causing local anesthetic cation trapping, and 3) effervescence of CO_2 when the vial is opened increases the pH of the solution from 6.5 to >7.0, making more free base available for nerve penetration. The first two of these mechanisms are predicated on the rapid diffusion of CO_2 through the nerve membrane into the axoplasm.

Investigations in man demonstrate that lidocaine~carbonate solutions produce a more rapid onset of brachial plexus and epidural blockade compared to the use of lidocaine~hydrochloride solutions (13, 14). However, another epidural block study failed to confirm this (15). It has been reported also that bupivacaine~carbonate given epidurally produces faster onset than bupivacaine~HCl. However, double-blind studies of brachial plexus or epidural blockade, failed to confirm these earlier reports of shorter onset with carbonated solutions (16, 17). Thus it is not clear that carbonation of local anesthetics consistently decreases onset time. However, it appears that epidurally injected carbonated solutions improve the quality of sensory anesthesia and the depth of motor blockade. The major advantage of carbonated local anesthetics may be in brachial plexus anesthesia, where they cause more profound conduction blockade in the radial, median and ulnar nerves.

pH Adjustment. Alkalization of local anesthetic solutions is used also to quicken the onset of conduction blockade. The addition of sodium bicarbonate increases the pH of the local anesthetic solution, in turn increasing the amount of drug in the uncharged ***base*** form. Thus, the local anesthetic should diffuse across the nerve sheath and nerve membrane faster and hasten the onset of anesthesia. Indeed, some clinical studies show that the addition of sodium bicarbonate to solutions of lidocaine or bupivacaine speeds the onset of brachial plexus or epidural blockade. In addition, the ***duration*** of brachial plexus block was prolonged also by increasing the pH of bupivacaine (18).

Wong et al.(19) studied the mechanistic basis of the potentiation of impulse inhibition by local anesthetic solutions containing bicarbonate-carbon dioxide ($HCO_3 \bullet CO_2$), relative to the inhibition in $HCO_3 \bullet CO_2$-free solutions at the same pH, by assaying compound action potential amplitudes in desheathed frog sciatic nerves. They compared the potencies of 12 different impulse-blocking agents in Ringer's buffered with $HCO_3 \bullet CO_2$

and in Ringer's containing only atmospheric CO_2 and buffered by MOPS, a zwitterionic compound (3-(N-morpholino)propanesulfonic acid-Ringer's). The relative inhibition produced by an agent in $HCO_3 \bullet CO_2$ divided by the inhibition produced in MOPS, was defined as the potentiation factor (PF). Only nominal potentiations occurred with charged local anesthetics (PF = 1.15), showing that little direct potentiation of the cationic local anesthetic species occurs, *per se*. Among the tertiary amine local anesthetics, potentiation of ester-linked drugs (procaine, RAG505; PF = 3.9, 5.4, respectively), exceeded that of their amide-linked homologues (procainamide, lidocaine; PF = 1.3, 2.8, respectively), which have higher pK_a values. This result is consistent with an ion trapping mechanism whereby CO_2 acidifies the axoplasm and thereby increases the concentration of protonated local anesthetic inside the nerve fibers. However, slight differences in the molecular structure of tertiary-amine local anesthetics with similar pK_a values resulted in significantly different potentiations (e.g., procaine, PF = 3.9; chloroprocaine, PF = 8.7), suggesting that the HCO_3 or CO_2 molecules interact specifically with the local anesthetic molecule or with local anesthetic binding sites in the nerve membrane. The authors concluded that $HCO_3 \bullet CO_2$ potentiates the impulse-blocking action of local anesthetics by the combined action of a) a nonspecific reduction in margin of conduction safety, b) ion trapping, and c) direct modification of local anesthetic binding at sites on the sodium channel.

Ackerman, et al. (20) did a similar study in patients. The purpose of their study was to determine the effect of pCO_2 on the onset of epidural analgesia with 2% chloroprocaine buffered to pH 7.7. They studied four groups consisting of ten patients each (see Table 3):

GROUP S—saline placebo
GROUP B—buffered with $NaHCO_3$
GROUP T—buffered with THAM (TROMETHAMINE)
GROUP BT—buffered with $NaHCO_3$ + THAM.

The time to the onset of analgesia was significantly faster in Group B (2.7 ± 0.8 min), while the onset of analgesia was significantly slower for Group T (5.4 ± 0.4 min) than either Group S (4.2 ± 0.8 min) or Group BT (3.4 ± 0.3 min). Regression analysis revealed that the onset times of the buffered solutions were significantly related to pCO_2 (r^2 = 0.81). On the other hand, the duration of analgesia of Group T (55.7 ± 4.29 min) and

Table 3. Effect of pH and PCO_2 on onset of epidural anesthesia with 2% chloroprocaine.

Group	Drug	pH	pCO2 (torr)	Onset (min)
S	Saline	4.35	11.8 ± 1.5	4.2 ± 0.8
B	$NaHCO_3$	7.7	113.0 ± 1.4	2.7 ± 0.8
T	THAM (tromethamine)	7.7	3.0 ± 0.3	5.4 ± 0.4
BT	$NaHCO_3$ + THAM	7.7	74.1 ± 1.0	3.4 ± 0.3

Data from reference 20.

Group BT (47.5 ± 5.1 min) were significantly longer than either Group S (27.0 ± 6.1 min) or Group B (26.2 ± 4.2 min). Thus, the onset of buffered epidural chloroprocaine was influenced by changes in pCO_2, while the duration was affected by the choice of the alkalinizing agent. This study shows also that while buffering chloroprocaine with $NaHCO_3$ statistically significantly decreases the onset of epidural anesthesia, the actual gain (1.5 min) is so small that the clinical usefulness of such a maneuver is questionable.

In the study by DiFazio, et al. (21), a pH adjustment of lidocaine from 4.6 to 7.2 hastened the onset of epidural anesthesia only 2.5 minutes. This is intriguing, because this pH change results in a 332-fold increase in the amount of base present in solution at the higher pH. This is equivalent to doing epidural anesthesia with 455% lidocaine at pH 4.6! Why isn't the onset of anesthesia hastened more than it is? The answer may be that the effect of increasing the amount of base in solution on the onset of anesthesia has limits. Rud (22) determined that, as the amount of lidocaine base increases, the concomitant speed of onset of nerve block is less than would be achieved with a linear relationship. It is possible that the concentrations of local anesthetics that we use clinically provide enough base (even at a low pH) so that the speed of onset expected from increasing the pH is blunted because the increase in the amount of base due to the pH change occurs on the plateau portion of the curve, as illustrated in Figure 7.

There is a limit to the amount of sodium bicarbonate that can be added to local anesthetics, because high pH causes many local anesthetics

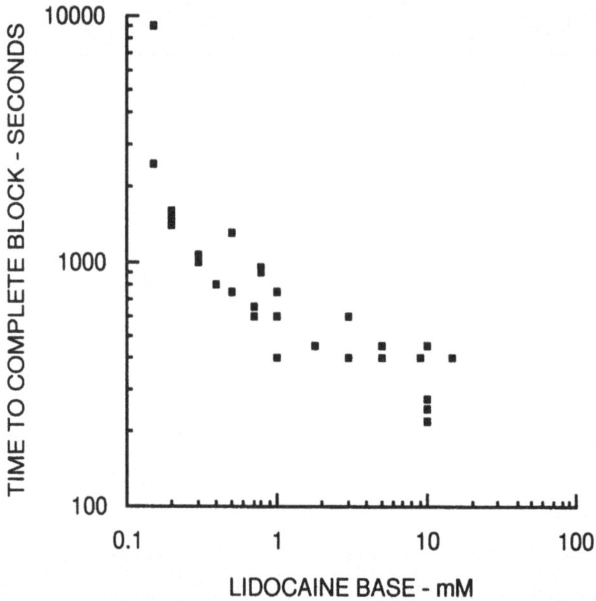

Figure 7. Relationship of time to block in isolated nerve to the concentration of lidocaine in the bathing solution. A 10 mM concentration of lidocaine ≅ 0.25% solution. Since the ratio of base/cation for lidocaine at pH = 7.4 is 1/3, then a solution, which is 10 mM in terms of base concentration, is ≅ to a 0.75% solution of lidocaine that is used clinically. (Data from Ref. 22, page 63)

to precipitate. Table 4 provides guidelines for adding sodium bicarbonate to the various local anesthetics (23). Another beneficial aspect of increasing the pH of local anesthetic solutions is that less pain is felt during injection (24).

Gassing with CO_2. In isolated nerve preparations, "gassing" local anesthetics with carbon dioxide enhances their diffusion through nerve sheaths, resulting in a more rapid onset (Figure 8) and a decrease in the minimum concentration (Cm) (1). The enhanced onset and depth of conduction blockade is believed to be due to the diffusion of carbon dioxide through the nerve membrane and a decrease in the axoplasmic pH. The lower pH increases the intracellular concentration of the active cationic form of the local anesthetic, which binds to a receptor in the sodium channel. In addition, the local anesthetic cation does not readily diffuse through membranes, such that the drug is trapped within the axoplasm, a situation referred to as ion trapping.

Table 4. Suggested amounts of $NaHCO_3$ to add to local anesthetics to adjust pH.

Local Anesthetic	ml of 4% $NaHCO_3$ per 20 ml of Local Anesthetic	pH after $NaHCO_3$
2% Chloroprocaine	4	7.51
3% Chloroprocaine	4	7.43
1% Mepivacaine	4	7.26
1.5% Mepivacaine	2	7.00
1% Etidocaine	0.015	5.90
1% Etidocaine (EPI)	0.1	5.73
1.5% Etidocaine (EPI)	0.1	5.76
0.25% Bupivacaine	1	6.97
0.5% Bupivacaine	0.05	6.62
0.75% Bupivacaine	0.05	6.56
0.5% Bupivacaine (EPI)	0.3	6.37
0.75% Bupivacaine (EPI)	0.3	6.32
1% Lidocaine	4	7.43
1.5% Lidocaine	4	7.31
2% Lidocaine	4	7.24
1% Lidocaine (EPI)	4	7.21
1.5% Lidocaine (EPI)	4	7.16
2% Lidocaine (EPI)	4	7.08

(EPI) = Commercially prepared epinephrine solution
Data from reference 23.

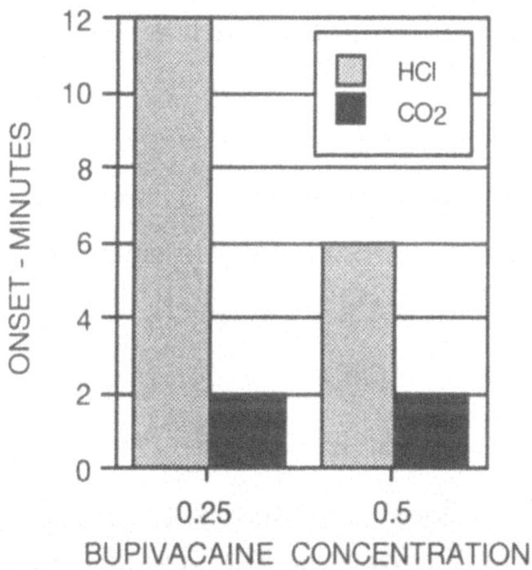

Figure 8. Onset time of conduction block in an isolated nerve following exposure to bupivacaine-HCl and bupivacaine-CO_2.

While carbonation of local anesthetic ***base*** solutions decreases onset, enhances spread and improves quality of conduction blockade, attempts to produce similar results by bubbling CO_2 through hydrochloride local anesthetic solutions (gassing) are not as effective. This is because gassing the non-carbonated local anesthetic solutions, prepared from the hydrochloride salt, with CO_2 reduces the pH from 6.5 to 4.9, decreasing the amount of base available for diffusion, and this slows the onset.

Solutions Containing Epinephrine. Local anesthetic solutions containing epinephrine have a pH of 4.5 to prevent oxidation of the epinephrine. Therefore, a larger increase in pH can be produced by adding sodium bicarbonate to these solutions compared to non-epinephrine containing solutions, which have a pH = 6.5. As a result, solutions containing epinephrine show the greatest decrease in onset when their pH is adjusted with sodium bicarbonate. An alternative to adjusting the pH with sodium bicarbonate is to add fresh epinephrine to the plain local anesthetic just before injection. This produces an epinephrine containing solution with pH 6.5, which increases the amount of base 100-fold without having to add sodium bicarbonate.

Additives. Attempts have been made to prolong the duration of anesthesia by adding substances like dextran to local anesthetic solutions (25). The effectiveness of dextran in prolonging the duration of regional anesthesia is uncertain. In one intercostal nerve block study, comparing bupivacaine with and without dextran, there was a prolongation of duration in some patients. But, the mean duration was not significantly prolonged by dextran (26).

Differences in results of the various investigations may be related to the pH of the dextran solution used. Dextran solutions with a pH of 8.0 significantly prolonged the duration of bupivacaine induced coccygeal nerve blocks in rats whereas the duration of block was not altered when dextran with a pH of 4.5 to 5.5 was added to bupivacaine. These results indicate that alkalinization of the anesthetic solution may be responsible for prolonged conduction blockade rather than the dextran itself.

Mixtures of Local Anesthetics

The popularity of using mixtures of local anesthetics for regional anesthesia has waxed and waned. The rationale for mixing local anesthetics is to compensate for the short duration of agents like chloroprocaine or lidocaine and the long latency of other agents like tetracaine and bupivacaine. Mixtures of chloroprocaine and bupivacaine theoretically offer advantages of rapid onset and low systemic toxicity (chloroprocaine) and long duration (bupivacaine). Brachial plexus blockade with a mixture of chloroprocaine and bupivacaine results in quick onset and prolonged duration (27). However, this is not true of epidural anesthesia, where the duration of anesthesia with a mixture of chloroprocaine and bupivacaine is shorter than that owing to bupivacaine alone (28). Thus, the kind of regional anesthetic block influences whether or not mixtures of local anesthetics have the intended effect. Furthermore, data from isolated nerve studies indicate that a metabolite of chloroprocaine may inhibit the binding of bupivacaine to membrane receptor sites (29). Another explanation for the shorter duration of bupivacaine when it is mixed with or given after chloroprocaine, relates to pH. Mixing a low pH solution like chloroprocaine (pH = 3.56) with bupivacaine (pH = 5.6) results in a mixture that has a pH of 3.6. This decreases the amount of un-ionized bupivacaine by 100-fold, lessening the amount of bupivacaine that penetrates the nerve and shortening its duration. In one study, the duration of bupivacaine blockade was unaffected by chloroprocaine when the pH of the mixture was increased from 3.6 to 5.6 (30).

Systemic toxicity is a concern when mixtures of local anesthetics are used for regional anesthesia. Early animal studies suggested that some mixtures may cause synergistic toxic effects. Yet, more recent data indicate that the toxicity of local anesthetics mixtures are additive and this is true of amide/amide or ester/amide mixtures (31). Since mixing local anesthetics dilutes the components, this should not change the toxicity of the injected solution. For example, the toxic dose of bupivacaine is believed to be between 175 to 225 mg, while that of chloroprocaine is 1000 mg. Doing an axillary block with 40 ml of 0.5% bupivacaine alone means injecting 200 mg of bupivacaine. The same block done with 40 ml of 3% chloroprocaine delivers 1200 mg of chloroprocaine. Mixing 0.5% bupivacaine and 3% chloroprocaine in equal amounts and injecting 40 ml of the mixture delivers 100 mg of bupivacaine (40 ml of 0.25% bupivacaine) and 600 mg of chloroprocaine (40 ml of 1.5% chloroprocaine).

Since the toxicities are additive, the potential systemic toxic effect of the mixture should be the same as either solution alone. However, because the convulsive effect of local anesthetics is related to their potency, the mixture may be more or less toxic than either solution alone. If bupivacaine is 8 times more potent than chloroprocaine (see Table 2), then the mixture has a relative potency of 1.167 compared to chloroprocaine alone (8 X 100 mg bupivacaine ≅ 800 mg chloroprocaine + 600 mg chloroprocaine ≅ 1400 mg chloroprocaine, in contrast to 1200 mg in the chloroprocaine alone solution), On the other hand, the mixture is only 0.875 times as potent as bupivacaine alone (600 mg chloroprocaine/8 ≅ 75 mg bupivacaine + 100 mg bupivacaine ≅ 175 mg bupivacaine , in contrast to 200 mg in the bupivacaine alone solution). The net result, however, is that the mixture is equivalent to either unmixed solution.

Currently, there appears to be no advantage to using mixtures of local anesthetic agents. Etidocaine and bupivacaine produce acceptable onsets of action and prolonged duration of anesthesia. Additionally, epidural and brachial plexus catheter techniques make it possible to repeatedly inject rapidly acting agents (chloroprocaine or lidocaine) thus providing anesthesia of indefinite duration. Alternatively, catheters can be used to quickly initiate anesthesia and prolong duration by injecting a rapidly acting agent, followed by low dose continuous infusions and/or infrequent bolus injections of long acting drugs.

Eutectic Mixtures of Local Anesthetics (EMLA). EMLA is a topical anesthetic, primarily intended for use on intact skin. It is a mixture of **crystalline** 5% lidocaine and 5% prilocaine ***base***, which becomes fluid at room temperature. This is caused by a lowering of the melting points of the constituents, similar to that produced when crystalline salt and ice are mixed. Other combinations of crystalline local anesthetics produce similar effects. Because of the high concentration gradients of the ***bases*** of lidocaine and prilocaine in EMLA cream, it is useful for anesthetizing intact skin. EMLA is intended for use in starting IVs in children, minor dermatologic operations like split-thickness skin grafting and the treatment of certain skin disorders. Unfortunately, it takes a fair amount of time for it to penetrate the cornified epithelium and it must be applied under an occlusive dressing, up to 60 to 90 minutes before the intended painful procedure is carried out (32).

Pregnancy

The spread of epidural or spinal anesthesia is greater in pregnant patients compared to nonpregnant patients. This exaggerated spread was attributed to mechanical factors (dilated epidural veins supposedly decrease the diameter of the epidural and subarachnoid space resulting in more extensive longitudinal spread of local anesthetic solution). Recent studies indicate that the increased local anesthetic sensitivity during pregnancy may be due to physiologic factors. For example, the spread of epidural anesthesia is similar during the first trimester of pregnancy and at term. This indicates that mechanical factors alone cannot explain the enhanced spread of anesthesia (33). Studies done in isolated **sheathed** vagus nerves reveal a more rapid onset and an increased sensitivity to local anesthetic induced conduction blockade in nerves obtained from pregnant rabbits (34, 35). A similar increased sensitivity to median nerve block with 1% lidocaine was observed in pregnant women (third trimester) compared to nonpregnant women (36). Recent experiments with isolated **desheathed** nerves indicate that the enhanced neuronal sensitivity owing to pregnancy may be due to fewer diffusion barriers instead of an increased sensitivity of the nerve membrane. A and B desheathed nerve fibers from pregnant animals are actually more resistant to local anesthetic block than those from nonpregnant animals (Lambert, unpublished, abstract pending). Since **sheathed** nerve fibers are more sensitive to local anesthetics, this implies that pregnancy decreases the diffusion barriers that the local anesthetic must penetrate to reach the receptor sites in the nerve where the block occurs. All in all, these results suggest that hormonal changes associated with pregnancy alter the basic responsiveness of the nerves to local anesthetics. Thus, the dosage for regional anesthetic procedures probably should be reduced during all stages of pregnancy.

SPECIFIC LOCAL ANESTHETIC AGENTS

Amino-Ester Agents (Table 5)

Cocaine. Isolated from the *Erythroxylon coca* bush, cocaine was the first drug successfully used for local anesthesia. Its high potential for

Table 5. Clinical uses of local anesthetics.

Agent	*Primary Use*	*Comments*
Amino-Esters		
Cocaine	TOP	Limit use due to addictive potential
Procaine	INFIL, SPIN	Limited—slow onset, short duration, allergy potential
Chloroprocaine	PNB, EPID	Fast onset, short duration, low toxicity
Tetracaine	SPIN	Limited—slow onset, toxicity
Amino-Amides		
Lidocaine	INFIL, IV REG, PNB, EPID, SPIN, TOP	Most versatile
Mepivacaine	INFIL, PNB, EPID, SPIN	Similar to lidocaine
Prilocaine	INFIL, IV REG, PNB, EPID	Methemoglobinemia at high dose, least toxic amide
Bupivacaine	INFIL, PNB, EPID, SPIN	Sensory-motor separation
Etidocaine	INFIL, PNB, EPID	Profound motor block
Miscellaneous		
Dibucaine	TOP, SPIN	Not available in USA
Benzocaine	TOP	Limited to topical

TOP = topical; INFIL = infiltration; SPIN = spinal; PNB = peripheral nerve block; EPID = epidural; IV REG = intravenous regional anesthesia

systemic toxicity and its addictive properties have limited its usefulness. However, cocaine is an excellent topical anesthetic and it is the only local anesthetic that produces vasoconstriction at clinically used concentrations. Because of its topical anesthetic and vasoconstrictor properties, it is still used by anesthesiologists to anesthetize and constrict the nasal mucosa prior to naso-tracheal intubation and by otolaryngologists during nasal surgery .

Procaine. Procaine was the first synthetic local anesthetic agent. It is a relatively weak local anesthetic with slow onset and short duration of action. Procaine's relatively low potency and rapid plasma hydrolysis is responsible for its low systemic toxicity. However, procaine is hydrolyzed to para-aminobenzoic acid, which causes allergic reactions in some patients. Procaine is primarily used for infiltration anesthesia, diagnostic differential spinal blocks in certain pain states, and for spinal anesthesia.

Chloroprocaine. This agent has a rapid onset, a short duration, and low systemic toxicity. Chloroprocaine is used mainly for epidural analgesia and anesthesia in obstetrics where its rapid onset and low systemic toxicity are beneficial in mother and fetus. However, frequent injections are necessary to produce adequate pain relief during labor. Often, epidural analgesia in the pregnant patient is started with chloroprocaine and continued with a longer acting agent such as bupivacaine. Chloroprocaine is useful also for regional anesthesia in ambulatory patients, when the duration of surgery is anticipated to be 30 to 60 minutes.

There are reports of prolonged sensory/motor deficits following the accidental intrathecal injection of large doses of chloroprocaine. These local irritant effects are believed to be due to the low pH and the sodium bisulfite contained in chloroprocaine solutions. After these injuries, sodium bisulfite was removed from the formulation.

Tetracaine. This agent is primarily used for spinal anesthesia. It is used as an isobaric, hypobaric or hyperbaric solution. Tetracaine provides a relatively rapid onset of spinal anesthesia, good sensory anesthesia and a profound motor block. Isobaric solutions of tetracaine last two to three hours, but the addition of epinephrine or phenylephrine can extend the duration to four to six hours.

Tetracaine is used rarely for other types of regional anesthesia because of its slow onset and its potential to cause systemic toxicity when large doses are used. Tetracaine is a good topical anesthetic and it is used for endotracheal surface anesthesia. Absorption of tetracaine from the tracheo-bronchial tree is extremely rapid and fatalities have occurred after aerosolizing tetracaine into the trachea.

Amino-Amide Agents (Table 5)

Lidocaine. Lidocaine was the first of the amino-amides to be introduced into clinical practice. Because of its inherent potency, rapid onset, moderate duration, and topical anesthetic activity, lidocaine is the most versatile and most commonly used local anesthetic. Solutions of lidocaine are available for infiltration, peripheral nerve block, spinal and epidural anesthesia. Lidocaine is used also as an ointment, jelly, viscous and aerosol for topical anesthesia.

Lidocaine is frequently given intravenously for treatment of ventricular arrhythmias. In addition, intravenous lidocaine is used as an anti-epileptic agent, as an analgesic for certain chronic pain states and as an intravenous supplement to general anesthesia.

Mepivacaine. The anesthetic profile of prilocaine is similar to lidocaine's. It produces profound anesthesia with rapid onset and moderate duration. Mepivacaine is used for infiltration, peripheral nerve blocks and epidural anesthesia. In some countries, 4% hyperbaric mepivacaine is used for spinal anesthesia.

Because mepivacaine is not effective as a topical anesthetic it is less versatile than lidocaine. In addition, the metabolism of mepivacaine is markedly prolonged in the fetus and newborn. Therefore, it is not usually employed for obstetrical anesthesia. On the other hand, in adults mepivacaine appears to be somewhat less toxic than lidocaine. In addition, the vasodilation caused by mepivacaine is less than that caused by lidocaine. Thus, mepivacaine produces longer duration anesthesia than lidocaine when the two agents are used without epinephrine.

Prilocaine. The anesthetic profile of prilocaine is similar also to lidocaine's. Prilocaine has a rapid onset, moderate duration, and a profound depth of anesthesia. It causes significantly less vasodilation than lidocaine. The duration of prilocaine without epinephrine is similar to that of lidocaine with epinephrine. Thus, prilocaine is useful in patients in whom epinephrine is contraindicated. Prilocaine is used for infiltration, peripheral nerve blocks and epidural anesthesia.

Prilocaine is the least toxic of the amino-amide local anesthetics. Thus, prilocaine is particularly useful for intravenous regional anesthesia. CNS toxic effects are rarely seen following tourniquet deflation even after early accidental release of the tourniquet occurs.

Methemoglobinemia occurs with large doses of prilocaine. This side effect is a relative contraindication to the use of this drug in obstetrics, even though prilocaine has not caused any adverse effects in mother, fetus or newborn. However, cyanosis owing to methemoglobinemia in newborns delivered to mothers who received prilocaine for epidural anesthesia during labor contradicts using this potentially valuable drug for labor analgesia.

Bupivacaine. Bupivacaine was the first local anesthetic to combine the properties of acceptable onset, long duration, profound anesthesia, and separation of sensory and motor blockade. This agent is used for infiltration, peripheral nerve blocks, and for epidural and spinal anesthesia. Depending on the site of injection, its duration of surgical anesthesia varies from 3 to 10 hours. The longest duration occurs with major peripheral nerve blocks such as brachial plexus blockade.

Bupivacaine is advantageous in epidural labor analgesia where pain relief lasting 2 to 3 hours decreases the frequency of top-up injections. Moreover, analgesia occurs with little motor block so that the laboring patient is better able to "push" at delivery. This differential sensory and motor block is also the basis for using bupivacaine for postoperative epidural analgesia, and for certain chronic pain states.

Ropivacaine. This is a new amide local anesthetic that is currently undergoing clinical trials. Ropivacaine is similar to mepivacaine and bupivacaine. The only difference between these drugs is in the group attached to the nitrogen atom of the piperidine ring (Table 1). Mepivacaine has a methyl group, ropivacaine a propyl group and bupivacaine a butyl group. These groups are believed to contribute to the cardiotoxic effect of these local anesthetics (see section on toxicity). Ropivacaine is being explored because it has properties that are similar to bupivacaine's. However, because of its shorter piperidine side chain (propyl group), it is hoped that ropivacaine might be less cardiotoxic than bupivacaine.

Clinical studies indicate that while ropivacaine is slightly less potent, than bupivacaine, the two agents are very similar. Ropivacaine and bupivacaine have similar pK_a and protein binding, but ropivacaine's lipid solubility is less than bupivacaine's. Thus, the onset and duration of the two drugs is similar. However, ropivacaine is less potent and will likely be used in 0.75% to 1% concentrations compared to 0.5% to 0.75% for bupivacaine. Like bupivacaine, ropivacaine causes good separation of sensory and motor block. It should be very useful, therefore, in obstetric anesthesia.

Etidocaine. This agent is characterized by very rapid onset, prolonged duration, and profound sensory and motor blockade. Etidocaine is used for infiltration, peripheral nerve blocks and epidural anesthesia. Its onset is significantly faster than bupivacaine's. Concentrations of etidocaine that are required for adequate sensory anesthesia also produce profound motor blockade. As a result, etidocaine is used mostly for long operations requiring good muscle relaxation. Etidocaine is of no use for labor analgesia or for postoperative pain relief because it does not differentially block sensory and motor fibers.

Miscellaneous

Dibucaine. This agent is used for spinal and topical anesthesia. For spinal anesthesia, dibucaine is formulated as an isobaric, hypobaric, or hyperbaric solution. If we compare dibucaine and tetracaine spinal anesthesia, the onset and spread of the two agents is similar, but the duration is slightly longer with dibucaine, and the degree of hypotension and the profoundness of motor blockade is less with dibucaine.

Benzocaine. This local anesthetic is used only for topical anesthesia. It is available in a variety of proprietary and non-proprietary preparations. Benzocaine is most commonly used in the operating room as an aerosol solutions for endotracheal anesthesia and as an ointment to lubricate endotracheal tubes.

REFERENCES

1. Gissen AJ, Covino BG, Gregus J: Differential sensitivities of mammalian nerve fibers to local anesthetic agents. Anesthesiology 53:467-474, 1983
2. Wildsmith JA, Gissen AJ, Gregus J, Covino BG: Differential nerve blocking activity of amino-ester local anaesthetics. Br J Anaesth 57:612-620, 1985
3. Wildsmith JA, Gissen AJ, Takman B, Covino BG: Differential nerve blockade: Esters v. amides and the influence of pKa. Br J Anaesth 59:379-84, 1987
4. Covino BG: Pharmacology of local anaesthetic agents. Br J Anaesth 58:701-716, 1986
5. Johns RA, DiFazio CA, Longnecker DE: Lidocaine constricts or dilates rat arterioles in a dose-dependent manner. Anesthesiology 62:141-144, 1985

6. Johns RA, Seyde WC, DiFazio CA, Longnecker DE: Dose-dependent effects of bupivacaine on rat muscle arterioles. Anesthesiology 65:186-191, 1986
7. Rosenberg PH, Heinonen E, Jansson SE, Gripenberg J: Differential nerve block by bupivacaine and 2-chloroprocaine. An experimental study. Br J Anaesth 52:1183-1189, 1980
8. Scott DB, McClure JH, Giasi RM, et al: Effects of concentration of local anaesthetic drugs in extradural block. Br J Anaesth 52:1033-1037, 1980
9. Gissen AJ, Covino BG, Gregus J: Differential sensitivity of fast and slow fibers in mammalian nerve. III. Effect of etidocaine and bupivacaine on fast/slow fibers. Anesth Analg 61:570-575, 1982
10. Concepcion M, Maddi R, Francis D, et al: Vasoconstrictors in spinal anesthesia with tetracaine—A comparison of epinephrine and phenylephrine. Anesth Analg 63:134-138, 1984
11. Chambers WA, Littlewood DG, Logan MR, Scott DB: Effect of added epinephrine on spinal anesthesia with lidocaine. Anesth Analg 60:417-420, 1981
12. Chambers WA, Littlewood DG, Scott DB: Spinal anesthesia with hyperbaric bupivacaine: Effect of added vasoconstrictors. Anesth Analg 61:49-52, 1982
13. Bromage PR: A comparison of the hydrochloride and carbon dioxide salts of lidocaine and prilocaine in epidural analgesia. Acta Anaesthesiol Scand (Suppl) 16:55-69, 1965
14. Bromage PR, Gertel M: An evaluation of two new local anaesthetics for major conduction blockade. Can Anaesth Soc J 17:557-564, 1970
15. Morison DH: A double-blind comparison of carbonated lidocaine and lidocaine hydrochloride in epidural anaesthesia. Can Anaesth Soc J 28:387-389, 1981
16. Brown DT, Morison DH, Covino BG, Scott DB: Comparison of carbonated bupivacaine and bupivacaine hydrochloride for extradural anaesthesia. Br J Anaesth 52:419-422, 1980
17. McClure JH, Scott DB: Comparison of bupivacaine hydrochloride and carbonated bupivacaine in brachial plexus block by the interscalene technique. Br J Anaesth 53:523-526, 1981
18. Hilgier M: Alkalinization of bupivacaine for brachial plexus block. Reg Anesth 10:59-61, 1985
19. Wong K, Strichartz GR, Raymond SA: On the mechanisms of potentiation of local anesthetics by bicarbonate buffer: Drug structure-activity studies on isolated peripheral nerve. Anesth Analg 76:131-143, 1993
20. Ackerman WE, Denson DD, Juneja MM, et al: Alkalinization of chloroprocaine for epidural anesthesia: Effects of pCO_2 at constant pH. Reg Anesth 15:89-93, 1990
21. DiFazio CA, Carron H, Grosslight KR, et al: Comparison of pH-adjusted lidocaine solutions for epidural anesthesia. Anesth Analg 65:760-764, 1986

22. Rud J: Local anesthetics. An electrophysiological investigation of local anesthesia of peripheral nerves, with special reference to xylocaine. Acta Physiol Scand (Suppl) 178 51:1-171, 1961
23. Peterfreund RA, Datta S, Ostheimer GW: pH adjustment of local anesthetic solutions with sodium bicarbonate: Laboratory evaluation of alkalinization and precipitation. Reg Anesth 14:265-270, 1989
24. Morris R, McKay W, Mushlin P: Comparison of pain associated with intradermal and subcutaneous infiltration with various local anesthetic solutions. Anesth Analg 66:1180-1182, 1987
25. Loder RE: A local anesthetic solution with longer action. Lancet 2:346-347, 1960
26. Bridenbaugh LD: Does the addition of low molecular weight dextran prolong the duration of action of bupivacaine? Reg Anesth 3:6, 1978
27. Cunningham NL, Kaplan JA: A rapid-onset, long-acting regional anesthetic technique. Anesthesiology 41:509-511, 1974
28. Cohen SE, Thurlow A: Comparison of a chloroprocaine—Bupivacaine mixture with chloroprocaine and bupivacaine used individually for obstetric epidural analgesia. Anesthesiology 51:288-292, 1979
29. Corke BC, Carlson CG, Dettbarn WD: The influence of 2-chloroprocaine on the subsequent analgesic potency of bupivacaine. Anesthesiology 60:25-27, 1984
30. Galindo A, Witcher T: Mixtures of local anesthetics: Bupivacaine-chloroprocaine. Anesth Analg 59:683-685, 1980
31. Spiegel DA, Dexter F, Warner DS, et al: Central nervous system toxicity of local anesthetic mixtures in the rat. Anesth Analg 75:922-928, 1992
32. Juhlin L, Evers H: EMLA: A new topical anesthetic. Adv Dermatol 5:75-91, 1990
33. Fagraeus L, Urban B, Bromage P: Spread of epidural analgesia in early pregnancy. Anesthesiology 58:184-187, 1983
34. Datta S, Lambert D, Gregus J, et al: Differential sensitivities of mammalian nerve fibers during pregnancy. Anesth Analg 62:1070-1072, 1983
35. Flanagan HL, Datta S, Lambert DH, et al: Effect of pregnancy on bupivacaine-induced conduction blockade in the isolated rabbit vagus nerve. Anesth Analg 66:123-126, 1987
36. Butterworth JF 4th, Walker FO, Lysak SZ: Pregnancy increases median nerve susceptibility to lidocaine. Anesthesiology 72:962-965, 1990

PAIN RESEARCH AND BASIC SCIENCE: PAIN AND THE SYMPATHETIC NERVOUS SYSTEM

P. G. Fine

INTRODUCTION

Our current understanding of the mechanisms involved in most chronic pain states is embryonic. This generalization holds true for the role played by the sympathetic nervous system (SNS) during initiation, propagation or maintenance of nociception and neuropathic pain, especially on a chronic basis. It is not surprising, then, that indications and rates of success for specific therapies are equally vague.

Therapeutic plans and outcomes tend to reflect individual practitioner's anecdotal experience, particular training, or opinions rather than a scientifically derived foundation or epidemiologically sound data base, which do not exist at this time. Most experts in the field (i.e., clinicians and basic scientists with a track record of commitment to clinical or bench research) seldom agree on diagnostic criteria for these clinical syndromes (1).

Historically, most assumptions and conclusions regarding a causal relationship between certain chronic pain states and the SNS have arisen from observational data. These observations consist of clinical features of autonomic dysregulation and dysfunction (usually evidencing SNS overactivity) coupled with pain relief resulting from sympathetic blocks. A circular logic has developed, linking physical signs of autonomic dysregulation and a therapeutic intervention (sympathetic block) with a hypothetical pathophysiological mechanism (SNS malfunction). However, the true underlying pathophysiology of these pain states has remained elusive.

Traditionally, these clinical conditions have been given the names "reflex sympathetic dystrophy" (RSD), "causalgia" and the like. In an effort to decrease ambiguity and confusion, there has been a recent trend to

T. H. Stanley and M. A. Ashburn (eds.), Anesthesiology and Pain Management, 65–75.

avoid descriptive names in favor of categorical names to label these clinical conditions. These are based upon putative mechanisms or responses to specific interventions. Thus, under the larger category of "Neuropathic Pain" would come the sub-categories of "sympathetically maintained pain" (SMP) or "sympathetically independent pain" (SIP), based upon whether the patient's pain could be attenuated by sympatholysis.

The bottom line is that we are left with a poorly understood condition or group of conditions which are extremely difficult to treat. This chapter will review the historical path we have taken to arrive at our present understanding of pain and the SNS followed by a summary of current thinking regarding underlying mechanisms. Hopefully, this will help to provide rational approaches toward diagnosis and treatment for anesthesiologists who practice in a variety of settings, who may be interested or otherwise called upon to see these patients.

THE PAST

Toward the end of the 16th century, Galen characterized his concept of harmony between bodily structures and functions as "sympathy of parts." Although he is credited for anatomical descriptions of the SNS, he never ascribed this (ephemeral) concept of "sympathy" to it (2). In the 17th century, Willis (3) refined this thesis, believing that "sympathy" indeed did relate to a particular function of the nervous system. He viewed all involuntary actions and reactions to pain and pleasure as phenomena of "sympathy."

Winslow (4) accurately described the SNS in the next century. He introduced the term "sympathetic" to describe the role of this part of the nervous system in maintaining "harmony" or "sympathy" between portions of the viscera. It wasn't until the 19th century that a sensory processing role was ascribed to the SNS by Bichat (5) and Bernard (6). Later in that century, Mitchell et al (7) introduced the term "causalgia" to describe the burning pain associated with nerve injuries in American Civil War soldiers.

During the first half of the 20th century, LeRiche (8) asserted that the SNS has a fundamental sensory processing role. He promoted the concept of a sympathetic afferent limb to anatomically substantiate his view. This concept remains controversial to this day. He applied his ideas clinically by administering local anesthetic sympathetic blocks for the treatment of angina and causalgia.

Livingston (9) postulated the "vicious circle" theory in 1943 to explain the phenomena of dystrophic changes and pain reinforcement observed in causalgia. He reiterated, in a refined manner, the notion that a self-perpetuating reflex arc is established that extends from the periphery to the spinal cord to the sympathetic efferent system back to the periphery. Shortly thereafter, Doupe (10) and Granit (11) suggested that "ephaptic" transmission (an artificial synapse forming a short circuit between sympathetic and sensory fibers) could account for this type of reflex self-perpetuating activity. Although there is now supporting evidence that ephaptic transmission occurs, there is little to implicate this as a SNS mechanism responsible for the maintenance of chronic pain states (12). Moving up to the current era, Bonica (13) is credited with expanding the premise concerning the etiology of SNS mediated pain syndromes to include both traumatic and nontraumatic causes and the role of sympathetic blocks for diagnosis and treatment. Furthermore, a full elaboration of this history can be appreciated in his recent comprehensive text (14).

THE PRESENT

Theories

In 1986, Roberts (15) published a synthesis of most of the recent animal model experiments investigating the role of the SNS as a component of nociceptive neuromodulation. With this empiric data, he put forth a hypothesis that allowed for the observation that ongoing tissue damage, and thus ongoing nociceptor stimulation-discharge, is not apparent (or necessary) in many chronic pain states where the SNS seems to be involved in the maintenance of painful sensations. His theory contends that the SNS, even in its normative state of functioning, maintains a condition of central nervous system sensitization by supporting the ongoing "activated" state of spinal receiving neurons whose firing thresholds have been lowered (sensitized) as a result of afferent discharges. The SNS facilitates the firing of peripheral mechanoreceptors whose afferent impulses impinge upon these receiving neurons which in turn signal, by virtue of their sensitized state, pain sensations (Figure 1).

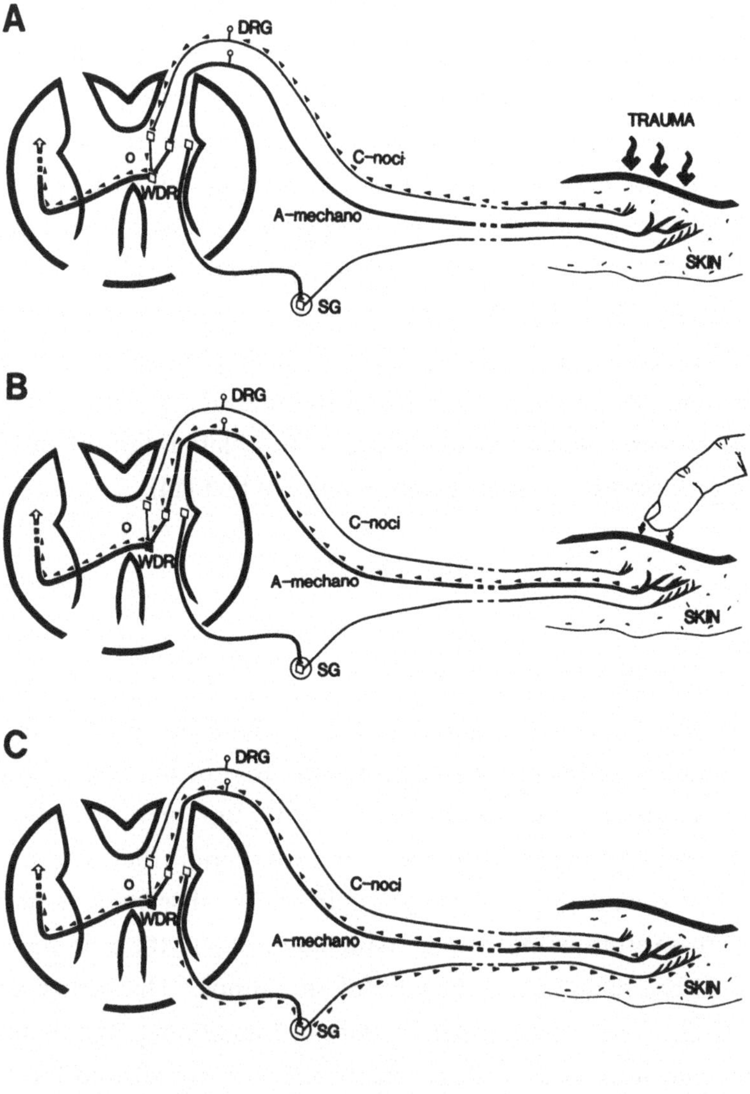

DRG = dorsal route ganglion
SG = sympathetic ganglion
WDR = wide dynamic range neuron

Figure 1. The sequence of events leading to SNS maintenance of pain perception, through sustained activation of sensitized spinal (sensory) receiving neurons. Adapted from Roberts (15).

At the time of his writing, it was considered that the SNS acted on mechanoreceptors in this way but not nociceptors and so the reflex arc, wherein the SNS was involved, was exclusive of nociceptor involvement. This explained the pain that is perceived after non-noxious mechanical stimulation (so-called allodynia) such as gently rubbing the skin over the affected part, but not the frequently reported symptom of spontaneous burning pain. Nevertheless, Robert's hypothesis suggests that blocking the SNS allows for normalization of the sensitized spinal neurons, over time, by decreasing their continual peripheral (low threshold) bombardment.

More recently, however, it has been demonstrated that when nociceptors are activated by injury, sympathetic stimulation can maintain tonic firing of the involved peripheral nociceptors, even after the noxious stimulus is removed (16). This finding may be quite important in furthering an explanation of the spontaneous burning pain that is virtually pathognomonic for causalgia and reflex sympathetic dystrophy. Again, blocking the SNS would allow for nociceptors to regain their resting state (**not** firing when **not** stimulated by a noxious event) and interrupt the pain-producing reflex.

Campbell et al (17) have elaborated a theory, based upon clinical responses to sympatholytic drugs, invoking up-regulation of peripheral alpha-1 receptors impacting activity of nociceptors. Crucial pieces of evidence for this hypothesis are the analgesic responses of patients to topical application of the alpha-2 (presynaptic) agonist clonidine (18) and intravenous phentolamine, an alpha-1 blocker (Figure 2) (19,20).

Compelling as these studies seem, it is important to note that skepticism (the key ingredient in healthy scientific evaluation) has been voiced by Ochoa regarding the interpretation of the data (21). Questions are raised about the specificity of the drug effects compared to placebo in similarly "afflicted" patients. This shadow of doubt has been substantiated in a just-completed study investigating the effects of intravenous phentolamine on chronic low back pain (22). In this study, we gave several placebo injections prior to the "active drug", and pain relief reports (placebo response) preceded active drug (Figure 3). Without these repeated injections, we would have been misled into concluding that the phentolamine was responsible for the resultant change in pain report. Clearly,

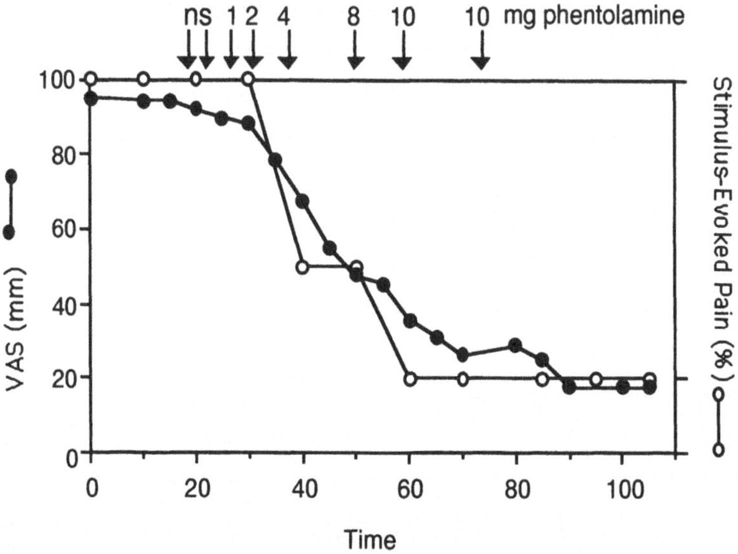

Figure 2. Responses of patients with a presumptive diagnosis of sympathetically maintained pain to intravenous phentolamine. Adapted from Raja et al (20).

more studies of this type are needed to define the role of sympatholytic drugs as diagnostic tools for the purpose of differentiating mechanisms of pain.

The connection between the SNS and opioid-receptor mediated neuromodulation is only now becoming apparent. The curious finding of opioid receptors within sympathetic ganglionic tissue (23) has not only led to a therapeutic tool for the reduction of symptoms associated with sympathetically maintained pain (24,25) (Figure 4), but now opens a world of inquiry as to the ontogeny of the pain perception and internal regulation system.

Pertinent to this discussion is a novel theory recently proposed by Hannington-Kiff (26). He poses the hypothesis that the sympathetically maintained pain syndromes result from failed opioid modulation of sympathetic and sensory function within autonomic ganglia, reminiscent of the more global abstinence syndrome observed in people undergoing acute opioid withdrawal.

This proposition is anecdotally supported by his clinical observations using opioids targeted at stellate and lumbar sympathetic

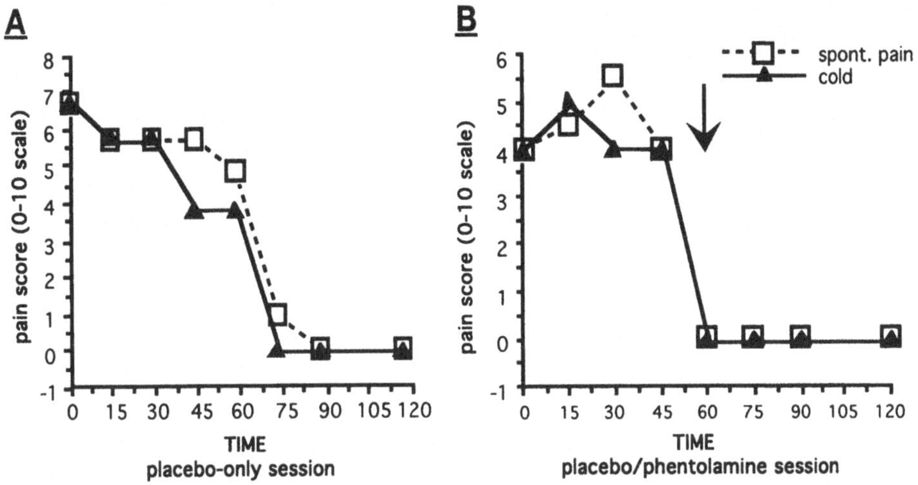

Figure 3a & b. Representative (and typical example) of placebo response paralleling phentolamine response in a placebo controlled double blind trial of intravenous phentolamine effects on chronic low back pain. In this model, blinded intravenous infusions are administered every 15 minutes, with only one of the infusions containing phentolamine 30 mg on one of two separate sessions. The arrow on Fig. 3b identifies the time when the phentolamine 30 mg infusion was begun (source: Fine PG).

ganglia in patients with characteristic sympathetically maintained pain. These findings are provocative but lack scientific corroboration as of yet.

In addition to these basic mechanistic insights and hypotheses, it is becoming increasingly clear that the SNS plays a role in the modulation of pain perception in a variety of clinical settings beyond the classical paradigms typically thought of as causalgia and reflex sympathetic dystrophy. The finding that sympathetic block decreases the symptomatology associated with myofascial pain (27) serves as clinically substantiating evidence that the SNS supports pain-producing peripheral-central reflex circuits. Coupled with data that suggests that trigger point injection analgesia for myofascial pain is naloxone reversible (implicating a central endogenous opioid mechanism), it appears that the SNS is not necessarily the perpetrator in these various self-perpetuating pain states, but serves as a vital link in the maintenance of them. Thus, the term "Sympathetic Maintained Pain" coined by Roberts (15) is fitting.

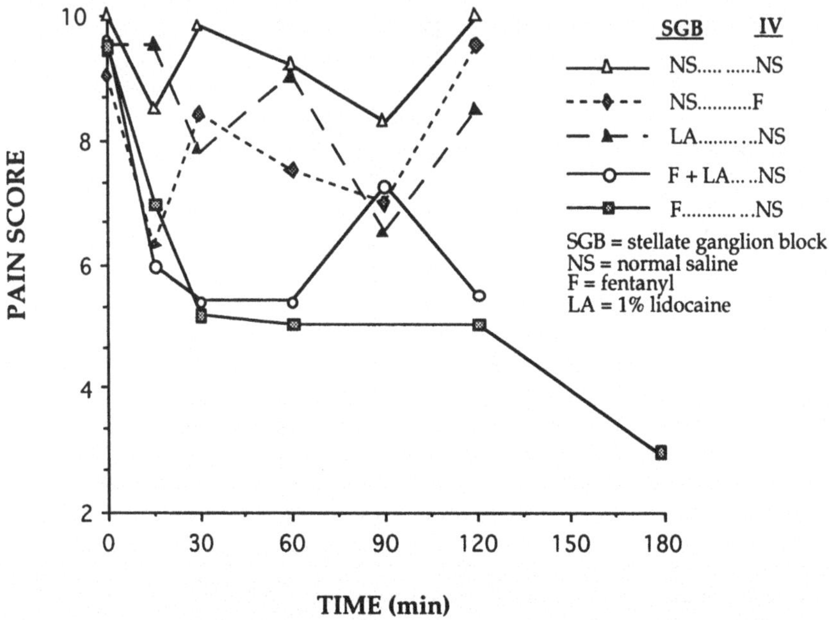

Figure 4. Demonstration of opioid-mediated analgesia resulting from fentanyl stellate ganglion "block" in a patient with sympathetically maintained pain. Comparison is made to other injections as noted, with all injections performed in a double blind randomized fashion. Adapted from Fine et al (24).

CONCLUSION

It is hoped that anesthesiologists (and other physicians) who evaluate and treat patients with pain syndromes thought to involve the SNS will consider the mechanisms and theories summarized in this chapter while formulating their diagnostic work-ups and plans of therapy. These thought processes will help direct therapies and, if good data is kept, help to give insight into the pathophysiology of these processes.

In evaluating and treating all patients with persistent pain syndromes, the assessment and treatment plan should "fit" the context of the whole patient. Simply casting therapies at body parts or "pieces" of the patient's pain syndrome will usually result in therapeutic failure. Table 1 (28) is provided in order to help you, the clinician, frame your approach, regardless of the theories or types of interventions to which you subscribe, as they may pertain to the SNS and persistent pain states.

Table 1. A scheme for anticipating treatment outcome from pretreatment information.

Level I. Anesthesia Only/Limited Rehabilitation (Outpatient)

Evaluation

- Duration of pain less than 3 months;
- Good correlation of physical findings and complaints;
- Medication use appropriate;
- Disability commensurate with physical findings;
- Psychosocial disruption is minimal or short-term;

Treatment

- Good compliance with prescribed treatment;

Objective improvement is matched with subjective improvement.

Level II. Anesthesia with Intensive Rehabilitation (Outpatient/Day Treatment)

Evaluation

- Duration of pain less than 1 year;
- Good correlation of physical findings and complaints;
- Medication appears to be greater than can be accounted for by physical findings alone;
- Psychosocial disruption is significant

Treatment

- Reasonable compliance with prescribed treatment;

Objective improvement is equal to or greater than subjective improvement.

Level III. Anesthesia with Comprehensive Interdisciplinary Team Management (Inpatient/Day Treatment)

Evaluation

- Duration of pain greater than 1 year;
- Poor or no correlation between physical findings and complaints;
- Medication use is usually problematic;
- Disability is obviously greater than can be accounted for by physical findings alone;
- Psychosocial disruption is severe and is often more long-standing than the pain complaints.

Treatment

- Poor to good compliance with prescribed treatment;

Objective improvement does not match subjective response (i.e., function increases, but complaints don't change much).

Adapted from Fine PG and Hare BD (28).

REFERENCES

1. Wilson PR: Reflex? Sympathetic? Dystrophy? Paradigm Shift? Clin J Pain 8:281-284, 1992
2. Procacci P, Maresca M: Reflex sympathetic dystrophies and algodystrophies: Historical and pathogenic considerations. Pain 31:137-146, 1987
3. Willis T: De Anima Brutorum. London, Davis, 1672
4. Winslow JB: Exposition Anatomique de la Structure du Corps Humain. Paris, Duprez et Desessartz, 1732
5. Bichat MFX: Anatomie Generale, Applique a la Physiologie et la Medicine. Paris, Brosson, 1801
6. Bernard C: Lecons sur la Physiologie et la Pathologie du Systeme Nerveux. Paris, Bailliere, 1858
7. Mitchell SW, et al: Gunshot Wounds and Other Injuries of Nerves. Philadelphia, J. B. Lippincott, 1864
8. LeRiche R: La Chirurgia de la Couleur. Paris, Masson, 1949
9. Livingston WK: Pain Mechanisms. New York, Macmillan, 1943
10. Doupe J, Cullen CH: Post-traumatic pain and the causalgic syndrome. J Neurol Neurosurg Psychiatry 7:33-48, 1944
11. Granit R, Leksell L, Skoglund CR: Fibre interaction in injured or compressed region of nerve. Brain 67:125-140, 1944
12. Devor M: Nerve pathophysiology and mechanisms of pain in causalgia. J Auton Nerv Syst 7:371-384, 1983
13. Bonica JJ: The Management of Pain. Philadelphia, Lea and Febiger, 1953
14. Bonica JJ: The Management of Pain, 2nd ed. Philadelphia, Lea and Febiger, 1990
15. Roberts WJ. A hypothesis on the physiological basis for causalgia and related pains. Pain 24:297-311, 1986
16. Hu SJ, Zhu J: Sympathetic facilitation of sustained discharges of polymodal nociceptors. Pain 38:85-90, 1989
17. Campbell JN, Meyer RA and Raja SN: Is nociceptor activation by alpha-1 adrenoreceptors the culprit in sympathetically maintained pain? APS Journal 1:3-11, 1992
18. Davis KD, Treede R-D, Raja SN, et al: Topical application of clonidine relieves hyperalgesia in patients with sympathetically maintained pain. Pain 47:309-317, 1991
19. Arnér S: Intravenous phentolamine test: Diagnostic and prognostic use in reflex sympathetic dystrophy. Pain 46:17-22, 1991
20. Raja SN, Treede R-D, Davis KD, Campbell JN: Systemic alpha-adrenergic blockade with phentolamine: A diagnostic test for sympathetically maintained pain. Anesthesiology 74:691-698, 1991
21. Ochoa JL: Reflex sympathetic dystrophy: A disease of medical understanding. Clin J Pain 8:363-366, 1992

22. Fine PG, Roberts WJ, Gillette RG, Child TR: A new approach to the placebo-controlled phentolamine test applied to chronic low back pain. Pain (in press)
23. Prosdocimi M, Finesso M, Gorio A: Enkephalin modulation of neural transmission in the cat stellate ganglion: Pharmacological actions of exogenous opiates. J Auton Nerv Syst 17:217-230, 1986
24. Fine PG, Ashburn MA: Effect of stellate ganglion block with fentanyl on postherpetic neuralgia with a sympathetic component. Anesth Analg 67:897-899, 1988
25. Arias LM, Bartkowski R, Grossman KL, et al: Sufentanil stellate ganglion injection in the treatment of refractory reflex sympathetic dystrophy. Reg Anesth 14:90-92, 1989
26. Hannington-Kiff JG: Does failed natural opioid modulation in regional sympathetic ganglia cause reflex sympathetic dystrophy. Lancet 338(8775):1125-1127, 1991
27. Bengtsson A, Bengtsson M: Regional sympathetic blockade in primary fibromyalgia. Pain 33:161-167, 1988
28. Fine PG, Hare BD: Introduction to chronic pain, Problems in Anesthesia: Chronic Pain. Edited by Hare BD and Fine PG. Philadelphia, J. B. Lippincott, 1990, pp. 553-560

LOCAL ANESTHESIA TOXICITY

D. H. Lambert

When properly given, local anesthetics are relatively free of side effects. However, systemic and localized toxicity occur with accidental intravascular injection or with excessive doses injected intrathecally. Additionally, other adverse effects occur with certain agents, e.g., allergic reactions to the amino-esters, and methemoglobinemia with high doses of prilocaine.

SYSTEMIC TOXICITY

Systemic toxicity affects the central nervous and the cardiovascular systems. The central nervous system (CNS) is more susceptible to local anesthetic toxicity than is the cardiovascular system. The dose and blood level of local anesthetic required to produce CNS toxicity is lower than the dose that causes circulatory collapse. Although local anesthetic cardiovascular toxicity occurs less frequently than CNS toxicity, it is more serious and more difficult to treat.

CENTRAL NERVOUS SYSTEM TOXICITY

Signs and Symptoms

The initial symptoms of CNS toxicity include feelings of lightheadedness and dizziness followed by visual and auditory disturbances such as difficulty in focusing and tinnitus. Other subjective CNS symptoms are disorientation and feelings of drowsiness. Objective signs of CNS toxicity are excitatory in nature. Those include shivering, muscular twitching and tremors initially involving muscles of the face and distal parts of the extremities. Later, tonic-clonic convulsions occur. If a

T. H. Stanley and M. A. Ashburn (eds.), Anesthesiology and Pain Management, 77–97.

sufficiently large dose or a rapid intravenous injection of local anesthetic is given, the initial signs of CNS excitation are followed rapidly by CNS depression. Ultimately, seizure activity ceases and respiratory depression is followed by respiratory arrest. In some patients, CNS depression occurs without the preceding excitatory phase, particularly if other CNS depressant drugs were given.

CNS excitation is believed to be due to local anesthetic blockade of inhibitory pathways in the cerebral cortex (1). The blockade of inhibitory pathways disinhibits facilitatory neurons, resulting in convulsions, owing to unopposed excitatory nerve activity. Further, increases in the administered dose of local anesthetic causes inhibition of both inhibitory and facilitatory pathways resulting in generalized CNS depression.

Anesthetic Potency

There is a correlation between local anesthetic potency and CNS toxicity (2). For example, in cats, the convulsive dose of procaine is approximately seven times the convulsive dose of bupivacaine and bupivacaine is approximately eight times more potent than procaine. A similar study in dogs indicates that the relative CNS toxicity of bupivacaine, etidocaine and lidocaine is 4:2:1. This is similar also to their relative local anesthetic potencies (3). Intravenous infusion studies in human volunteers show a similar relationship between the intrinsic anesthetic potency and the dosage that causes CNS symptoms (4,5).

RATE OF INJECTION

The rate of injection and, therefore, the rapidity that toxic blood levels are reached alters the toxicity of local anesthetics. For example, when etidocaine is infused into human volunteers at the rate of 10 mg/ml, CNS symptoms occur when the venous blood level reaches 3.0 μg/ml (mean dose = 236 mg). Increasing the infusion rate to 20 mg/ml causes CNS symptoms when the venous blood level is only 2.0 μg/ml (mean dose = 161 mg) (6).

ACID BASE STATUS

The acid base status effects the CNS toxicity of local anesthetic. In cats, the convulsive threshold of various local anesthetics is related to the arterial pCO_2 (Figure 1). For example, increasing the pCO_2 from 25-40 torr to 65-81 torr decreases the convulsive threshold of procaine, mepivacaine, prilocaine, lidocaine and bupivacaine by approximately 50%. Decreasing the arterial pH also decreases the convulsive threshold of these agents. In fact, the pH is probably more important than the pCO_2 in terms of the CNS toxicity of local anesthetics. Respiratory acidosis (increased pCO_2, decreased pH) decreases the convulsant threshold of local anesthetics. However, compensated metabolic alkalosis (increased pCO_2, <u>increased</u> pH) does not decrease the convulsive threshold as much as the increased pCO_2 owing to respiratory acidosis.

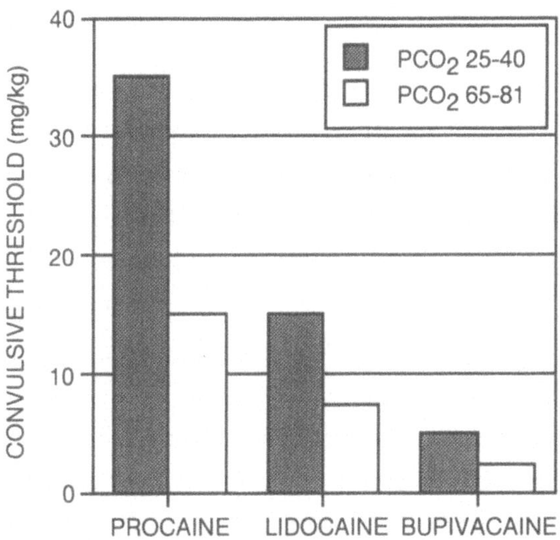

Figure 1. Effect of hypercarbia on the convulsive threshold of procaine, lidocaine and bupivacaine.

This potentiating effect of acidosis and/or hypercarbia may be due to several factors. Hypercarbia increases cerebral blood flow. Therefore, more local anesthetic is delivered to the brain. Additionally, hypercarbia may increase the diffusion of CO_2 across the nerve membrane, causing intracellular pH to fall. Intracellular acidosis promotes the conversion of the base form of the local anesthetic to the cationic (active) form. Since the cation does not diffuse across the nerve membrane, ionic trapping occurs, increasing CNS toxicity of the local anesthetic.

Hypercarbia and/or acidosis also decreases the binding of local anesthetics by plasma protein. Therefore, elevating the pCO_2 or decreasing the pH increases the proportion of free drug available for diffusion into the brain. On the other hand, acidosis increases the cationic form of the local anesthetic and this should decrease diffusion into the nerve.

In summary, local anesthetics greatly affect the CNS. Signs of CNS excitation leading to frank convulsions are the most common manifestation of systemic local anesthetic toxicity. Excessive doses or rapid intravenous injection of these drugs may lead also to CNS depression and respiratory arrest. The CNS toxicity of local anesthetics correlates with their anesthetic potency and this toxicity can be affected by factors such as rate of injection, hypercarbia and acidosis.

CARDIOVASCULAR SYSTEM TOXICITY

Direct Cardiac Effects

Electrophysiology. The primary cardiac electrophysiological effect of local anesthetics is a decrease in the maximum rate of depolarization, which is believed to be due to a decrease in sodium conductance in the fast sodium channels. The action potential duration and the effective refractory period are also decreased by local anesthetics. However, the ratio of the effective refractory period to the action potential duration is increased in Purkinje fibers and in ventricular muscle cells. This predisposes the patient to re-entry type arrhythmias.

Effects on the Electrocardiogram. Qualitative differences exist between the electrophysiological effects of the various agents. Bupivacaine depresses the rapid phase of depolarization (V_{max}) in Purkinje fibers and ventricular muscle cells to a greater extent than lidocaine (7). In addition, compared to lidocaine, the rate of recovery from steady-state block is slower in bupivacaine treated papillary muscles. This slow rate of recovery results in an incomplete restoration of V_{max} between action potentials, particularly at high heart rates. In contrast, recovery from lidocaine is complete, even at rapid heart rates. The different effects of lidocaine and bupivacaine are believed to be responsible for the antiarrhythmic activity of lidocaine and the arrhythmogenic potential of bupivacaine. Recent studies comparing ropivacaine to lidocaine and bupivacaine show ropivacaine to be intermediate in suppressing V_{max} and recovery from steady-state block (8).

Electrophysiologic studies in intact dogs and in man corroborate the findings observed in isolated cardiac tissue. As the dose and blood levels of lidocaine increase, so, too, does the conduction times through various parts of the heart. This is reflected in the electrocardiogram as an increase in the PR interval and QRS duration. Extremely high concentrations of local anesthetics depress spontaneous pacemaker activity in the sinus node resulting in sinus bradycardia and sinus arrest.

Effects on Inotropy. Local anesthetics also depress the mechanical activity of cardiac muscle. All local anesthetics exert a dose-dependent negative inotropic action in isolated cardiac tissue, which is proportional to their potency (9). Thus, the more potent local anesthetics depress cardiac contractility at lower concentrations than the less potent drugs (Table 1). Local anesthetics can be divided into three groups in terms of their myocardial depressant effect. The more potent agents, bupivacaine, tetracaine and etidocaine depress cardiac contractility at the lowest concentrations. The agents of moderate anesthetic potency, lidocaine, mepivacaine, and prilocaine, are intermediate in terms of myocardial depression. Finally, procaine and chloroprocaine, the least potent local anesthetics, require the highest concentrations to decrease cardiac contractility.

Table 1. Comparative effects of local anesthetics on cardiac contractility and cardiac output.

Agent	Relative Potency	50 % Decrease in Isolated Atria (µg/ml)	50 % Decrease in Canine Cardiac Output (mg/kg)
Procaine	1	277	100
Chloroproc	1	102	30
Cocaine	2	56	—
Lidocaine	2	67	30
Prilocaine	2	42	40
Mepivacaine	2	55	40
Etidocaine	8	—	20
Bupivacaine	8	6	10
Tetracaine	8	6	20

Studies in intact dogs in which a strain gauge arch was sutured to the right ventricle show that all local anesthetic agents are negative inotropes (10). As in the isolated cardiac tissue studies, there is a relationship between the potency of local anesthetics and their myocardial depressant effect (Figure 2). For example, tetracaine which is approximately eight times more potent than procaine is approximately 8 times more potent in depressing myocardial contractility than procaine. Hemodynamic studies in closed-chest anesthetized dogs show that tetracaine, etidocaine and bupivacaine cause a 50% decrease in cardiac

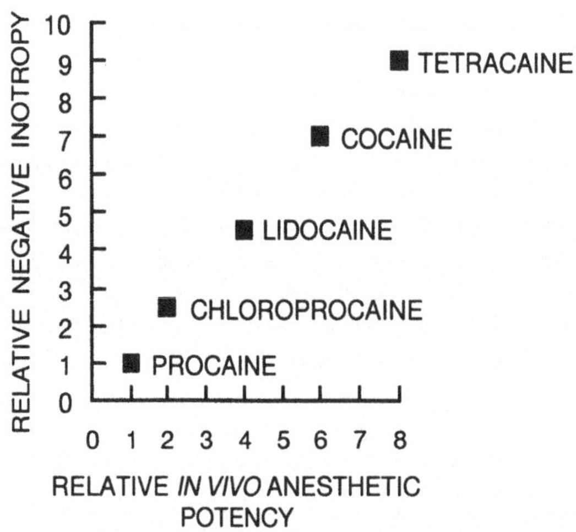

Figure 2. Relationship between myocardial depressant effect and relative anesthetic potency of various local anesthetics.

output at doses of 10 to 20 mg/kg. On the other hand, it takes 30 to 40 mg/kg of lidocaine, mepivacaine, prilocaine and chloroprocaine and 100 mg/kg of procaine to cause the same decrease in cardiac output.

The mechanism by which local anesthetics depress myocardial contractility is not precisely known, but it may involve an interaction with calcium. Both procaine and tetracaine increase the release of calcium from skeletal muscle. The relative potency of tetracaine and procaine in terms of their ability to increase the rate of calcium efflux from sartorius muscle is proportional to their local anesthetic potency. Displacement of calcium from cardiac muscle should result in a decrease in myocardial contractility. However, studies with isolated guinea pig hearts show that increasing the extracellular calcium concentration does not reverse the negative inotropic action of bupivacaine or lidocaine.

Direct Peripheral Vascular Effects. Local anesthetics exert a biphasic effect on peripheral vascular smooth muscle. Direct measurements of the arteriolar diameter of rat cremasteric muscle reveal that 10^0 to 10^3 μg/ml lidocaine causes a dose related 60 to 88% vasoconstriction (11). However, increasing the concentration of lidocaine to 10^4 μg/ml produces a 27% increase in arteriolar diameter, which indicates vasodilation. Isolated rat portal vein studies show also that low concentrations of local anesthetics stimulate spontaneous myogenic contractions and augment basal tone (vasoconstriction), while higher concentrations inhibit myogenic activity (vasodilation).

In vivo studies confirm the biphasic effect of local anesthetics on the peripheral vasculature. Blood flow studies in animal and man show that low doses of local anesthetics decrease peripheral arterial flow without changing blood pressure, indicating an increase in peripheral vascular resistance. Higher doses of local anesthetics increase blood flow in peripheral arteries, indicating vasodilation. Owing to its ability to inhibit the uptake of norepinephrine by storage granules, cocaine is the only local anesthetic that causes vasoconstriction. The non-reabsorbed norepinephrine is responsible for cocaine's vasoconstriction. A comparison of the various local anesthetics fails to demonstrate a good correlation between their potency and their vasodilating effects. However, there is a correlation between their duration of action and the duration of vasodilation. Thus, the duration of canine femoral artery vasodilation due to lidocaine, mepivacaine, and prilocaine (intermediate duration drugs) lasts approximately 5 minutes, but is much longer with bupivacaine, tetracaine and etidocaine (long duration drugs).

The pulmonary vasculature is particularly sensitive to the effects of local anesthetics. Procaine markedly increases pulmonary vascular resistance in the Starling heart-lung preparation. Studies in anesthetized dogs using pulmonary artery catheters show also that esters and amides increase pulmonary artery pressure and pulmonary vascular resistance. Relatively large intravenous doses of procaine, chloroprocaine and tetracaine increase pulmonary vascular resistance by approximately 300%. Three mg/kg of bupivacaine causes the pulmonary vascular resistance to increase 100 to 200%. Ten mg/kg of mepivacaine, lidocaine or prilocaine increases pulmonary vascular resistance 50 to 100%. On the other hand, near lethal doses of esters or amides, decrease pulmonary vascular resistance.

The biphasic peripheral vascular effect of local anesthetics may be related to changes in smooth muscle calcium. There is competitive antagonism between local anesthetic drugs and calcium ions in smooth muscle. Local anesthetics displace calcium from smooth muscle membrane binding sites into the cytoplasm. The increase in cytoplasmic calcium stimulates contraction, increasing myogenic tone, which causes vasoconstriction. However, further increasing the concentration of local anesthetic displaces more and more membrane-bound calcium. Eventually, there is little calcium to displace and this decreases cytoplasmic calcium, resulting in smooth muscle relaxation and vasodilation.

COMPARATIVE CARDIOVASCULAR TOXICITY OF LOCAL ANESTHETICS

There is a direct relationship between local anesthetic potency and cardiovascular depression. The more potent drugs, bupivacaine and etidocaine, can cause rapid and profound cardiovascular depression in certain patients after accidental intravascular injection. This is associated with severe cardiac arrhythmias and the cardiac depression is often resistant to treatment. Thus, the more potent and highly lipid soluble drugs like bupivacaine and etidocaine are more cardiotoxic than less potent and less lipid soluble agents like lidocaine, mepivacaine and, possibly, ropivacaine.

The cardiotoxicity of bupivacaine appears to differ from that of lidocaine and mepivacaine in the following ways:

1. The ratio of the dosage required for irreversible cardiovascular collapse to the dosage for CNS toxicity (convulsions), i.e., the CC/CNS ratio, is lower for bupivacaine and etidocaine compared to lidocaine, mepivacaine and ropivacaine.
2. Ventricular arrhythmias and fatal ventricular fibrillation may occur following the rapid intravenous administration of a large dose of bupivacaine but not lidocaine.

3. Pregnant animals or patients may be more sensitive than nonpregnant animals or patients to the cardiotoxic effects of bupivacaine.
4. Cardiac resuscitation is more difficult following bupivacaine-induced cardiovascular collapse.
5. Acidosis and hypoxia potentiates the cardiotoxicity of bupivacaine.

CC/CNS Ratio

In sheep, the CC/CNS ratio for bupivacaine and etidocaine is lower than that of lidocaine (12). For example, the mean CC/CNS dose ratio for lidocaine is 7.1 indicating that seven times as much lidocaine is necessary to cause irreversible cardiovascular collapse than is needed to cause convulsions (Figure 3). On the other hand, the CC/CNS ratio averages 3.7 for bupivacaine, 4.4 for etidocaine, 7.6 for mepivacaine, and 1.9 for ropivacaine. Although the central nervous system is more sensitive to the toxic effects of all agents than the cardiovascular system, there is a smaller difference between the dose of bupivacaine, etidocaine, and ropivacaine that caused convulsions and cardiovascular collapse compared to lidocaine and mepivacaine. The arterial drug concentration associated with CNS and cardiovascular toxicity (CC/CNS blood level ratio) averages 3.6 for lidocaine, 1.6 for bupivacaine, 1.7 for etidocaine, 2.5

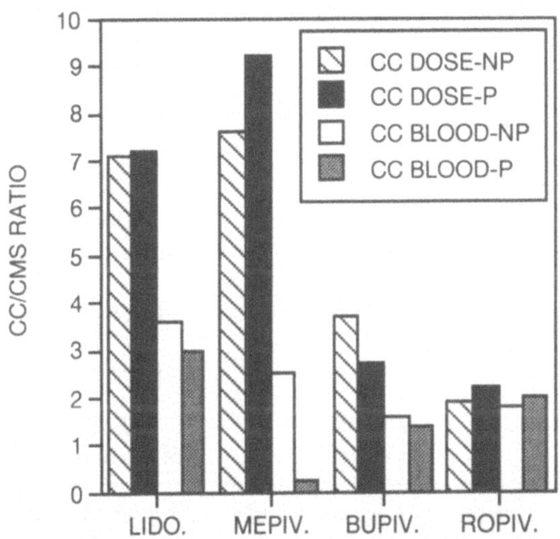

Figure 3. CC/CNS dose and blood level ratio for lidocaine, mepivacaine, bupivacaine, and ropivacaine in pregnant and non-pregnant sheep.

for mepivacaine, and 1.8 for ropivacaine (Figure 3). At the time of cardiovascular collapse, the mean myocardium to blood concentration ratio was 3.5 for bupivacaine, 3.2 for etidocaine, 3.7 for ropivacaine, 2.2 for lidocaine, and 6.4 for mepivacaine. Thus, the greater myocardial sensitivity owing to bupivacaine, etidocaine, and ropivacaine appears to be due to a combination of myocardial uptake and drug potency.

Ventricular Arrhythmias

A number of animal studies show that toxic doses of bupivacaine cause ventricular arrhythmias (13) (Table 2). A study in dogs determined the ability of various local anesthetics to cause ventricular fibrillation at convulsant and supra-convulsant doses. Ventricular fibrillation did not occur with lidocaine, mepivacaine or tetracaine. On the other hand, ventricular fibrillation occurred in approximately 20% of the animals given etidocaine and in 50% given bupivacaine (14). In another study of cardiac toxicity in dogs at two and three times the convulsive dose,

Table 2. Ventricular arrhythmias owing to lidocaine and bupivacaine in various animal models.

	Arrhythmias	
Animal Model	**Lidocaine**	**Bupivacaine**
Unanesthetized Paralyzed Cat	6% PVC	100% PVC
Anesthetized Dog	0	0
Unanesthetized Dog	0	40% - VT, VF
Unanesthetized Sheep	0	80 - 100% PVC, VT
Hypoxic, Acidotic Sheep	0	17 - 50% VT, VF
Isolated Guinea Pig Heart	0	33 - 50% PVC bigeminy, trigeminy
Intracoronary Injection—Anesthetized Pig	VF AT 64 mg	VF AT 4 mg
Intracranial Injury —Cat	17% VT	100% VT
Intracranial Injury —Rat	55% VT no deaths	55% VT 50% deaths

PVC = Premature ventricular contraction; VT = Ventricular tachycardia; VF = Ventricular fibrillation lidocaine caused death in 83% of animals but no ventricular arrhythmias compared to 100% death and 100% ventricular arrhythmias with bupivacaine and 66% deaths but only 50% ventricular arrhythmias with ropivacaine (15). These results suggest that ventricular fibrillation is not caused by the piperidine ring structure of bupivacaine because mepivacaine also contains the piperidine group and it did not cause ventricular arrhythmias. However, ventricular ectopy may be caused by the side chain on the piperidine ring since increasing the length of the side chain is associated with a higher incidence of arrhythmias -- bupivacaine > ropivacaine > mepivacaine = 0. In addition, there does not appear to be a correlation between the frequency of ventricular arrhythmias and the lipid solubility or protein binding of local anesthetics. Large doses of etidocaine, which is more lipid soluble than bupivacaine and equally protein bound, causes fewer ventricular arrhythmias and fibrillation than bupivacaine.

It is uncertain whether the bupivacaine-induced cardiac arrhythmias are due to a direct cardiac effect or are secondary to a CNS effect or both. Perfusing isolated guinea pig hearts with bupivacaine causes conduction block, bigeminy and trigeminy, which does not occur with lidocaine perfusion (16). Ventricular fibrillation occurs in intact pigs when bupivacaine is injected directly into the left anterior descending coronary artery (17). These results suggest that the ventricular arrhythmias are the result of a direct action on the heart. On the other hand, injecting bupivacaine directly into certain regions of the brain also causes cardiac arrhythmias (18, 19). Moreover, bupivacaine does not cause cardiac arrhythmias in dogs given pentobarbital, indicating a potential relationship between the CNS and the cardiotoxicity of bupivacaine.

Enhanced Cardiotoxicity in Pregnancy

A number of the cardiotoxic reactions owing to bupivacaine occurred in pregnant patients. As a result, the 0.75% solution is not recommended for obstetric anesthesia in the U.S.A. Studies in pregnant and non-pregnant sheep show that the CC/CNS dosage ratio for bupivacaine decreases from 3.7 ± 0.5 in non-pregnant sheep to 2.7 ± 0.4 in pregnant animals (20). Nevertheless, there was little difference in the CC/CNS blood level ratio, which varied from 1.6 ± 0.1 in non-pregnant animals to 1.4 ± 0.1 in pregnant ewes. However, the blood level of bupivacaine when circulatory collapse occurred was lower in pregnant animals. The corresponding CC/CNS dose and blood level ratios and blood concentration at cardiovascular collapse for ropivacaine, lidocaine and mepivacaine appear in Table 3. There was no difference in the myocardial uptake of bupivacaine in pregnant and non-pregnant sheep at the time of cardiovascular collapse. Thus, if the pregnant patient is more susceptible to the cardiotoxic effects of bupivacaine, it apparently is not due to myocardial uptake of drug.

Cardiac Resuscitation

It is difficult to resuscitate patients from bupivacaine cardiac toxicity. Studies in acidotic and hypoxic sheep confirm that cardiac resuscitation is difficult following bupivacaine toxicity (21). Studies in bupivacaine toxic cats and dogs show that resuscitation is possible but requires large doses of epinephrine and atropine. In addition, bretylium but not lidocaine reverses the cardiodepressant effects of bupivacaine and raises the ventricular tachycardia threshold (22, 23).

Effect of Acidosis and Hypoxia

Acid-base status affects the cardiovascular toxicity of local anesthetics (21). Isolated atrial tissue studies show that hypercarbia, acidosis and hypoxia potentiate the negative chronotropic and inotropic action of lidocaine and bupivacaine. The combination of hypoxia and acidosis markedly potentiates bupivacaine's cardiodepressant effects. In sheep, hypoxia and acidosis increase cardiac arrhythmias and the mortality rate due to bupivacaine toxicity. Acidosis does not increase myocardial tissue uptake of local anesthetic. On the contrary, investigations in rabbits show that the heart takes up less bupivacaine during acidosis. Hypercarbia, acidosis and hypoxia occur quickly during seizure activity caused by rapid intravascular injection of local anesthetics. Thus, the rapid cardiovascular depression seen after accidental intravenous injection of bupivacaine may be partly due to severe acid-base changes.

Table 3. Toxicity of various local anesthetics in non-pregnant and pregnant sheep.

	CC/CNS Dose		CC/CNS Blood		CC Blood (μg/ml)		Myocardial Conc. (μg/g)	
Drug	**Non-Preg**	**Preg**	**Non-Preg**	**Preg**	**Non-Preg**	**Preg**	**Non-Preg**	**Preg**
Bupivacaine	3.7 ± 0.5	2.7 ± 0.4	1.6 ± 0.1	1.4 ± 0.1	8.0 ± 0.9	5.5 ± 0.8	25	19
Etidocaine	4.4 ± 0.9		1.7 ± 0.2					
Ropivacaine	1.9 ± 0.1	2.2 ± 0.3	1.8 ± 0.1	2.0 ± 0.05	7.3 ± 0.3	9.6 ± 2.1	26.7 ± 2.8	30.5 ± 1.2
Lidocaine	7.1 ± 1.1	7.2 ± 0.6	3.6 ± 0.3	3.0 ± 0.3	35.1 ± 3.2	41.2 ± 6.7		
Mepivacaine	7.6 ± 1.4	9.2 ± 1.3	2.5 ± 0.2	2.4 ± 0.3	41.6 ± 2.4	45.6 ± 6.2	268 ± 12.3	317 ± 26.2

CC/CNS Dose = ratio of the dose of local anesthetic that caused cardiovascular collapse (CC) to the dose that caused seizures (CNS).

CC/CNS Blood = ratio of the blood level of local anesthetic that caused cardiovascular collapse (CC) to the dose that caused seizures (CNS).

CC Blood = the blood level of local anesthetic at the time of cardiovascular collapse.

Myocardial Conc. = the amount of drug in the myocardium after cardiovascular collapse.

MISCELLANEOUS SYSTEMIC EFFECTS

Membrane Stabilization

Local anesthetics cause a number of miscellaneous systemic effects. Most of these are due to their membrane stabilizing actions. For example, local anesthetics block cholinergic receptors at the neuromuscular junction, ganglia and other sites Normally, these miscellaneous effects are clinically insignificant.

Methemoglobinemia

A unique side effect is methemoglobinemia, owing to prilocaine (24,25). There is a dose-response relationship between the dose of epidural prilocaine and the degree of methemoglobinemia. The development of clinically significant methemoglobinemia requires injecting more than 600 mg of prilocaine. The formation of methemoglobinemia is related to prilocaine's chemical structure. Prilocaine lacks a methyl group in the benzene ring. Hepatic metabolism of prilocaine produces O-toluidine which oxidizes hemoglobin to methemoglobin. Methemoglobinemia caused by prilocaine is spontaneously reversible, or it can be treated with intravenous methylene blue (1 mg/kg).

Allergic Effects

The amino-esters such as procaine are derivatives of the allergen para-aminobenzoic acid (PABA). Consequently, the amino-esters sometimes cause allergic reactions. Allergic reactions to the amino-amides are extremely rare. Intradermal injections of amino-esters and amino-amides, in patients with and without a history of local anesthetic allergy, caused positive skin reactions in 25 of 60 patients without history of allergy (26, 27). In all cases, the intradermal reactions occurred with amino-ester agents—procaine, tetracaine and chloroprocaine. The amino-amides, lidocaine, mepivacaine or prilocaine caused no reactions. Eight of eleven patients with a history of local anesthetic allergy developed a positive skin reaction to procaine, tetracaine or chloroprocaine, but not to lidocaine, mepivacaine or prilocaine. In these studies, no subject developed anaphylaxis. Although the amino-amides do not usually cause allergic reactions, amino-amide solutions may contain the preservative, methylparaben, which is structurally similar to PABA. Because patients injected intradermally with methylparaben develop a positive skin reaction, it may appear that the skin reaction is due to the amino-amide when in fact it is due to the methylparaben.

Local Tissue Toxicity

Local anesthetics rarely cause nerve damage. Studies on isolated frog sciatic nerve show that concentrations of procaine, cocaine, tetracaine and dibucaine that cause irreversible conduction blockade are in excess of the concentrations used clinically. Intrathecal injections of lidocaine, tetracaine or etidocaine in rabbits show that spinal cord damage occurred only with 2% tetracaine, which is greater than the maximum 1% concentration used for spinal anesthesia in man (28). Prolonged sensory motor deficits occurred in some patients after the accidental subarachnoid injection of large doses of chloroprocaine intended for epidural anesthesia (29, 30). Animal studies regarding the neurotoxicity of chloroprocaine are contradictory (Table 4). The etiology of the neural injury owing to chloropro-

Table 4. Potential neurotoxicity of chloroprocaine and other local anesthetics in animal models.

Animal Model	*Results*
In vitro Rabbit Vagus Nerve	Local irritation with CP but not LIDO or BUPIV
In vivo Rat Sciatic Nerve	No irritation with CP or LIDO
In vitro Rabbit Vagus Nerve	Irreversible block with commercial CP and Na BISULFITE but not with pure CP
Spinal - Dog	Paralysis with CP but not with BUPIV or low pH saline
Spinal - Rabbit	Paralysis with commercial CP and Na BISULFITE but not with pure CP
Spinal - Sheep	Minimal toxicity with CP, LIDO, BUPIV and control solutions
Spinal - Monkey	Minimal toxicity with CP and BUPIV

CP = chloroprocaine; LIDO = lidocaine; BUPIV = bupivacaine

caine is now known to be due to the low pH and the antioxidant, sodium bisulfite, contained in chloroprocaine solutions. Paralysis occurred only in rabbits injected intrathecally with chloroprocaine solutions that contained sodium bisulfite (31). Pure solutions of chloroprocaine (no sodium bisulfite) did not cause paralysis. On the other hand, solutions of sodium bisulfite alone (no chloroprocaine) caused paralysis.

A detailed study in the isolated rabbit vagus nerve investigated the neurotoxicity of the components of commercial chloroprocaine solutions (32). These solutions contain 2 to 3% chloroprocaine, 0.2% sodium bisulfite, and have a pH around 3.0. Bathing isolated vagus nerves for 30 minutes with commercial 3% chloroprocaine results in irreversible conduction blockade. However, bathing the nerves with commercial 3% chloroprocaine buffered to pH 7.0 causes <u>reversible</u> conduction block. A 3% chloroprocaine solution with pH of 3.0 but without sodium bisulfite also causes reversible blockade. Bathing the nerves with a 0.2% sodium bisulfite solution at a pH of 3.0 causes irreversible conduction block, whereas, a 0.2% sodium bisulfite solution with a pH of 7.0 causes no conduction block. The results of these studies (Table 5) indicate that the combination of pH< 3.0 and 0.2% sodium bisulfite is responsible for the potential neurotoxicity of commercial chloroprocaine solutions; 2 to 3% chloroprocaine itself does not appear to be neurotoxic.

Table 5. Chloroprocaine toxicity in isolated vagus nerve.

			Recovery Time (min)	
Drug	**pH**	**% Bisulfite**	**A Fibers**	**C Fibers**
3% Nesacaine	**3.0**	**0.2**	**infinite**	**infinite**
3% Nesacaine	7.3	0.2	60	120
3% Chloroprocaine	**3.0**	**0.2**	**infinite**	**infinite**
3% Chloroprocaine	7.3	0.2	60	120
3% Chloroprocaine	3.2	none	60	120
3% Chloroprocaine	7.2	none	60	120
None	7.0	0.2	no	block
None	**3.3**	**0.2**	**infinite**	**infinite**

Data from reference (32).

As a result of these *in vitro* studies, the manufacturers of chloroprocaine removed the sodium bisulfite from the solution. Unfortunately, they substituted sodium ethylenediaminetetraacetic acid (EDTA). EDTA is a calcium chelating agent. It may be responsible for the recent reports of severe back pain after epidural anesthesia with the EDTA-containing chloroprocaine solution (33). The pain may be due to tetanic contractions of the back muscles owing to localized hypocalcemia from calcium sequestration. An alternative explanation is that the EDTA is neurotoxic, *per se*. *In vivo* rat experiments show that EDTA (in concentrations slightly higher than that present in the commercial chloroprocaine solution) is neurotoxic (34).

There are recent reports of cases of cauda equina syndrome after continuous spinal anesthesia (35,36). Most, but not all, occurred with so-called microcatheters and large doses of 5% hyperbaric lidocaine (Table 6). There is another case report of cauda equina syndrome that occurred after the accidental intrathecal injection of 32 ml of 2% lidocaine intended for epidural anesthesia (37). These cases indicate that commonly used local anesthetics, while safe when used in appropriate amounts and in appropriate locations, can be neurotoxic under certain circumstances.

A new study in the isolated frog sciatic nerve, similar to the one described above for chloroprocaine, shows that some of the local anesthetics routinely used for spinal anesthesia cause irreversible or partially reversible conduction block (38). The study consists of recording the block of the compound action potential amplitude before and after

Table 6. Cauda equina syndrome after continuous spinal anesthesia.

Catheter Gauge	Drug	Number of Injections	Total Dose (mg)	Duration of Injury (mo)
28	Lidocaine	4	175	>7
28	Lidocaine	>3	300	>1
28	Lidocaine	7	190	>10
20	Tetracaine	5	37	>31
28	Lidocaine	8	285	>3
28	Lidocaine	9	215	>9

All solutions hyperbaric. Data from reference (35, 36).

bathing the nerves for 15 minutes with the local anesthetic solutions (or components of the solution, e.g., dextrose), after washing the drug out for 2 to 3 hours, and, finally, after soaking the nerves over night in Ringer's solution. Table 7 shows the results and indicates that 5% lidocaine and 0.5% tetracaine caused irreversible block, while 1.5% lidocaine and 0.75% bupivacaine caused partially reversible block and 0.06% tetracaine caused total recovery. Thus, we know from years of clinical practice that these local anesthetic solutions are safe for spinal anesthesia, when given as a single injection and in small doses. However, when they are injected through a spinal catheter and given repeatedly in large doses, they can displace the CSF, come directly in contact with the cauda equina nerves, and damage them (38). Furthermore, a recent case study indicates that single injection spinal anesthesia with 5% lidocaine can cause transient neurotoxicity (39).

Skeletal muscle is more sensitive to local irritation owing to local anesthetics than other tissues. Skeletal muscle changes occur with most of

Table 7. Percent of control (before drug) compound action potential amplitude (mean ± SEM).

Drug	After 15 Min in Drug	After 2-3 Hr in Drug	After Overnight Soak
Ringer's†	109 ± 2	105 ± 6	27 ± 6
5% L, 7.5% D†	0	0	0
5% LIDO	0	0	0
1.5% L, 7.5% D	0	54 ± 5	28 ± 7
1.5% LIDO	0	67 ± 10	30 ± 7
7.5% DEXT‡	89 ± 4	107 ± 4	46 ± 11
7.5% DEXT*	84 ± 4	99 ± 18	59 ± 16
0.75% BUPIV†	0	76 ± 3	44 ± 8
0.5% TETRA	0	0	0
0.06% TETRA†	0	93 ± 2	64 ± 0.6

L and LIDO = Lidocaine, D and DEXT = Dextrose, BUPIV = Bupivacaine, TETRA = Tetracaine. †These local anesthetics are equipotent and are 200X the dose required for 50% block in isolated nerve. ‡10% dextrose diluted with Ringer's. *Dextrose dissolved in Ringer's. n = 5 for all experiments, except for BUPIV and TETRA, where n = 3. Data from reference (38).

the clinically used local anesthetics (40, 41). The more potent longer acting agents like bupivacaine and etidocaine cause a more localized skeletal muscle damage than the less potent agents like lidocaine and prilocaine. The skeletal muscle damage is reversible. Muscle regeneration is usually complete two weeks after the local anesthetic injection. These skeletal muscle changes are not accompanied by overt clinical signs of local irritation.

REFERENCES

1. DeJong RH: Physiology and Pharmacology of Local Anesthesia. (2 ed.) Springfield, Charles C. Thomas, 1977
2. Englesson S: The influence of acid-base changes on central nervous system toxicity of local anaesthetic agents. I. An experimental study in cats. Acta Anaesthesiol Scand 18:79-87, 1974
3. Liu PL, Feldman HS, Giasi R, et al: Comparative CNS toxicity of lidocaine, etidocaine, bupivacaine, and tetracaine in awake dogs following rapid intravenous administration. Anesth Analg 62:375-379, 1983
4. Scott DB: Evaluation of the toxicity of local anaesthetic agents in man. Br J Anaesth 47:56-61, 1975
5. Scott DB, Lee A, Fagan D, et al: Acute toxicity of ropivacaine compared with that of bupivacaine. Anesth Analg 69:563-9, 1989
6. Scott DB: Toxicity caused by local anaesthetic drugs (editorial). Br J Anaesth 53:553-554, 1981
7. Clarkson CW, Hondeghem LM: Mechanism for bupivacaine depression of cardiac conduction: Fast block of sodium channels during the action potential with slow recovery from block during diastole. Anesthesiology 62:396-405, 1985
8. Arlock P: Actions of three local anaesthetics: Lidocaine, bupivacaine and ropivacaine on guinea pig papillary muscle sodium channels (Vmax). Pharmacol Toxicol 63:96-104, 1988
9. Block A, Covino BG: Effect of local anesthetic agents on cardiac conduction and contractility. Reg Anesth 6:55-61, 1982
10. Stewart DM, Rogers WP, Mahaffrey JE, et al: Effect of local anesthetics on the cardiovascular system of the dog. Anesthesiology 24:620-624, 1963
11. Johns RA, DiFazio CA, Longnecker DE: Lidocaine constricts or dilates rat arterioles in a dose-dependent manner. Anesthesiology 62:141-144, 1985
12. Morishima HO, Pedersen H, Finster M, et al: Etidocaine toxicity in the adult, newborn, and fetal sheep. Anesthesiology 58:342-346, 1983
13. Reiz S, Nath S: Cardiotoxicity of local anaesthetic agents. Br J Anaesth 58:736-746, 1986

14. Eicholzer AW, Feldman HS: Acute toxicity of etidocaine following various routes of administration in the dog. Toxicol Appl Pharmacol 37:13-21, 1976
15. Feldman HS, Arthur GR, Covino BG: Comparative systemic toxicity of convulsant and supraconvulsant doses of intravenous ropivacaine, bupivacaine, and lidocaine in the conscious dog. Anesth Analg 69:794-801, 1989
16. Tanz RD, Heskett T, Loehning RW, Fairfax CA: Comparative cardiotoxicity of bupivacaine and lidocaine in the isolated perfused mammalian heart. Anesth Analg 63:549-556, 1984
17. Reiz S, Häggmark S, Johansson G, Nath S: Cardiotoxicity of ropivacaine—A new amide local anaesthetic agent. Acta Anaesthesiol Scand 33:93-98, 1989
18. Heavner JE: Cardiac dysrhythmias induced by infusion of local anesthetics into the lateral cerebral ventricle of cats. Anesth Analg 65:133-138, 1986
19. Thomas RD, Behbehani MM, Coyle DE, Denson DD: Cardiovascular toxicity of local anesthetics: An alternative hypothesis. Anesth Analg 65:444-450, 1986
20. Morishima HO, Pedersen H, Finster M, et al: Bupivacaine toxicity in pregnant and nonpregnant ewes. Anesthesiology 63:134-139, 1985
21. Covino BG: Toxicity of local anesthetics, Advances in Anesthesia. Vol. 3. Edited by Stoelting RK, Barash PG, Gallagher TJ. Chicago, Year Book Medical Publishers, Inc., 1986, pp. 37-65
22. Kasten GW, Martin ST: Bupivacaine cardiovascular toxicity: Comparison of treatment with bretylium and lidocaine. Anesth Analg 64:911-916, 1985
23. Chadwick HS: Toxicity and resuscitation in lidocaine- or bupivacaine-infused cats. Anesthesiology 63:385-90, 1985
24. Scott DB, Owen JA, Richmond J: Methæmoglobinæmia due to prilocaine. Lancet 2:728-729, 1964
25. Lund PC, Cwik JC: Propitocaine (Citanest) and methemoglobinemia. Anesthesiology 26:569-571, 1965
26. Aldrete JA, Johnson DA: Evaluation of intracutaneous testing for investigation of allergy to local anesthetic agents. Anesth Analg 49:173-183, 1970
27. Aldrete JA, O'Higgins JW: Evaluation of patients with history of allergy to local anesthetic drugs. South Med J 64:1118-1121, 1971
28. Adams HJ, Mastri AR, Eicholzer AW, Kilpatrick G: Morphologic effects of intrathecal etidocaine and tetracaine on the rabbit spinal cord. Anesth Analg 53:904-908, 1974
29. Ravindran RS, Bond VK, Tasch MD, et al: Prolonged neural blockade following regional analgesia with 2-chloroprocaine. Anesth Analg 59:447-451, 1980
30. Reisner LS, Hochman BN, Plumer MH: Persistent neurologic deficit and adhesive arachnoiditis following intrathecal 2-chloroprocaine injection. Anesth Analg 59:452-454, 1980

31. Wang BC, Hillman DE, Spielholz NI, Turndorf H: Chronic neurological deficits and Nesacaine-CE—An effect of the anesthetic, 2-chloroprocaine, or the antioxidant, sodium bisulfite? Anesth Analg 63:445-457, 1984
32. Gissen AJ, Datta S, Lambert D: The chloroprocaine controversy. II. Is chloroprocaine neurotoxic? Reg Anesth 9:135-145, 1984
33. Fibuch EE, Opper SE: Back pain following epidurally administered Nesacaine-MPF (see comments). Anesth Analg 69:113-115, 1989
34. Wang BC, Li D, Hiller JM, et al: Lumbar subarachnoid ethylenediaminetetraacetate induces hindlimb tetanic contractions in rats: Prevention by $CaCl_2$ pretreatment; observation of spinal nerve root degeneration. Anesth Analg 75:895-899, 1992
35. Rigler ML, Drasner K, Krejcie TC, et al: Cauda equina syndrome after continuous spinal anesthesia. Anesth Analg 72:275-281, 1991
36. Schell RM, Brauer FS, Cole DJ, Applegate RA II: Persistent sacral nerve root deficits after continuous spinal anaesthesia. Can J Anaesth 38:908-911, 1991
37. Drasner K, Rigler ML, Sessler DI, Stoller ML: Cauda equina syndrome following intended epidural anesthesia. Anesthesiology 77:582-585, 1992
38. Lambert DH, Lambert LA, Strichartz GP: Potential neurotoxicity of lidocaine solutions used for spinal anesthesia (abstract). Anesthesiology 77:A898, 1992
39. Schneider M, Ettlin T, Kaufmann M, et al: Transient neurologic toxicity after hyperbaric subarachnoid anesthesia with 5% lidocaine. Anesth Analg 76:1154-1157, 1993
40. Benoit PW, Belt WD: Some effects of local anesthetic agents on skeletal muscle. Exp Neurol 34:264-278, 1972
41. Libelius R, Sonesson B, Stamenović BA, Thesleff S: Denervation-like changes in skeletal muscle after treatment with a local anaesthetic (Marcaine®). J Anat 106:297-309, 1970

EFFECT OF POSTOPERATIVE PAIN ON SURGICAL STRESS RESPONSE.

H. Kehlet

Pain is one of the sequelae of acute injury and may participate in the release and maintenance of the surgical stress response. Furthermore, pain-induced reflex responses may adversely influence respiratory function, increase cardiac demands, decrease intestinal motility and initiate skeletal muscle spasm. Therefore, there is a common belief that alleviation of acute pain may also reduce the surgical stress response and improve outcome.

It is well documented that inhibition of nociceptive stimuli is most effectively achieved with neural blockade using local anesthetics (1-3). Such a nociceptive blockade also provides pain relief and may inhibit various aspects of the endocrine metabolic response, such as the catabolic hormone response, hypermetabolism, negative nitrogen balance, etc. A single shot spinal or epidural analgesia has only a short-lasting inhibitory effect on the surgical stress response compared to a pronounced inhibition following a 24-hour blockade, which may have long lasting metabolic effects into the subsequent postoperative days (1,3-5). The effect of a "preemptive" neural blockade on the hyperglycemic and cortisol response is more pronounced compared to a similar blockade administered after surgical incision (1). The stress reducing effect of epidural local anesthetic blockade is pronounced in lower body operations, but less so in upper abdominal/thoracic procedures, probably due to insufficient afferent blockade (1-3,6-8).

The protein sparing effect of a nociceptive blockade with epidural analgesia may be clinically important, since postoperative fatigue and convalescence is related to loss of muscle tissue and function (9). Again, in lower body procedures, epidural local anesthetics may improve nitrogen balance, attenuate the pronounced postoperative changes in

T. H. Stanley and M. A. Ashburn (eds.), Anesthesiology and Pain Management, 99–103.

muscle amino acid composition and nitrogen turn over (1-5). These effects are most pronounced in lower body procedures and less so in major upper abdominal procedures (3), where the effect on the catabolic hormonal response is also small. In a study with a combination of thoracic epidural analgesia plus etomidate for inhibition of the cortisol response and somatostatin for inhibition of the glucagon response, the catabolic hepatic protein response was prevented in patients undergoing cholecystectomy (10).

Pain relief by epidural opioids has only a moderate inhibitory effect on the surgical stress response (1-3,11). Similarly, pain relief by epidural alpha-2-agonist administration (clonidine), providing about the same analgesia as after epidural opioids, also has minimal modifying effect on the surgical stress response (3,11). There is a lack of sufficient information on the effect of PCA opioid administration on the stress response, but so far this technique does not provide a stress-free postoperative period (12).

Improved analgesia with combined low-dose epidural with opioid and local anesthetic has not resulted in major inhibition of the cortisol response to thoracic surgery (13), but has been demonstrated to reduce the catecholamine release and to improve hemodynamics after coronary artery by-pass (14).

Pain relief by intercostal blockade has not been demonstrated to inhibit the pituitary hormone response to thoracotomy or abdominal surgery (3,15).

Pain relief by administration of non-steroidal anti-inflammatory drugs may have some positive metabolic effects with reduction of postoperative nitrogen balance and hemodynamic responses to mesenteriale traction (16), but further studies are needed before definite conclusions can be made.

Pain relief by interpleural local anesthetics has no important effect on the surgical stress response (17).

Acupuncture and transcutaneous stimulation has no inhibitory effect on surgical stress (18,19). In addition, an approach with high-dose continuous celiac plexus blockade plus intermittent wound infiltration with local anesthetics was ineffective (20).

Most importantly, elimination of pain after classical chole-cystectomy by a multi-modal regimen with high-dose epidural local anesthetics and morphine together with systemic non-steroidal anti-inflammatory drugs, did not lead to a pronounced inhibition of the cortisol response, hyperthermia, fatigue, or improvement of pulmonary function (21). Thus, pain relief *per se* may not necessarily result in modification of the surgical stress response. Again, the explanation to these negative findings may be the insufficient afferent blockade of nociceptive pathways other than those conducting pain.

Recent studies have found improved pain relief by a single high-dose of preoperative prednisolone, together with an effective epidural regimen. This regimen reduced the hyperthermic, IL-6, prostanoid and acute phase protein response, and improved pulmonary function and fatigue (22,23). These findings suggest a combined neural and humoral blockade enhances analgesia and inhibits the global stress response. However, further studies regarding the potential side effects of such a strategy are obviously needed.

So far, the most effective nociceptive blockade to reduce the adrenocortical response to major abdominal surgery has been continuous spinal anesthesia or combined spinal-epidural anesthesia (24,25), probably due to a more efficient afferent neural blockade (26).

In summary, pain relief *per se* does not necessarily inhibit the surgical stress response since the nociceptive block is incomplete with most techniques. Presently, neural blockade with local anesthetics is the most effective. Continuous efforts to improve pain relief and to modify the surgical stress response are warranted, since the evidence so far suggests a subsequent improvement in outcome (3).

REFERENCES:

1. Kehlet H: Modification of responses to surgery and anesthesia by neural blockade: Clinical implications, Neural Blockade in Clinical Anesthesia and Management of Pain. Edited by Cousins MJ, Bridenbaugh PO, Philadelphia, J. B. Lippincott, 1987, pp. 145-188
2. Kehlet H: Role of neural stimuli and pain, Mediators of Sepsis. Edited by Lamy M, Thijs LG. Berlin, Springer Verlag, 1992, pp. 196-205
3. Kehlet H: General vs. regional anesthesia, Principles and Practice of Anesthesiology. Edited by Rogers MC, Tinker JH, Covino BG, Longnecker DE. St. Louis, C.V. Mosby, 1993, pp. 1218-1234
4. Carli F, Emery PW: Intra-operative exttrdural block with local anaesthetic. Acta Anaesthesiol Scand 34:263-266, 1990

5. Carli F, Webster J, Pearson M, et al: Protein metabolism after abdominal surgery: Effect of 24-h extradural block with local anaesthetic. Br J Anaesth 67:729-734, 1991
6. Dahl JB, Rosenberg J, Kehlet H: Effect of thoracic epidural etidocaine 1.5% on somatosensory evoked potentials, cortisol and glucose during cholecystectomy. Acta Anaesthesiol Scand 36:378-382, 1992
7. Naito Y, Tamai S, Shingu K, et al: Responses of plasma adrenocorticotropic hormone, cortisol and cytokines during and after upper abdominal surgery. Anesthesiology 77:426-431, 1992
8. Watters JM, March RJ, Desai D, et al: Epidural anaesthesia and analgesia do not affect energy expenditure after major abdominal surgery. Can J Anaesth 40:314-319, 1993
9. Christensen T, Kehlet H: Postoperative fatigue. World J Surg 17:220-225, 1993
10. Heindorff H, Schulze S, Mogensen T, et al: Hormonal and neural blockade prevents the postoperative increase in amino acid clearance and urea synthesis. Surgery 111:543-590, 1992
11. Kehlet H: Surgical stress—The role of pain and analgesia. Br J Anaesth 63:189-195, 1989
12. Møller IW, Dinesen K, Søndergård S, et al: Effect of patient-controlled analgesia on plasma catecholamine, cortisol and glucose concentrations after cholecystectomy. Br J Anaesth 61:160-164, 1988
13. Zwarts SJ, Hasenbos MAMW, Gielen MJM, Kho H-G: The effect of continuous epidural analgesia with sufentanil and bupivacaine during and after thoracic surgery on the plasma cortisol concentration and pain relief. Reg Anesth 14:183-188, 1989
14. Liem TH, Booij LH, Gielen MJ, et al: Coronary artery bypass grafting using two different anesthetic techniques. Part III: Adrenergic responses. J Cardiothorac Vasc Anesth 6:162-167, 1992
15. Sheinin B. Sheinin M, Asantila R, et al: Sympatho-adrenal and pituitary hormone responses during and immediately after thoracic surgery—Modulation by four different pain treatments. Acta Anaesthesiol Scand 31:762-767, 1987
16. Dahl JB, Kehlet H: Non-steroidal anti-inflammatory drugs—Rationale for use in severe postoperative pain. Br J Anaesth 66:703-712, 1991
17. Rademaker BMP, Sih IL, Kalkman CJ, et al: Effects of intrapleurally administered bupivacaine 0.5% on opioid analgesic requirements and endocrine response during and after cholecystectomy: A randomized double-blind controlled study. Acta Anaesthesiol Scand 35:108-112, 1991
18. Kho HG, van Egmond JV, Eijk RJR, Kapteyns WM: Lack of influence of acupuncture and transcutaneous stimulation on the immunoglobulin levels and leucocyte counts following upper abdominal surgery. Eur J Anaesthesiol 8:39-45, 1991
19. Kho HG, Kloppenborg PWC, van Egmond J: Effects of acupuncture and transcutaneous stimulation analgesia on plasma hormone levels

during and after major abdominal surgery. Eur J Anaesthesiol 10:197-208, 1993

20. Hamid SK, Scott NB, Sutcliffe NP, et al: Continuous coeliac plexus blockade plus intermittent wound infiltration by bupivacaine following upper abdominal surgery: A double-blind randomised study. Acta Anaesthesiol Scand 36:534-539, 1992
21. Schulze S, Roikjær O, Hasselstrøm L, et al: Epidural bupivacaine and morphine plus systemic indomethacin eliminates pain but not systemic response and convalescence after cholecystectomy. Surgery 103:321-327, 1988
22. Schulze S, Møller IW, Bang U, et al: Effect of combined prednisolone, epidural analgesia and indomethacin on pain, systemic response and convalescence after cholecystectomy. Acta Chir Scand 156:203-209, 1990
23. Schulze S, Sommer P, Bigler D, et al: Effect of combined prednisolone, epidural analgesia and indomethacin on the systemic response after colonic surgery. Arch Surg 127:325-331, 1992
24. Dahl JB, Rosenberg J, Dirkes WE, et al: Prevention of postoperative pain by balanced analgesia. Br J Anaesth 64:518-520, 1990
25. Webster J, Barnard M, Carli F: Metabolic response to colonic surgery: Extradural vs. continuous spinal. Br J Anaesth 67:467-469, 1991
26. Dirkes WE, Rosenberg J, Lund C, Kehlet H: The effect of intrathecal lidocaine and combined intrathecal lidocaine and epidural bupivacaine on electrical sensory thresholds. Reg Anesth 16:262-264, 1991

POSTOPERATIVE PAIN ASSESSMENT AND CHOICE OF METHODS OF TREATMENT

L. B. Ready

MEASUREMENT OF ACUTE PAIN

Sound approaches to acute pain treatment must include appropriate assessment. There are a number of instruments that can be used at the bedside to evaluate pain and thereby gauge the success or failure of a particular treatment plan. These include subjective reports from patients, both qualitative and quantitative, as well as objective observations by the pain therapist, including the effect of therapy on important functions such as the ability to breathe deeply, cough, move in bed, or ambulate. Additional insight can be gained by asking the simple question: "Are you satisfied with the treatment of your pain?" It is important that any measurement scale be applied both before and after treatment so that the effects of treatment (success or failure) can be measured.

THERAPEUTIC PRINCIPLES

Any treatment plan should include consideration of the natural history of acute pain, and should be flexible with regard to changing needs. The following four principles of therapy for acute pain should be identified and applied to all treatment plans:

1. Determine the source and magnitude of nociception.
2. Understand the relationship between ongoing nociception and other components of suffering (anxiety, ethnocultural components, meaning of pain, etc.) and provide therapy for these components as necessary.
3. Establish adequate drug levels to achieve and maintain analgesia.
4. Re-evaluate and refine therapy regularly based on the needs of individual patients.

T. H. Stanley and M. A. Ashburn (eds.), Anesthesiology and Pain Management, 105–115.

OPTIONS FOR THE TREATMENT OF ACUTE PAIN

Systemic Opioids

Opioids produce analgesia as a result of their agonist effects on opiate receptors in the central nervous system. Effective doses of appropriate drugs can be administered by the oral, rectal, transdermal, or sublingual route, or by subcutaneous, intramuscular, or intravenous injection or infusion. Because intramuscular opioid injection is such an unpredictable delivery system, effective and safe analgesia requires careful ongoing assessment of patients, with adjustments in doses and frequency of administration until individual care is optimized. Intravenous opioid infusions can abolish wide swings in drug concentration and permit prompt titration to the needs of individual patients.

Oral opioids in appropriate doses are remarkably effective. Frequently they can be used in place of parenteral drugs 12 to 24 hours after superficial surgery, and after some intraabdominal procedures as soon as oral intake is established. Placing oral analgesics at the bedside can improve analgesia by permitting patients to choose the dose and frequency of administration best suited to their individual needs.

Transdermal delivery of fentanyl, a synthetic opioid, after surgery has been demonstrated to be effective (1). This method of opioid administration avoids the discomfort of injections and offers a useful alternative for patients unable or unwilling to swallow oral medications. Therapeutic blood levels are achieved, and the usual side effects associated with opioid administration are seen.

Patient-Controlled Analgesia

Patient-controlled analgesia (PCA), the self-administration of small doses of opioids by patients when they experience pain, was conceived and developed to minimize the effects of pharmacokinetic and pharmacodynamic variability among individual patients (2,3). This approach is based on the premise that a negative feedback loop exists; when pain is reduced, there will be no further demand for analgesics until the pain returns. PCA devices consist of a microprocessor-controlled pump triggered by depressing a button. When triggered, a preset amount of opioid is delivered into the patient's intravenous line. A timer in the pump prevents administration of an additional bolus until a specified period has elapsed. Thus individual patients titrate opioids to their own needs within safe clinical parameters. A variety of devices are now commercially available for this purpose.

Quality of analgesia with PCA has been reported consistently as superior or equal to that with intramuscular opioids. Less PCA opioid use compared with intramuscular control groups is observed frequently. Satisfaction of patients and nurses is high. The principle advantages of PCA to patients are; high quality analgesia, autonomy, elimination of delay in decisions to medicate for pain, and freedom from painful intramuscular injections. It may take nurses less time to provide for the analgesic needs of postoperative patients using PCA.

Optimal efficacy and safety using PCA, as with other forms of treatment for postoperative pain, requires careful planning, establishment of appropriate policies and procedures, education of physicians and nurses, and frequent medical assessment of individual patients. Preoperative patient teaching will facilitate further optimal results. A number of opioid analgesics can be used in PCA therapy. Those best suited are the potent opioids with a rapid onset and intermediate duration of action. Morphine and meperidine are widely used.

Regional Anesthetic Techniques

A variety of neural blockade techniques continued into the postoperative period can result in effective and safe analgesia. These include topical application, local infiltration of incisions with long-acting local anesthetics, blockade of peripheral nerves or plexuses, and continuous block techniques at various sites in the periphery or neuraxis. Postoperative local anesthetic infusions into the brachial plexus sheath, femoral sheath, lumbar plexus, and sciatic nerve have been used to maintain analgesia and sympathetic blockade after a variety of surgical procedures. Spinal anesthesia can provide analgesia for several hours after the completion of surgery if long-acting agents are used. Continuous epidural anesthesia through a catheter offers several options for postoperative analgesia. Local anesthetic boluses or infusions can provide profound analgesia, improved bowel function, higher arterial oxygen tension, and

Psychological and Other Methods

Following surgery, patients may suffer "discomfort" from causes unrelated to their incisions. Some of these may be physical, such as headaches or sensations arising from nasogastric tubes, surgical drains, and intravenous catheters. Others will be the result of non-organic causes such as anxiety, fear, or insomnia. Therapy for these latter problems can enhance patients' overall sense of well-being and, in some cases, result in less "pain" being reported.

A number of studies have shown that psychological support in the form of discussion, reassurance, and the provision of information pre-operatively result in less anxiety, less opioid use after surgery, and a shorter hospital stay compared with control groups (7-9). Hospitals are designed usually for the convenience of the staff, and sometimes leave patients feeling "depersonalized" and helpless. Measures which restore freedom, control, and participation in care, even involving simple self-care tasks, are likely to be beneficial.

No currently available approach to postoperative pain control achieves these goals in all patients after all kinds of surgery. Regardless of how analgesia is provided, compromises are frequently necessary.

MAKING THE CHOICE

Needless to say, the optimal use of any technique requires knowledge, skill, experience, and attentiveness to individual patient responses. With these elements, a variety of approaches to the treatment of postoperative pain can produce satisfactory results. By contrast, even with the most modern and sophisticated techniques, ordering the same analgesic doses and administration intervals for all patients while failing to regularly assess their efficacy will yield sub-optimal results. It is beyond the scope of this section to consider all available forms of therapy for post-operative pain. Major emphasis will be given to factors which should influence the choice between two of the newer methods of pain control—patient-controlled analgesia (PCA) and epidural opioid analgesia (EOA). In choosing the best technique, a number of factors must be considered.

fewer pulmonary complications. Many regional anesthetic techniques can be adapted for use in infants and children.

Intrathecal and Epidural Opioids

Following initial reports in 1979 of the clinical efficacy of intrathecal and epidural opioids, they have been used to control pain following a wide variety of surgical procedures (4). Intrathecal opioids have the appeal of ease of administration, either at the time of intrathecal local anesthetic injection for surgical anesthesia, or as a separate technique when general anesthesia is administered. Many patients will remain comfortable for 24 hours or more after a single injection of intrathecal morphine.

The epidural route has been used much more extensively for postoperative pain control. Reasons include popularity of the technique alone or in combination with light general anesthesia during surgery, willingness to leave an epidural catheter in place for extended periods to maintain analgesia, familiarity with postoperative analgesia using epidural local anesthetics, and freedom from the risk of post-lumbar puncture headache.

In a randomized double-blinded study by Rawal et al. (5) of obese patients undergoing gastroplasty for weight reduction, the effects of intramuscular and epidural morphine were compared with respect to analgesia, ambulation, gastrointestinal motility, early and late pulmonary function, duration of hospitalization, and occurrence of deep vein thrombosis in the postoperative period. With a protocol designed to provide adequate analgesia by either route, the average dose of intramuscular morphine was up to seven times greater than that required by the epidural route. Patients receiving epidural morphine reported superior analgesia, ambulated sooner, had fewer pulmonary complications, had earlier return of bowel function, and were discharged from hospital earlier than patients receiving intramuscular morphine.

Yeager et al. (6) randomized high-risk surgical patients to two groups: the first received general anesthesia and conventional postoperative analgesia (i.e., IM or IV opioids), while the second group received combined epidural/general anesthesia and epidural opioids for postoperative pain. Mortality, overall complication rate, infection rate, time to extubation, and hospital costs were significantly lower in the epidural group.

A variety of drugs and combinations are currently used to provide postoperative epidural analgesia. Tables 1-3 provide some clinically relevant comparisons among several popular choices.

Table 1. Relative efficacy of epidural agents.

Effective	More Effective	Most Effective
Fentanyl ≤ 75 μg/h	Fentanyl ≥ 100 μg/h	Morphine
Meperidine ≤ 10 mg/h	Meperidine ≤ 20 mg/h	Bupivacaine 0.125% + fentanyl 4 μg/ml
Bupivacaine 0.0625% + fentanyl 2 μg/ml	Bupivacaine 0.0625% + fentanyl 4 μg/ml	Bupivacaine 0.25%
	Bupivacaine 0.125%	

Table 2. Possible problems with epidural local anesthetic techniques.

Function Blocked	Possible Problem
Sympathetic	Hypotension (thoracic > lumbar)
Proprioception	Difficulty ambulating
Sensory	Pressure injury Mask a complication
Motor	Loss of function (cough, ambulation)

Table 3. Epidural bupivacaine - 0.0625% vs. 0.125%.

Item	Bupivacaine 0.0625%	Bupivacaine 0.125%
Hypotension	absent	rare
Loss of proprioception	subtle effect (lumbar > thoracic)	marked effect (lumbar > thoracic)
Sensory block	variable	present
Motor block	rare	common
Application	high volume infusion	low volume infusion (segmental block)

By contrast, some patients enter the hospital with the belief and expectation that their needs should be evaluated and met by their doctors and nurses. Such patients are likely to be threatened by PCA and the responsibility they must assume to treat their own pain. Their fears and concerns are likely to lead to inadequate pain control. Such patients are likely to be more comfortable receiving EOA or other forms of therapy that require the doctors and nurses to regularly assess pain and administer doses of drugs as they judge them to be necessary.

Institutional Factors

New services developed to improve the treatment of acute pain in hospitalized patients have been described and are of current interest to anesthesiologists. Establishing such a service involves a considerable administrative commitment. It includes a close liaison with nurses to develop appropriate educational and procedural standards, as well as interactions with surgeons, hospital pharmacists, and those providing the surgical anesthetics. A well-planned and organized service is essential to optimal comfort and safety using EOA, PCA, and other methods of therapy. Until such organized care is possible, it may be best to delay introduction of sophisticated methods of pain control.

REFERENCES

1. Caplan RA, Ready LB, Oden RV, et al: Transdermal fentanyl for postoperative pain management: A double-blind placebo study. JAMA 261:1036-1039, 1989
2. Harmer M, Rosen M, Vickers MD: Patient-Controlled Analgesia. London, Blackwell Scientific Publications, 1985
3. Ferrante FM, Ostheimer GW Covino BG: Patient-Controlled Analgesia. Boston, Blackwell Scientific Publications, 1989
4. Cousins MJ, Mather LE: Intrathecal and epidural administration of opiates. Anesthesiology 61:276-310, 1984
5. Rawal N, Sjöstrand U, Christoffersson E, et al: Comparison of intramuscular and epidural morphine for postoperative analgesia in the grossly obese: Influence on postoperative ambulation and pulmonary function. Anesth Analg 63:583-592, 1984
6. Yeager MP, Glass DD, Neff RK, Brinck-Johnsen T: Epidural anesthesia and analgesia in high-risk surgical patients. Anesthesiology 66:729-736, 1987

These can be categorized as: 1) clinical, 2) patient-related, and, 3) institutional factors.

Clinical Factors

It is well known that certain surgical procedures result in more pain than others. Incisions involving the upper abdomen or thorax are expected to cause more pain than operations on the hand or foot. The postoperative pain therapist should be aware of the growing evidence that although PCA produces analgesia that is frequently superior to intramuscular opioids given on an "as needed" basis, it may not produce as much pain relief as EOA. Two studies report this finding in women following cesarean section (10,11), while the same observation has been made after open-knee surgery (12) and after cholecystectomy (13). For some patients, the additional analgesia available with EOA may be of critical importance. This is particularly true when severe pain may compromise pulmonary function leading to atelectasis and pneumonia. Examples include patients with rib fractures or pain resulting from abdominal and thoracic incisions. Those with underlying medical conditions such as respiratory insufficiency or obesity may also derive particular benefit from the best available analgesia. In these situations, the need for profound analgesia is of major importance and may make EOA the preferred choice.

Other factors may favor the selection of PCA for analgesia. It does not require the extra time and skill that is necessary for the anesthesiologist to place epidural catheters. The question of who will re-inject epidural catheters during the day and night does not apply. The time required to educate ward nurses is less for PCA than for EOA. In some patient populations, side effects such as nausea, pruritus, and urinary retention are more common and more severe with EOA than with PCA.

Certain clinical issues in patient selection remain controversial. What approach for postoperative pain control should be recommended in patients with opioid tolerance and/or drug-seeking behavior? In the author's experience, EOA frequently is not successful in patients who demonstrate major opioid tolerance. The combination of dilute local anesthetics and opioids infused through an epidural catheter has been more effective. A commonly used combination is 0.0625% bupivacaine and fentanyl 2 μg/ml. Following an initial loading bolus of 15-20 ml, the infusion is started at a rate of 10-15 ml/hr and titrated to produce adequate analgesia. Concern has been expressed that drug-seeking patients after surgery might abuse the opportunity to self-medicate with a PCA pump containing an opioid. Although the management of this population is never easy, we have found it useful after surgery to provide for such patients' basic preoperative opioid requirements with long-acting oral opioids or fixed-dose intravenous opiate infusions while allowing them to use supplemental opioids from a PCA pump as needed for their incisional pain. Careful preoperative discussion assures a clear understanding of the reason for each component of therapy including its planned duration. Conflict and anger postoperatively, when it its time to remove the PCA pump, are thus reduced. Reported pain scores in this population are typically high, although objective observation shows adequate respiratory patterns, effective coughing, and the ability to tolerate early ambulation and physical therapy.

Another area of controversy involves the management of post-operative pain in patients with coagulopathies or who are scheduled to receive anticoagulants to facilitate vascular or cardiac surgery. EOA may be of great benefit to some of these patients, but is it safe? There is no clear scientific answer. Each patient should be considered individually with careful weighing of possible risks and expected benefits. Some anesthesiologists currently offer epidural anesthesia and analgesia to selected patients in this category; others do not. The interested reader is referred to a review of this subject (14). PCA offers an attractive alternative in those situations when it is deemed prudent to avoid an epidural catheter.

Although EOA and PCA can result in improved analgesia, both techniques are associated with a number of side effects. With EOA, pruritus, nausea and vomiting, and urinary retention are common. Sedation occurs infrequently. With PCA, the same side effects occur but in many situations they tend to be less frequent and less severe. Both techniques can result in respiratory depression which, if not recognized early, can be life-threatening. It is beyond the scope of this article to discuss these side effects in detail. Frequently they can be prevented or controlled, but when they occur they can be a major determinant of patient comfort and satisfaction with the management of their postoperative pain.

Effective methods for controlling pain are associated with risks. Traditional fears of addiction to opioids in hospitalized patients with acute pain are unfounded and are not a justifiable reason to withhold adequate analgesia (15). Lack of understanding of the nature of opioid-induced respiratory depression has also lead to inadequate analgesia in countless patients. With well organized clinical services established to provide modern analgesia, the risks associated with EOA and PCA may be no higher than with intramuscular opioid injections. Careful patient selection, appropriate choice of drugs and dosage, nurse education, and adequate medical supervision can result in the safe application of both these methods throughout a modern hospital (16).

Patient-related Factors

Each patient facing surgery is a unique human being. Many will harbor concerns, fears, expectations, recollections of previous experience with pain, preferences, and possibly, limitations. These factors alone or in combination may be of paramount importance when choosing a method of pain control. For example, although epidural morphine might produce superior analgesia after a major abdominal operation, a patient with a morbid fear of "a needle in the back" may be better treated in some other way. Or, a patient scheduled for a procedure ordinarily well suited to PCA will not obtain satisfactory analgesia if he or she is unwilling, or does not have the mental capacity to self-administer medication for pain.

Most people admitted to the hospital for surgery are accustomed to an independent lifestyle. On arrival in hospital, basic human rights involving eating, mobility, privacy, and even control over bodily functions may be taken over by hospital staff. Uncertainty about what to expect, fear about the surgery, and isolation from a familiar and controllable environment are compounded by the sudden experience of a new source of stress—postoperative pain. PCA allows patients to self-administer an analgesic, giving back, at least in one area, a sense of control over their care. Without having to negotiate with others for pain medication, more immediate pain relief is obtained. For people who are distressed by loss of "control" in the hospital setting, PCA will be greatly appreciated and viewed as superior to other methods that involve less control.

7. Egbert LD, Battit GE, Turndorf H, Beecher HK: The value of the preoperative visit by an anesthesiologist. JAMA 185:553-555, 1963
8. Egbert LD, Battit GE, Welch CE, Bartlett MK: Reduction of postoperative pain by encouragement and instruction of patients. N Engl J Med 270:825-825, 1964
9. Schmitt FE, Wooldridge PJ: Psychological preparation of surgical patients. Nurs Res 22:108-116, 1973
10. Eisenach JC, Grice SC, Dewan DM: Patient-controlled analgesia following cesarean section: A comparison with epidural and intramuscular narcotics. Anesthesiology 68:444-448, 1988
11. Harrison DM, Sinatra R, Morgese L, Chung JH: Epidural narcotic and patient-controlled analgesia for post-cesarean section pain relief. Anesthesiology 68:454-457, 1988
12. Loper KA, Ready LB: Epidural morphine following anterior cruciate ligament repair: A comparison with patient-controlled intravenous morphine. Anesth Analg 68:350-352, 1989
13. Loper KA, Ready LB, Nessly M, Rapp SE: Epidural morphine provides greater pain relief than patient-controlled intravenous morphine following cholecystectomy. Anesth Analg 69:826-828, 1989
14. Owens EL, Kasten GW, Hessel EA II: Spinal subarachnoid hematoma after lumbar puncture and heparinization: A case report, review of the literature, and discussion of anesthetic implications. Anesth Analg 65:1201-1207, 1986
15. Miller RR, Greenblatt DJ: Drug Effects in Hospitalized Patients. New York, John Wiley and Sons, 1976, pp. 151-152
16. Ready LB, Oden R, Chadwick HS, et al: Development of an anesthesiology-based postoperative pain management service. Anesthesiology 68:100-106, 1988

PATIENT-CONTROLLED ANALGESIA (PART I): HISTORICAL PERSPECTIVE

P. F. White

In designing patient-controlled analgesia (PCA) equipment, biomedical engineers have utilized negative feedback control technology. When feedback control is applied to the control of pain, the patient self-administers analgesic medication to decrease the error signal [i.e., the difference between the pain experienced and the acceptable (tolerable) level of pain] to zero (1,2). PCA techniques attempt to close the feedback loop without the necessity of nursing staff intervention, thereby, improving the effectiveness of the pain control system.

Since the first widely used PCA device was introduced into clinical practice in the United Kingdom in 1976, several more technologically advanced PCA delivery systems have been introduced in the United States. The major advantages of these newer PCA systems relate to their computerized programming features and fail-safe designs. This chapter will describe some of the important features of PCA systems which have been developed over the last twenty years.

Historical PCA Infusion Devices

The Cardiff Palliator™ (Graseby Dynamics) is a line-powered syringe pump which can be preprogrammed to deliver the desired dose of medication at a predetermined flow rate with a preselected minimum dose interval. The parameters are adjustable over a wide range to accommodate a variety of drugs and dosage regimens. To minimize the possibility of the button being pressed accidentally, the button must be pressed twice in rapid succession (within 1 sec) to achieve a successful demand. A disposable 20 ml syringe can be filled with the analgesic of choice. A yellow indicator lamp (which remains on during the lockout interval) and

T. H. Stanley and M. A. Ashburn (eds.), Anesthesiology and Pain Management, 117–125.

a tone sounds when a bolus dose is successfully infused. An audible alarm sounds whenever the syringe is empty. The thumbwheel switches are accessible on the front and rear of the device for controlling the incremental dose (range 1 to 999 mg), dilution control (range 1 to 99 mg/ml), interval time (range 1 to 99 minutes), and delivery rate (range 1 to 99 ml/hr). Unfortunately, these thumbwheel switches are not tamper proof and therefore the settings had to be frequently monitored. A "second generation" Cardiff Palliator containing the safety and security features present on the more recently developed PCA devices will be available for clinical use in the near future.

The Pharmacia Prominject™ pump is a microprocess-controlled, programmable infusion pump with three different modes of operation (namely, patient-controlled, consecutive infusions, and constant infusion). The consecutive infusion mode allows for the administration of a loading dose ("priming" infusion), followed by a constant maintenance infusion. This device is also capable of delivering split incremental doses (e.g., a bolus dose delivered over 1 minute followed by an infusion of the equivalent dose over 1 hour). After selecting the desired operational mode, the operator enters the drug concentration, dose, lock-out interval (in PCA mode), and time for infusion of the dose. The alphanumeric message panel guides the operator step-by-step through the programming procedure. The prescribed drug is delivered from a standard 20 ml B-D Luer lock disposable syringe which is covered by a clear tamper-proof Perspex cover. This cover is locked with a key which also electronically locks the keyboard. A hard copy of the drug usage record is produced by a built-in dot matrix printer. The time, date, and accumulated dose are printed simultaneously with the event or retrospectively from the microprocessor memory. Acoustic and diagnostic alarms and status messages will report line occlusion, empty syringe, low battery charge, and improper program settings. The device can be mounted on an infusion stand or placed on a table top.

The On Demand Analgesia Computer (ODAC™, Janssen Scientific Instruments) is a highly innovative experimental PCA device. This infusion device allows the patient to interact directly with the machine using a tape cassette. In addition to demand doses, this device can administer a background infusion based on the amount of analgesic drug which the patient demanded during the previous 16-minute interval. An integral pneumograph sensor prevents analgesic administration if the respiratory rate is depressed. With further technological refinement, the ODAC™ could become a clinically useful device in the management of postoperative pain. However, it would seem unlikely that any of the "second generation" pharmacokinetically-based, computer-controlled opioid infusion systems currently under investigation will be available for clinical use in the near future.

Commercially Available PCA Infusion Devices

The Abbott Life Care™ PCA Infusers (Abbott Laboratories, North Chicago, IL) combine microprocessor and stepping motor technology for the safe delivery of either intermittent bolus doses and/or a continuous infusion of narcotic analgesics from disposal cartridges. These relatively lightweight, portable, computerized volumetric infusion pumps have lockable security doors that prohibit unauthorized access to the analgesic drug or the controls while the unit is in operation. A liquid crystal display indicates the operational status, total cumulative dose, number of bolus doses administered, as well as other status and alarm messages. Pre-filled (e.g., morphine 1 mg/ml, meperidine 10 mg) or empty drug cartridges are available. After the cartridge has been inserted into the pump and the special "Y" tubing (containing a one-way check valve) has been primed, the device can be connected to an existing IV catheter.

With the first generation Life Care PCA device, the incremental (bolus) dose volume and lockout were set using thumbwheel switches. The newer (Life Care PCA PLUS) infuser is fully computerized and can be programmed to deliver either intermittent bolus doses, continuous infusions, or a continuous infusion which is supplemented by bolus injections on demand. When the door is closed and the key removed, the display reads "ready," indicating that the patient can activate the device by pressing the patient-control button. Immediately after a bolus dose is delivered, the device enters the mandatory "lockout" mode for a minimum of 5 minutes. The device can be programmed to signal when a successful dose is delivered, or every time the patient demand button is activated ("placebo" effect). The newer version has a 36-hour memory which records the administered dose as well as key events (e.g., changes in the dosage regimen). The optional printer can provide a 12-hour hard copy of the patient's history. While in operation, the PCA infusion pump is secured to an IV pole with a Duolock® locking mechanism.

The Bard Harvard PCA™ (C.R. Bard, Inc., Murray Hill, NJ) is a portable syringe infusion pump capable of both continuous and intermittent drug administration. In addition, this device can also be programmed to deliver a continuous background (basal) infusion which is supplemented with bolus doses on demand. The pump has a stepper motor and is microprocessor controlled to prevent faulty operation due to an empty drug syringe, low flow, runaway, excess pressure, low battery, or control circuit failure. The alphanumeric message panel guides the operator through the sequences necessary for correct pump operation. When the pump is in the operational mode, prescription and dosage data can be read and/or changed only after an authorized user enters a preassigned access code. A key switch allows the operator to unlock the cover over the syringe compartment. A 60 ml disposable plastic syringe can be filled with the desired concentration of the prescribed opiate analgesic. The syringe is connected to a Harvard "Y"-type extension set (containing a one-way antireflux valve), then it is placed in the syringe cradle and purged. The device's microprocessor-controlled memory records the total number of patient attempts during the lockout period as well as the number of successful injections to allow the operator to optimize the analgesic regimen. The memory also records key events (e.g., changes in the infusion rate).

The Bard PCA I is a simplified version of the original Harvard PCA device which provides added patient maneuverability. It has a simplified programming system which involves the use of dials to set the dose, the delay interval (i.e., minimum time between successive doses) and the "basal" infusion rate. Like the original Bard PCA device, this pump accepts standard 60 ml disposable plastic syringes. This battery-powered (four D-size alkaline batteries) device has a computerized display and memory which provides information about the number of injections and attempts as well as the total dose of analgesic medication.

The Bard Ambulatory PCA device is extremely useful in both inpatient and outpatient settings. This light weight portable device is fully computerized and battery powered (9V). Although this compact device is usually worn by the patient, it can be locked to an IV pole. It has essentially all the features available on the original Harvard PCA device, [e.g., intermittent, continuous infusion or continuous (basal) supplemented on demand] . In addition, it has a large drug volume capacity (either 100 ml or 250 ml disposable plastic containers). This PCA device also has all the fail-safe features of the larger infuser and the drug compartment is tamper proof. Special microbore tubing is available for use of the device with epidural or subcutaneous administration techniques.

The <u>IVAC PCA Infusor</u> is a portable, battery (four D-size) operated device. Although it is a fully computerized syringe-based pump, it has simplified programming features on its liquid crystal display. The alphanumeric message panel guides the operator step-by-step through the programming procedure. In the PCA mode, the patient can self-administer on demand or the staff can preset the infusion system to continuously deliver medication over an extended period of time. The prescribed drug can be delivered from a wide variety of standard 20-60 ml disposable plastic syringes and is covered by a clear tamper proof plastic cover. This cover is locked with a key which also electronically locks the keyboard. The standard microbore tubing with an antireflex valve is available for intravenous use. Analogous to the other computerized PCA devices, this device has a 24-hour memory (which remains operational for up to 99 hours even after the device is turned off), acoustic and diagnostic alarm features, and can be secured to an IV pole.

The <u>Pharmacia CADD-PCA</u> (Pharmacia Deltec, St. Paul, MN) is a small (15 oz), portable, programmable analgesic infusion device which can provide for the safe delivery of parenteral analgesics both in the hospital as well as outside the hospital environment. Although this PCA device has not been extensively evaluated for the treatment of acute postoperative pain, its compact size may allow for increased patient activity and mobility during the early postoperative period. The device delivers the analgesic drug on demand, with incremental doses ranging from 0.1 to 99.5 mg and a lockout interval from 5 to 99 min. The pump can also be used to continuously infuse analgesics, with a basal infusion rate of 0.1 to 99.5 mg/hr (depending on the concentration of the solution). Analgesic medication is contained in prefilled, sterilized disposable cassettes which are maintained in a locked compartment. Alarms warn the user when there is a low residual drug volume, low battery power, or a mechanical failure. The updated version of this PCA system has a lockable door and pole clamp, as well as a hand-held remote dose button.

The Baxter PCA Infusor™ (Baxter Healthcare Corp., Chicago, IL) is a small non-electronic device which is fully disposable. It consists of a light-weight plastic cylinder containing the analgesic medication inside an elastic balloon. The drug chamber holds a volume of 40 ml and the amount of drug delivered per injection is dependent upon the opioid concentration. The device is nonprogrammable, delivering a fixed 0.5 ml dose at intervals of 6 min or longer. As the balloon reservoir slowly deflates, solution flows through a small orifice (flow restrictor) which determines the time required to fill the injection reservoir (6 min). The injection reservoir is located on a wristband which is activated by pushing a button. There is no drug infusion between depressions of the medication demand button. Although its simplified design obviates the need for fail-safe features, it is less flexible than the other systems with respect to the administered dose.

The Abbott Provider™ 5000 is a lightweight portable PCA pump (14 oz.) which can deliver analgesic medication intermittently on demand or by continuous infusion. The pumping mechanism consists of a microprocessor-controlled eccentric/rotor peristaltic pump. The power supply consists of two 9V disposable lithium batteries which can deliver 4800 ml at a maximum rate of 250 ml/hr. The minimum drug infusion rate of 0.1 ml/hr will maintain the patency of the catheter and/or the vein. This device has a liquid crystal display, memory function, as well as audible and visual safety alarms. The software has been extensively revised in order to make it more user-friendly.

SUMMARY

The rational use of a PCA infusion device allows the patient to overcome variations in both pharmacokinetic and pharmacodynamic factors by carefully titrating the rate of opioid administration to meet their individual analgesic needs (3). The commercially-available PCA infusion pumps have been recently evaluated with respect to safety, security and overall ease of use (4). All the PCA pumps tested met the accuracy, electrical safety and performance criteria established by biomedical engineers (5). The Bard Ambulatory PCA, the Pharmacia CADD-PCA and the Baxter PCA infusor were all judged to be suitable for ambulatory use. However, the totally disposable Baxter device was not recommended for general hospital or home care bedside use because of its higher costs and lack of dose adjustment features.

Interestingly, in a recently published comparison of five commonly used PCA devices (6), the Baxter PCA infusor was consistently rated the highest by the nursing staff (Figure. 1). The reasons for the popularity of

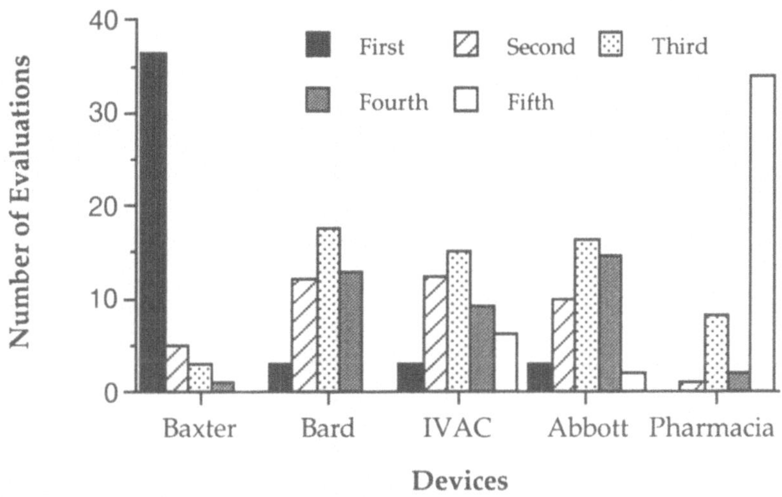

Figure 1. Overall ranking of the five patient-controlled analgesia devices (first = best to fifth = worst) by the nurses at the end of the 5-month trial period. [From Sawaki et al., 1992 (6)]

this device related to user-friendliness, reliability, ease of troubleshooting and documentation (Tables 1-3). Difficulties in programming and trouble-shooting the more sophisticated computerized devices by the nursing staff also raised concerns among the patients regarding their safety. Similar comparative evaluations among the second and third generation PCA devices are clearly needed.

In conclusion, the safe and effective delivery of opioid analgesic medications "on (patient) demand" is possible using a variety of delivery systems. When utilizing PCA to control acute pain, the physician can

Table 1. Overall nursing assessment of the five PCA devices.

	Ease of Documentation (%)			Frequency of Problems (%)			Ease of Troubleshooting (%)		
	Easy	Average	Difficult	Rare	Occasional	Frequent	Easy	Average	Difficult
Abbott	56	31a	13	49	45[a]	6	40	52[a]	8
Bard	50	42a	8	50	44[a]	6	35	57[a]	8
Pharmacia	20[a]	26	54[a]	29[a]	16	55[a]	4[a]	21	75[a]
Baxter	94	6	0	94	4	2	89	9	2
IVAC	61	29[a]	10	57	35a	8	40	52[a]	8

[a]Significantly different from Baxter device, $P > 0.05$.
From Sawaki et al., 1992 (6)

Table 2. Ward nurses' monthly assessments of the five PCA devices.

	Problems with power source (%)		Difficulty with memory function (%)			Interference with ambulation (%)		
	No	Yes	No	Yes	Never	Rarely	Occasionally	Frequently
Abbott	54	46[a]	62	38	35[b]	27	19	19
Bard	94	6	28	72[c]	18[b]	24	24	34[d]
Baxter	N/A	N/A	N/A	N/A	38[b]	24	28	10
Pharmacia	77	23[a]	30	70[c]	78	16	6	0
IVAC	100	0	76	24	33[b]	41	19	7

[a]Significantly different from Bard and IVAC, $P < 0.05$.; [b]Significantly different from Baxter, $P < 0.05$.; [c]Significantly different from Abbott and IVAC, $P < 0.05$; [d]Significantly different from Baxter and IVAC, $P < 0.05$.
From Sawaki et al., 1992 (6)

choose either a simplified, non-electronic disposable PCA device or an ultra-sophisticated computer-controlled infusion device with a wide variety of delivery modes. It would appear that future generations of PCA devices must be both safer for our patients and more cost-effective for the health care system.

Table 3. Patient assessment of PCA therapy with the five different PCA devices.

	Difficult to use at night (%)		Additional cost justified (%)		
	Yes	No	Yes	No	Uncertain
Abbott	6	94	43	32	25
Bard	8[a]	92	38	30	32
Baxter	1	99	48	31	21
Pharmacia	10[b]	90	40	30	30
IVAC	2	98	31	37	32

[a]Significantly different from the Baxter device, $P < 0.05$.
[b]Significantly different from the Baxter and IVAC devices, $P < 0.05$.
From Sawaki et al., 1992 (6).

REFERENCES

1. McCarthy JP: The Cardiff Palliator, Patient Controlled Analgesia. Edited by Harmer M, Rosen M, Vickers MD. Oxford, Blackwell Scientific Publications, 1985, p. 87
2. Jacobs OLR, Bullingham RES: Modelling, estimation and control for demand analgesia, Patient Controlled Analgesia. Edited by Harmer M, Rosen M, Vickers MD. Oxford, Blackwell Scientific Publications, 1985, p. 57
3. White PF: Patient-controlled analgesia: A new approach to the management of postoperative pain. Semin Anesth 4:255-266, 1985
4. Editorial. Patient-controlled analgesic infusion pumps (I). Health Devices 17:137, 1988
5. Editorial. Patient-controlled analgesia infusion pumps (II). Health Devices 17:368, 1988
6. Sawaki Y, Parker RK, White PF: Patient and nurse evaluation of patient-controlled analgesia delivery systems for postoperative pain management. J Pain Symptom Manage 7:443-453, 1992

PROBLEMS IN THE MANAGEMENT OF POSTOPERATIVE PAIN

L. B. Ready

I. INTRODUCTION

It is the obligation of all health care professionals to provide patients with effective relief of pain. In addition to basic humanitarian reasons, a growing number of reports are demonstrating that effective pain relief is associated with a reduced risk of certain postoperative complications, earlier mobilization, shortened hospital stay, and reduced costs. Regrettably, an examination of both older and more recent studies shows that major deficits have existed and still persist in this area of care.

In this presentation, reasons why these problems have occurred are discussed and some of the scientific findings that have been published on the subject are considered. Areas where deficits are well documented include postoperative pain, trauma and burns, acutely painful medical conditions, procedural pain, and pediatric acute pain. In order for effective and safe pain relief to be possible, there are a number of requirements. These include appropriate goals and attitudes, adequate knowledge and skills, regular assessment, availability of suitable treatment methods, and a commitment to quality assurance.

II. ATTITUDES ABOUT PAIN RELIEF

A number of inappropriate attitudes about pain relief are widely held and, along with associated knowledge deficits, they contribute to inadequate care (Table 1). They arise from a number of sources which include patients and their families, physicians, nurses, pharmacists, hospital administrators, health care systems, and drug regulatory agencies. In this presentation a number of studies are presented which help define

T. H. Stanley and M. A. Ashburn (eds.), Anesthesiology and Pain Management, 127–132.

Table 1. Knowledge deficits associated with acute pain management.

	Knowledge Deficit	Pervasive Attitude	Resultant Behavior
Health Care Professionals	Anatomy, physiology, psychology of acute pain	Hurting is normal and harmless	Low priority to treat pain
	Pharmacology of opioids	Fear—respiratory depression, cardiovascular instability, addiction	PRN treatment - dose too small: too infrequent
	Assessment of pain	Assume adequate care	Patients who complain of pain are "bad"
	Patient variability	Usual dose are effective	Inflexible prescribing
	Spectrum of treatment options	"One size fits all"	Wrong treatment
Patients and Families	Option for effective pain control	Pain can't be avoided	"Grin and bear it"
	Making the system respond	Staff are cruel, uncaring	Argue, cajole, demand - the "adversarial relationship"
	Doctors and nurses are busy	Other patients are more important	Avoid reporting pain
Health Care Systems, Administrators, Payors	Pain control is very important to patients	Superior pain relief is "unnecessary"	Resist providing personnel, equipment
	Reduction in rate of complications and cost of providing care with effective analgesia	Effective pain control is too expensive	Resist funding the costs of effective pain relief

some of these attitudes and related practice behaviors. For the interested reader, the bibliography lists a considerable number of publications which relate to deficits in treating acute pain .

III. THE FUTURE

There are encouraging signs that awareness of the importance of acute and postoperative pain is increasing. These include:

1. Clinical Practice Guideline for Acute Pain Management: Operative or Medical Procedures and Trauma. This document was commissioned by the Office of the Forum for Quality and Effectiveness in Health Care, of the Agency for Health Care Policy and Research (AHCPR), Department of Health and Human Services. The committee that developed the guidelines undertook a detailed, interdisciplinary clinic review of "current needs, therapeutic practices and principles, and emerging technologies for postoperative pain control." Information and opinion was obtained from 30 external consultants and through testimony presented at an open forum from concerned parties. A representative of the ASA provided testimony and endorsed the process as did a number of individual anesthesiologists. Interest in the subject from non-physician groups was also high. Additional information was collected through a comprehensive review and analysis of scientific publications on the subject of postoperative pain and its treatment.

The text of the guidelines is extensive. Important elements include recognition of historic inadequacies in postoperative pain management, clear acknowledgement of the importance of good pain control, and a statement of the need for the involvement of specialists in appropriate cases. The guidelines also emphasize the need for a process of accountability by institutions for the adequate provision of postoperative analgesia. They recommend responsibility for that activity be placed in the hands of those with the greatest knowledge and interest in postoperative pain. Overall, the AHCPR Guidelines are supportive of the efforts of anesthesiologists to provide postoperative analgesia, and they have now been endorsed publicly by the Federal Government. Copies can be obtained free of charge by calling 1-800-358-9295.

2. The International Association for the Study of Pain (IASP) task force on acute pain has published a document entitled MANUAL OF ACUTE PAIN: A PRACTICAL GUIDE. The book is written with an appreciation that interest in acute pain is multidisciplinary, and with the knowledge that clinical practice patterns and resources for providing care vary widely throughout the world. Consequently, considerable emphasis has been placed on principles of evaluation and therapy with tabulation of more specific technical and pharmacological information. Readers are guided through a process designed to assist in determining how best to provide optimal care for patients with acute pain in their particular practice situations.

In addition to information on adult postoperative pain, this book includes chapters on trauma and burn pain, acute pediatric pain, painful medical conditions, acute cancer pain, and pain in obstetrics. A case study approach is used to illustrate the evaluation and treatment of a variety of frequently encountered acute pain problems. This publication has been mailed free of charge to all IASP members and can be purchased for $15.00 by calling the IASP office at 206-547-6409.

3. The American Society of Anesthesiologists (ASA) has formed a committee to develop Pain Practice Guidelines for the specialty. When completed, these will further highlight the importance of adequate pain relief, therapeutic options, and the important role to be played in the future by anesthesiologists.

REFERENCES

1. Abbott FV, Gray-Donald K, Sewitch MJ, et al: The prevalence of pain in hospitalized patients and resolution over six months. Pain 50:15-28, 1992
2. Austin KL, Stapleton JV, Mather LE: Relationship between blood meperidine concentrations and analgesic response: A preliminary report. Anesthesiology 53:460-466, 1980
3. Austin KL, Stapleton JV, Mather LE: Multiple intramuscular injections: A major source of variability in analgesic response to meperidine. Pain 8:47-62, 1980
4. Banister EH: Six potent analgesic drugs. A double-blind study in post-operative pain. Anaesthesia 29:158-162, 1974
5. Beyer JE, DeGood DE, Ashley LC, Russell GA: Patterns of postoperative analgesic use with adults and children following cardiac surgery. Pain 17:71-81, 1983

6. Bonica JJ: Current status of postoperative pain therapy. Current Topics in Pain Research and Therapy. Edited by Yokota T, Dubner R. Amsterdam, Excerpta Medica, 1983, pp. 169-189
7. Cartwright PD: Pain control after surgery: A survey of current practice. Ann R Coll Surg Engl 67:13-16, 1985
8. Chapman PJ, Ganendran A, Scott RJ, Basford KE: Attitudes and knowledge of nursing staff in relation to management of postoperative pain. Aust N Z J Surg 57:447-450, 1987
9. Cohen FL: Postsurgical pain relief: Patients' status and nurses' medication choices. Pain 9:265-274, 1980
10. Cronin M, Redfern PA, Utting JE: Psychiatry and postoperative complaints in surgical patients. Br J Anaesth 45:879-886, 1973
11. Dahlström B, Tamsen A, Paalzow L, Hartvig P: Patient-controlled analgesic therapy, Part IV: Pharmacokinetics and analgesic plasma concentrations of morphine. Clin Pharmacokinet 7:266-279, 1982
12. Donald I: At the receiving end: A doctor's personal recollections of second-time valve replacement. Scott Med J 21:49-57, 1976
13. Donovan M, Dillon P, McGuire L: Incidence and characteristics of pain in a sample of medical-surgical inpatients. Pain 30:69-78, 1987
14. Donovan BD: Patient attitudes to postoperative pain relief. Anaesth Intensive Care 11:125-129, 1983
15. Editorial: Tight-fisted analgesia. Lancet 1(7973):1338, 1976
16. Eland JM, Anderson JE: The experience of pain in children. Pain: A Source Book for Nurses and Other Health Care Professionals. Edited by Jacox AK. Boston, Little, Brown and Co, 1977, pp. 453-473
17. Keats AS: Postoperative pain: Research and treatment. J Chronic Dis 4:72-83, 1956
18. Keeri-Szanto M, Heaman S: Postoperative demand analgesia. Surg Gynecol Obstet 134:647-651, 1972
19. Lasagna L, Beecher HK: The optimal dose of morphine. JAMA 156:230-234, 1954
20. MacInnes C: Cancer Ward. New Society 36:232, 1976
21. Marks RM, Sachar EJ: Undertreatment of medical inpatients with narcotic analgesics. Ann Intern Med 78:173-181, 1973
22. Mather L, Mackie J: The incidence of postoperative pain in children. Pain 15:271-282, 1983
23. Max MB: U.S. Government disseminates acute pain treatment guidelines: Will they make a difference? Pain 50:3-4, 1992
24. Melzack R, Abbott FV, Zackon W, et al: Pain on a surgical ward: A survey of the duration and intensity of pain and the effectiveness of medication. Pain 29:67-72, 1987
25. Nayman J: Measurement and control of postoperative pain. Ann R Coll Surg Engl 61:419-426, 1979
26. Owen H, McMillan V, Rogowski D: Postoperative pain therapy: A survey of patients' expectations and their experiences. Pain 41:303-307, 1990

27. Papper EM, Brodie BB, Rovenstine EA: Postoperative pain: Its use in the comparative evaluation of analgesics. Surgery 32:107-109, 1952
28. Puntillo KA: Pain experience in intensive care patients. Heart Lung 19:526-533, 1990
29. Rose DK, Cohn MM, Yee DA: Postoperative pain control—how are we doing (abstract)? Anesth Analg 76 :S355, 1993
30. Sriwatanakul K, Weis OF, Alloza JL, et al: Analysis of narcotic analgesic usage in the treatment of postoperative pain. JAMA 250:926-929, 1983
31. Tamsen A, Hartvig P, Fagerlund C, Dahlström B: Patient-controlled analgesia therapy, Part II: Individual analgesic demand and analgesic plasma concentrations of pethidine in postoperative pain. Clin Pharmacokinet 7:164-175, 1982
32. Tamsen A, Bondesson U, Dahlström B, Hartvig P: Patient-controlled analgesic therapy, Part III: Pharmacokinetics and analgesic plasma concentrations of ketobemidone. Clin Pharmacokinet 7:252-265, 1982
33. Tamsen A, Sakurada T, Wahlström A, et al: Postoperative demand for analgesics in relation to individual levels of endorphins and substance P in cerebrospinal fluid. Pain 13:171-183, 1982
34. Utting JE, Smith JM: Postoperative analgesia. Anaesthesia 34:320-332, 1979
35. Weis OF, Sriwatanakul K, Alloza JL, et al: Attitudes of patients, housestaff, and nurses toward postoperative analgesic care. Anesth Analg 62:70-74, 1983
36. Wilder-Smith CH, Schuler L: Postoperative analgesia: Pain by choice? The influence of patient attitudes and patient education. Pain 50:257-262, 1992
37. Wilson JF, Brockopp GW, Kryst S, et al: Medical students' attitudes toward pain before and after a brief course on pain. Pain 50:251-256, 1992

PATIENT CONTROLLED ANALGESIA (PART II): AN UPDATE ON CLINICAL USAGE[*]

P. F. White

In 1972, Mark et al. reported that medical inpatients were frequently undertreated with opioid analgesics. Since that time, there have been many other reports describing inadequate use of analgesics in the treatment of acute pain. Despite advances in our knowledge of the pathophysiology of pain and the pharmacology of analgesic drugs, as well as availability of more effective techniques for postoperative pain control, many patients do not receive optimal analgesic therapy. Until recently, a majority of hospitalized patients receiving parenteral opioid analgesics for moderate or severe pain failed to be adequately relieved by these drugs.

Why do patients continue to suffer from acute pain when effective opioid analgesics are available? The primary reasons may relate to a lack of information about analgesic medications and misconceptions about their potency, side effects and addictive potential. In no other area of medicine has such an extravagant concern for side effects limited treatment. The inherent pharmacokinetic and pharmacodynamic variability which exists among patients contributes to difficulty in determining the appropriate dose of analgesic medication. Individualization of analgesic therapy is crucial if one hopes to improve postoperative pain relief. Patient-controlled analgesia (PCA) is a system that is designed to accommodate the wide range of analgesic requirements that can be anticipated when managing postoperative pain. It is possible with PCA to allow the patient to vary the rate of analgesic drug administration. In this way, analgesic medication supply can be titrated to meet the patient's needs.

---

[*]Adapted from Reinhart DJ, White PF: Patient-controlled analgesia: An update on its clinical use, Pain Management. Edited by Paris PM, Brody M. Philadelphia, W.B. Saunders , 1993.

T. H. Stanley and M. A. Ashburn (eds.), Anesthesiology and Pain Management, 133–142.

The concept of a "demand analgesia" system began in the mid-1960's. Sechzer first described the intravenous (IV) administration of opioids for postoperative analgesia in small incremental doses on patient demand by a nurse observer. Sechzer observed that the postoperative analgesic requirement was cyclical and varied considerably among patients. Shortly thereafter, pain researchers began evaluating instruments that would allow patients to self-administer small IV doses of opioid drugs. Early PCA devices consisted of an electronically controlled infusion pump connected to a timing device which was activated by depressing a thumb button located on the end of a cord extending from the PCA machine. When activated, the machine delivered a preset amount of analgesic drug.

The first commercially available PCA device, known as the Cardiff Palliator (Graseby Dynamics Ltd.), was developed by investigators at the Welsh National School of Medicine. This research group subsequently described a wide range of clinical uses for PCA analgesia. After initial reports that patients could safely and reliably control their own analgesia, other investigative groups confirmed these findings. Since the mid-1970's, several microprocessor-controlled PCA devices have been developed, including the On-Demand Analgesia Computer (ODAC), the Pharmacia Prominject™, the Abbott LifeCare PCA™, the Bard Harvard PCA, the Leicester Micropalliator, and the Programmable On-Demand Analgesia Computer (PRODAC). These early PCA devices contained many of the features of a PCA present in modern PCA devices. The essential features of a PCA delivery system include the following:

1. A drug reservoir that allows repeated doses of analgesia without the intervention of a nurse or physician.
2. An infusion device able to accurately deliver a prescribed dose of analgesic medication.
3. A means by which the patient can trigger the device, referred to as a "demand."
4. The programming of a particular demand dose (bolus) which is the amount of analgesic agent delivered in response to the patient "demand."

5. A delay or lockout interval between successive doses to prevent the patient from administering a second dose until they perceived the effect of the previous dose.
6. A secure drug reservoir with a connecting tubing system which prevents drug siphoning (e.g., back-check value).

With an "on demand" delivery system for managing postoperative pain, the patient is allowed to self-administer opioid analgesic medication, minimizing the effects of pharmacokinetic and pharmacodynamic variability on the response to analgesic medication.

THE VERSATILITY OF PCA THERAPY

With the rapid growth in acute pain management services, we find ourselves dealing with an intriguing variety of analgesia techniques. The IV-PCA can be used with a variety of opioid analgesics, giving it enhanced flexibility in the management of individual patient's analgesic needs. In addition, on-demand analgesia has gained popularity as a result of its effectiveness when utilized via the IM, oral, subcutaneous and peridural routes.

The use of on-demand epidural analgesia has received significant attention with numerous reports concerning its efficacy in the treatment of postoperative pain. In the early investigations with this route of PCA therapy, there were some therapeutic failures when comparing it to IV-PCA. However, Parker and colleagues found no significant difference in pain relief when comparing IV-PCA to epidural PCA hydromorphone after obstetrical surgery. Although the epidural group required 70 to 80% less medication, they also suffered a higher incidence of nausea and pruritus. Nevertheless, the epidural PCA group was discharged earlier than the IV-PCA treated patients. In another study, utilizing the same analgesia medication but comparing on-demand epidural hydromorphone with a constant epidural infusion of hydromorphone, these investigators found that the on-demand group consumed significantly less drug than the continuous infusion group.

In a recent study, epidural PCA was compared to IV-PCA with fentanyl for post-thoracotomy pain. There was no difference between the two groups in respiratory rates, $PaCO_2$ values, pain scores or changes in bedside pulmonary function tests (i.e., FVC and FEV_1). However, fentanyl requirements were significantly less when given via the epidural route, supporting the concept of a direct spinal cord site of action for epidural fentanyl. Bustamante et al. reported that patients receiving epidural PCA morphine required significantly less morphine than the IV-PCA group following major vascular surgery. However, this opioid-sparing effect with the epidural route did not result in a decrease of opioid-related side effects or improved patient outcome.

Intramuscular PCA has been evaluated by placing a small-gauge cannula in the deltoid muscle of the non-dominant arm. The subcutaneous (SC) route of PCA administration has also been studied with morphine, hydromorphone and oxymorphone. SC-PCA represents a clinically acceptable alternative to IV-PCA in the treatment of postoperative pain in both inpatients and outpatients. Recently, Litman, et al, reported the successful use of oral PCA in adolescents by placing a limited number of analgesia tablets by the patient's bedside, giving them some degree of independence and self-control over their postoperative treatment while in the hospital.

Use of Background (Basal) Infusion with PCA Therapy

In addition to "on-demand" dosing, PCA devices are able to deliver a fixed-rate continuous infusion. In theory, a concurrent baseline (basal) opioid infusion with PCA should be helpful in maintaining a consistent therapeutic "analgesic" level of the analgesic medication, thus decreasing the need for supplemental injections of analgesic medication. Several investigators have advocated this technique as part of every standard PCA protocol.

Patients who are excessively sedated as a result of residual anesthetic effects or fatigued after surgery may underdose themselves with opioid medication when using PCA therapy. Furthermore, patients who are comfortable at rest may experience distressing pain with sudden increase in physical activity. The use of a continuous infusion at nighttime was thought to facilitate sleep. However, recent studies would suggest that there is no advantage to a continuous infusion of opioid medication. Several studies even suggested potential harmful effects of bolus plus infusion techniques. Finnegan reported a higher incidence of confusion in patients receiving a continuous infusion. Owen concluded that a continuous infusion does not decrease the number of bolus demands. Other studies suggested that patients receiving continuous infusion had a higher incidence of respiratory depression. Using continuous infusion PCA to enhance sleep may be ill-advised since sleep may enhance respiratory depression and sedation given at bedtime may further potentiate the opioid's central nervous system depressant effects. Recently, Parker et al. studied 230 adult women randomized to receive IV-PCA morphine alone or IV-PCA morphine with a continuous infusion of morphine, 0.5, 1.0 or 2.0 mg/hr. Patients receiving the 2.0 mg/hr infusion used significantly more morphine from 9 to 72 hours after their operation than the control group. The presence of a constant infusion did not significantly decrease the number of patient demands or supplemental bolus doses. These investigators concluded that the use of a continuous opioid infusion in combination with a standard PCA regimen did not improve pain management compared with PCA alone after abdominal hysterectomy. In more recent studies comparing patient-controlled epidural analgesia with and without a background continuous infusion, investigators have also concluded that although both groups had high quality analgesia, the addition of a continuous infusion conferred no additional benefit to the patient.

SELECTION OF PCA MEDICATION

The desirable pharmacologic properties of an opioid analgesic for PCA therapy include:

1. A rapid onset of analgesic action such that the patient can maintain control of their pain and does not have to wait for pain relief, or have to continually press the on-demand button;
2. High efficacy in providing pain relief. The potency of the drug is of less concern since the medication can be administered in varying size bolus doses as needed;
3. An intermediate duration of action to improve controllability;

4. Not producing tolerance or uncomfortable side effects, and
5. Having minimal side effects or adverse drug reactions.

Although the ideal PCA analgesic is not available, a wide variety of parenteral analgesics are used with PCA delivery systems. Of the many medications used in PCA therapy, morphine and meperidine were used the most extensively in clinical trials. The duration of analgesia produced by methadone and buprenorphine may be too long, whereas fentanyl and its newer analogs may be too short-acting when administered in incremental doses. However, alfentanil and sufentanil can also be effectively used as on-demand analgesics when combined with a background (or basal) infusion. Sufentanil, when given in 5 to 15 μg bolus doses, is effective in managing postoperative pain. However, the frequency of demands will be higher than with morphine, meperidine or hydromorphone due to its shorter duration of action.

The side effect profile of opioids at equianalgesic doses would be another rational basis for drug choice. Some reports have favored alfentanil because its use is alleged to be associated with less sedation than with other opioids. Recent reports by Hill and coworkers comparing morphine, alfentanil and fentanyl suggest no significant difference in depression of ventilatory drive or sedation. In another study comparing morphine and oxycodone, Sinatra et al. concluded that both agents offered similar pain relief but there was more nausea with oxycodone and more sedation with morphine. The agonist-antagonist analgesics, such as butorphanol and nalbuphine, produce "ceiling" or plateau effects with respect to both respiratory depression and analgesia. In clinical circumstances where agonist-antagonists could provide acceptable analgesia (i.e., less severe pain), these drugs may be less likely to produce clinically-significant respiratory depression than pure mu agonists. Currently, there is no one PCA opioid analgesic that is superior to the others. Until we gain better insights into PCA medication profiles, selection of the "right drug" for PCA control of postoperative pain will be made on theoretical, pharmacokinetic, economic or prejudicial grounds.

USE OF PCA THERAPY AFTER PEDIATRIC SURGERY

On-demand analgesia has been used effectively and safely in patients as young as 5 years of age, provided there is an appropriate level of nursing supervision. Compared to nurse controlled analgesia, children (>10 years old) undergoing spinal surgery were able to achieve superior pain control with a PCA delivery system. PCA has evolved into an important technique for pain control in the pediatric patient and suitable dosage regimens and monitoring procedures have been developed for these children. Recently, Irwin and colleagues reported that younger children may have difficulty activating PCA devices, especially when they are drowsy or when visual accommodation is affected by opioids. They found that children were better able to locate and activate the demand device when it was in the form of a wristwatch button worn on the palmar aspect of the wrist. However, most of the children needed initial reminders and encouragement to recognize when and how to activate the system.

USE OF PCA THERAPY FOR OBSTETRICAL ANALGESIA

Some of the earliest clinical trials with IV PCA were for the control of labor pain. In 1964, Scott described its use in laboring patients. However, PCA has not gained wide acceptance during labor despite the fact that opioid analgesia is still the most common form of pain relief offered to patients on the labor units. Compared to a continuous epidural infusion of bupivacaine, use of epidural PCA with bupivacaine was associated with improved outcome (e.g., fewer instrumented deliveries).

Several other investigators have recently evaluated PCA for labor analgesia. A major concern of obstetricians has been the potential effect of excessive systemic opioid administration, resulting in neonatal respiratory depression. Although this is a valid concern, preliminary studies have failed to document any neonatal compromise. When studies were carried out with opioid agonist-antagonists (e.g., nalbuphine and butorphanol), complete ablation of painful sensations was not possible. Systemic opioid analgesia with a PCA device is unlikely to replace epidural local anesthetic analgesia for labor pain.

OTHER APPLICATIONS OF PCA THERAPY

PCA has now expanded its uses outside the realm of acute postoperative pain. In addition to the control of cancer pain, PCA has been tried in the Intensive Care Unit (ICU). Lange and colleagues used PCA on postoperative ICU patients and concluded that PCA reduces pulmonary complications and demands on the ICU nursing staff. PCA has shown to be effective in titrating analgesia in burn patients. Recently, Gaukroger et al. published a study reporting on the successful use of PCA morphine sulfate in pediatric burn patients ranging in age from 4 to 14 years. A subsequent study of 24 adult burn patients concluded that PCA analgesia is a safer and more effective method for controlling pain in selected burn patients when compared to intermittent intravenous injections of morphine.

There have been several reports on the utilization of PCA to control the pain of sickle cell crisis. Recently, Mackie and colleagues used PCA in adolescents for the relief of pain from prolonged oropharyngeal mucositis pain following bone marrow transplantation. Another recent advance in PCA therapy is patient-controlled intraventricular analgesic administration for intractable pain syndromes. Twenty-eight patients underwent implantation of a patient-controlled device for intraventricular analgesic administration. The mean dose of morphine administered was 1.8 mg and the average duration of pain relief was 170 hours.

PCA has also been used on a limited basis for intraoperative conscious sedation and analgesia. Recently, Zelcer and colleagues utilized intraoperative PCA alfentanil for patients undergoing minor outpatient procedures associated with intermittent discomfort. This form of analgesia was comparable to physician-controlled administration of medication with respect to patient comfort and satisfaction during vaginal ovum pickup procedures. In a recent study, PCA alfentanil was successfully employed during extracorporeal shock wave lithotripsy. Using a PCA delivery system, Rudkin and colleagues found propofol to be more favorable than midazolam for intraoperative conscious sedation due to its more rapid response to fluctuating intraoperative sedation requirements, superior recovery characteristics and beneficial effects on mood. Ghouri et al. recently compared midazolam, propofol and alfentanil when administered using a PCA device for intraoperative sedation during procedures performed under local anesthesia. Midazolam produced more effective amnesia, propofol was associated with more pain on injection, and alfentanil produced more respiratory depression and postoperative nausea.

Loper et al. describe two cases in which the PCA device was utilized for the delivery of midazolam in ICU patients also receiving morphine PCA. These patients were intubated and used between 2 and 8 mg of midazolam per day for several days using this PCA technique. The patients reported less anxiety and required less ventilatory assistance. Patient acceptance of having a measure of control over their pharmacologic therapy in the ICU setting was excellent. In another double-blind, randomized, cross-over study, pain investigators concluded that PCA could be utilized to determine if a patient's pain was nociceptive *versus* neuropathic in origin. These data were useful in predicting if higher doses of opioid medication would produce improved analgesia.

In research, PCA has been used to document the morphine-sparing effects of other analgesics (e.g., ketorolac, diclofenac, nefopam, ibuprofen, and dihydrocodeine). Segal and colleagues used PCA morphine to demonstrate the morphine-sparing effect of oral-transdermal clonidine in elderly men undergoing radical prostatectomy procedures. In the first 48 hours following surgery, those receiving transdermal clonidine used between 50 and 65 mg of PCA morphine compared to 102 mg in the control (placebo) group.

THE FUTURE OF PCA

It is likely that PCA techniques and applications will continue to expand in the future. The availability of smaller on-demand devices have facilitated the use of ambulatory PCA. Very small PCA pumps have been used in clinical trials and may offer additional advantages in the future. Interchangeable microchips are now available that allow customization of the PCA program for unique patient populations (e.g., Bard PCA II device). There will likely be continued utilization of patient-controlled analgesia as long as it continues to enjoy a good safety record. However, the PCA device is only as safe and effective as the physicians and nurses who are prescribing and implementing the therapy. While PCA represents a major advance in the treatment of acute pain, its use may be associated with severe, even life-threatening complications. The efficacy and safety of the PCA depends upon proper programming of the PCA device and patients that are able to utilize the therapy in a rationale manner. User-friendly PCA devices will decrease the likelihood of operator errors. While the manufacturers assure us that their pumps are fail-safe, many more hours of patient use are required before these claims can be substantiated. Future studies with newer methods of PCA therapy need to focus on patient outcome and issues related to the cost-effectiveness of the therapy.

BIBLIOGRAPHY

1. White PF: Patient-controlled analgesia: A new approach to the management of postoperative pain. Semin Anesth 4:255-266, 1985
2. White PF: Use of patient-controlled analgesia for management of acute pain. JAMA 259:243-247, 1988
3. Urquhart ML, Klapp K, White PF: Patient controlled analgesia: A comparison of intravenous versus subcutaneous hydromorphone. Anesthesiology 69:428-432, 1988
4. White PF: Subcutaneous-PCA: An alternative to IV-PCA for postoperative pain management. Clin J Pain 6:297-300, 1990
5. Parker RK, Holtmann B, White PF: Patient-controlled analgesia. Does a concurrent opioid infusion improve pain management after surgery? JAMA 266:1947-52, 1991
6. Parker RK, Holtmann B, White PF: Effects of a nighttime opioid infusion with PCA therapy on patient comfort and analgesic requirements after abdominal hysterectomy. Anesthesiology 76:362-367, 1992
7. Parker RK, White PF: Epidural patient-controlled analgesia: An alternative to intravenous patient-controlled analgesia for pain relief after cesarean delivery. Anesth Analg 75:245-251, 1992
8. Zelcer J, White PF, Chester S, et al: Intraoperative patient-controlled analgesia: An alternative to physician administration during outpatient monitoring anesthesia care. Anesth Analg 75:41-4, 1992
9. Sawaki Y, Parker RK, White PF: Patient and nurse evaluation of patient-controlled analgesia delivery systems for postoperative pain management. J Pain Symptom Manage 7:443-453, 1992
10. Ghouri AF, Taylor E, White PF: Patient-controlled drug administration during local anesthesia: A comparison of midazolam, propofol and alfentanil. J Clin Anesth 4:476-479, 1992
11. Weldon BC, Connor M, White PF: Pediatric PCA: The role of concurrent opioid infusions and nurse-controlled analgesia. Clin J Pain 9:26-33, 1993

ORGANIZATION AND OPERATION OF AN ACUTE PAIN SERVICE

L. B. Ready

INTRODUCTION

The optimal care of surgical patients includes effective control of incisional pain. Despite advances in knowledge of pathophysiology, pharmacology of analgesics, and the development of more effective techniques for postoperative pain control, many patients do not receive adequate analgesia. The reasons for inadequate treatment are many. These include deficiencies in knowledge and skills on the parts of health care providers, patients, and those responsible for the management of health care systems, including governmental agencies. It has only recently been recognized that there are wide variations from patient to patient in the amount of pain that is experienced in response to a particular insult. There are also great differences in responsiveness to particular therapeutic approaches.

Attention is beginning to focus on in-hospital services created to improve the management of acute pain. We and others have described the development and experience of postoperative pain management services (1-15). The purpose of this presentation is to provide additional detail regarding the organizational and operational aspects of this type of service.

One of the most important and effective therapeutic modalities to become available to control postoperative pain has been epidural opioid analgesia (EOA). Unfortunately, a number of factors have limited its widespread use. These include the time required by anesthesiologists to initiate and supervise treatment, lack of structured interdisciplinary programs in hospitals to treat postoperative pain, and fear of life-threatening respiratory depression. Any program planning to offer EOA must deal with these issues.

T. H. Stanley and M. A. Ashburn (eds.), Anesthesiology and Pain Management, 143–150.

Patient-controlled analgesia (PCA) also represents a major improvement over intramuscular opioids for treating postoperative pain. The cost of PCA pumps and unfounded fears about safety are reasons why there has not been more widespread use of this technology. By optimizing pump use and development of safe protocols and procedures, an organized acute pain service can overcome these problems and can offer care in ways that benefit both patients and the institution.

ORGANIZATION

Hospital Locations Where Care Is Provided

Our initial experience with postoperative pain control was using epidural opioid analgesia (EOA) in patients following extensive thoracic surgery. These were typically patients who, because of their age and a variety of underlying medical problems, were scheduled for postoperative admission to our intensive care unit. It soon became apparent that the benefits of superior analgesia to these patients extended beyond the time that ICU care was needed. It was also clear that there were many additional patients undergoing painful surgical procedures who could benefit from postoperative EOA, but who did not require ICU admission. We, therefore, gradually expanded availability of EOA to all post-surgical wards in the hospital, preceded in all cases by the development of nursing protocols and procedures and by careful and detailed nurse training. Patient-controlled analgesia (PCA) was similarly introduced gradually to all post-surgical wards, also preceded by the development of nursing protocols and appropriate nurse training. Standard orders have been developed for use throughout our institution both for EOA and PCA. Their purpose is to provide a consistent and familiar approach to care in all areas while minimizing the risk of errors of omission or duplication in the orders.

Safety Issues

1. Monitoring: Although early reports mentioned the occurrence of sudden respiratory arrest in patients receiving EOA, all recent reports of which we are aware describe slowly increasing ventilatory insufficiency.

Our experience now exceeds 6,500 surgical patients treated with a variety of epidural opioids (some with local anesthetics added) and an additional 2,700 patients who received a single injection of epidural or subarachnoid morphine following cesarean section. In the few cases of respiratory depression we have observed, gradually increasing somnolence was a prominent feature. Our current monitoring practice relies primarily on well trained nurses who check both respiratory rate and a simple beside sedation scale hourly for the first 24 hours in all patients receiving an epidural or intrathecal opioid.

2. Order-writing: To avoid potentially dangerous duplication, it is necessary to establish that all pain-related orders, including orders for sedatives, hypnotics, and other CNS depressants, come from one source. In our case it is the Acute Pain Service. Responsibility for analgesic therapy reverts to the surgeon when patients can obtain satisfactory pain relief with oral analgesics.

3. Medical Support: Clinical rounds on all patients on the Acute Pain Service are made each morning and thereafter throughout the day as necessary. For each patient, quality of analgesia and side effects are assessed, effective opioid dose is noted, the epidural catheter site is inspected, and chart documentation of care is completed. Acute Pain Service physicians are available at all times to answer questions from ward nurses, to consult with surgeons, or to see patients who are experiencing problems with any aspect of their pain relief.

Nursing Policies and Procedures

Developing hospital-wide nursing policies and procedures helps standardize clinical practice using techniques such as EOA and PCA. Standardization promotes safety and creates a framework from which individualized patient care follows. Policies, the foundation or "ground rules" for practice, accompanied by step-wise procedures which outline the "how to" are located in manuals on each nursing unit. The polices and procedures (alternately called nursing protocols) also serve as ongoing educational and informational references.

MANPOWER AND TRAINING

Pain Management Physicians

A postoperative pain management service makes considerable demands, both administrative and clinical, on those responsible for its operation. Initial administrative duties include liaison with nursing services in the development of policies and protocols, standard orders, monitoring practice, and medical responsibility. Hospital administration must be consulted to initiate the purchase or leasing of equipment (e.g., PCA pumps). Teaching programs for ward nurses must be developed, updated as needed, and frequently offered. Mechanisms for disseminating information to surgeons and surgical patients are necessary. An educational program is also needed for the operating room anesthesiologists. In an academic department, the education of medical students, anesthesiology residents, and fellows must be planned. Appropriate research should be encouraged and supported early in the evolution of a new service.

Once a program has been established, physicians must be available to provide daily patient care and a call response capability. In a busy hospital this can easily become a full-time activity.

Operating Room Anesthesiologists

Close cooperation and communication are essential between the operating room anesthesiologist and the postoperative pain management team which assumes responsibility for analgesia when surgery is completed. Recommendations for postoperative analgesia including benefits, risks, and alternatives are best made to patients at the time of the preanesthetic visit.

Nurses

1. EOA: Ongoing education is integral to patient safety. Nursing education must precede implementation of EOA or PCA in the clinical setting. Our education program for nursing management of patients receiving EOA consists of a video program accompanied by written material and practical experience under supervision. The nurse education video is entitled *Epidural Analgesia: The Basics and Beyond.* Those interested in

more information should call the Health Sciences Center for Educational Resources, University of Washington, Seattle, WA (206) 685-1186.

2. PCA: The educational thrust for nurses when introducing PCA is the set-up and operation of PCA pumps. Most companies marketing PCA devices provide educational resources and inservice training for nursing staff. We use a videotape to assist in educating new nursing staff.

Surgeons

For reasons of patient safety, the standard orders for EOA and PCA specify that all orders for pain control and sedatives are to be given by the pain service. Responsibility for analgesic therapy reverts to the surgeon when patients can obtain satisfactory pain relief with an oral analgesic. To facilitate a smooth transition, the surgeon is asked to write oral analgesic orders immediately after surgery to become effective when EOA or PCA are discontinued.

Pharmacists

To facilitate prompt, safe care, the hospital pharmacy must become familiar with special preparations of opioids for epidural injection or infusion, and the loading and operating procedures for a number of pumps sometimes used for administering them. They can assure drug compatibility when local anesthetics and opioids are mixed and can alert physicians if they identify the possibility of adverse drug interactions. They must develop reliable stocking and dispensing procedures for opioids administered by PCA pumps. Controlled substance regulations must be followed while using these new methods of opioid administration.

ACUTE PAIN SERVICE ACTIVITY

The University of Washington Medical Center is a 430 bed referral center providing most types of surgical care. It has no pediatric beds. Figure 1 shows the annual number of patients treated by the Acute Pain Service during its first 7 years of operation. Figure 2 shows the proportion of surgical patients treated by the Acute Pain Service in a recent year. In most cases, patients having outpatient surgery or major cardiac procedures were not treated. Sources of patients treated by the Acute Pain Service are shown in Figure 3.

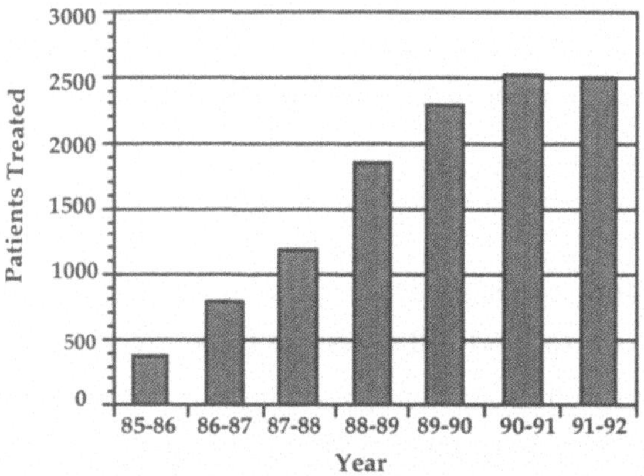

Figure 1. Total number of patients treated by the Acute Pain Service during each of its first 7 years of operation.

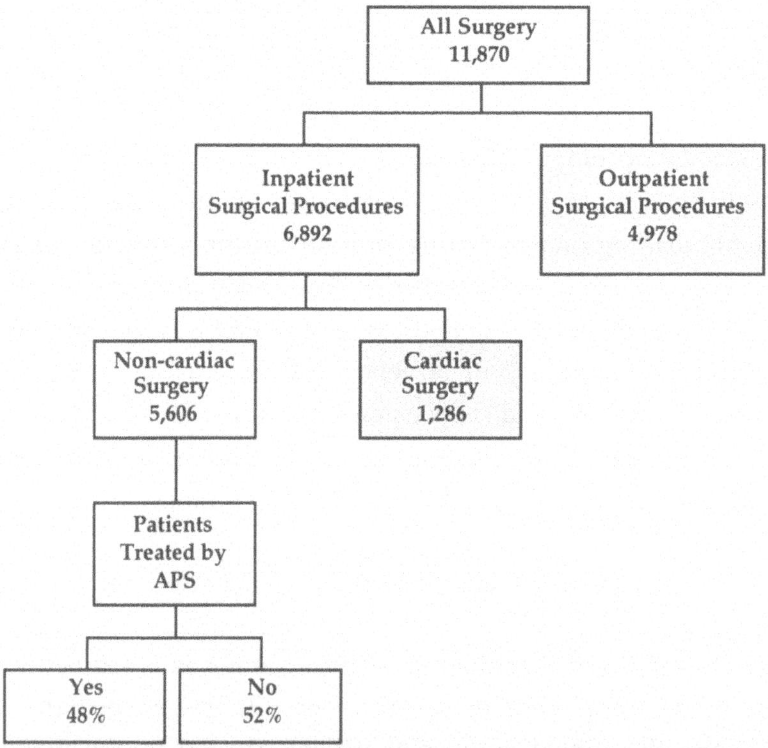

Figure 2. Proportion of all surgical patients treated by the Acute Pain Service during a typical year. In most cases, patients having outpatient surgery or major cardiac procedures were not treated.

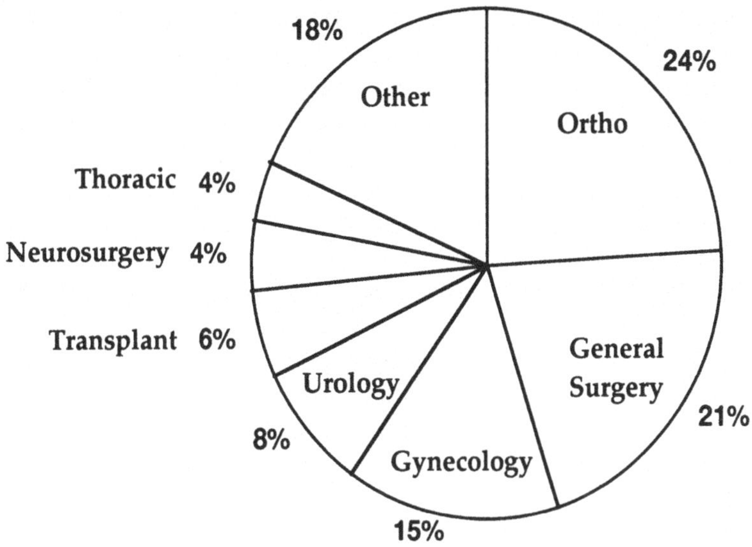

Figure 3. Sources of patients treated by the Acute Pain Service.

REFERENCES

1. Ready LB, Oden R, Chadwick HS, et al: Development of an anesthesiology-based postoperative pain management service. Anesthesiology 68:100-106, 1988
2. Ramsey DH: Perioperative pain: Establishing an analgesia service,, Problems in Anesthesia: Perioperative Analgesia. Edited by Brown DL. Philadelphia, J. B. Lippincott, 1988, pp. 321-326
3. Ready LB, Wild LM: Organization of an acute pain service: Training and manpower, Anesthesiology Clinics of North America: Postoperative Pain. Edited by Oden RV. Philadelphia, Saunders, 1989, pp. 229-239
4. Berde C, Sethna NF, Masek B, et al: Pediatric pain clinics: recommendations for their development. Pediatrician 16:94-102, 1989
5. Macintyre PE, Runciman WB, Webb RK: An acute pain service in an Australian teaching hospital: The first year. Med J Aust 153:417-421, 1990
6. Chien BB, Burke RG, Hunter DJ: An extensive experience with postoperative pain relief using postoperative fentanyl infusion. Arch Surg 126:692-695, 1991
7. Cross DA, Hunt JB: Feasibility of epidural morphine for postoperative analgesia in a small community hospital. Anesth Analg 72:765-768, 1991
8. Rawal N: Postoperativ Smärta Och Dess Behandling. Örebro: Kabi Pharmacia, 1991

9. Smith G: Pain after surgery (editorial). Br J Anaesth 67:233-234, 1991
10. Wheatley RG, Madej TH, Jackson IJ, Hunter D: The first year's experience of an acute pain service. Br J Anaesth 67:353-359, 1991
11. Domsky M, Kwartowitz J: Efficacy of subarachnoid morphine in a community hospital. Reg Anesth 17:279-282, 1992
12. Gould TH, Crosby DL, Harmer M, et al: Policy for controlling pain after surgery: Effects of sequential changes in management. Br Med J 305:1187-1193, 1992
13. Ready LB: The acute pain service. Acta Anaesthesiol Belg 43:21-27, 1992
14. Ready LB, Loper KA, Nessly M, Wild L: Postoperative epidural morphine is safe on surgical wards. Anesthesiology 75:452-456, 1991
15. Schug SA, Haridas RP: Development and organizational structure of an acute pain service in a major teaching hospital. Aust N Z J Surg 63:8-13, 1993

ROLE OF NON-OPIOID ANALGESICS IN THE PERI-OPERATIVE PERIOD

G. P. Joshi, B. Fredman, and P. F. White

INTRODUCTION

"Slapping the patient on the face and telling him or her that it's all over' is a complete inversion of the truth. As far as the patient is concerned, it is often just the beginning" (1). Although the currently available armamentarium of analgesic drugs and techniques is impressive (2), we have not fully exploited it for the benefit of patients undergoing outpatient operations (3). Management of acute postoperative pain is one of the primary responsibilities of anesthesiologists, however, it poses some unique problems following ambulatory surgery (4). The increasing number and complexity of operations being performed on an outpatient basis are presenting the practitioner with new challenges with respect to acute pain management. Outpatients undergoing day-care procedures require an analgesic technique that is effective, has minimal side effects, is intrinsically safe, and can be easily managed away from the hospital or surgery center (5).

The adequacy of postoperative pain control is one of the most important factors in determining when a patient can be safely discharged from the outpatient facility. Since inadequately treated pain is a major cause of unanticipated hospital admissions after ambulatory surgery, the ability to provide adequate pain relief by simple methods that are readily available to the day-care patient in his or her home environment is one of the major challenges for providers of outpatient surgery and anesthesia. Unfortunately, there are very few well-controlled studies that have examined the incidence and severity of pain after outpatient surgery, or the adequacy of its treatment. Even in the majority of postsurgical inpatients, parenteral opiate analgesics administered for moderate or

T. H. Stanley and M. A. Ashburn (eds.), Anesthesiology and Pain Management, 151–169.

severe pain fail to achieve adequate pain relief. Not surprisingly, inadequate analgesia is the most common surgically-related cause of unanticipated hospital admission after ambulatory surgery.

Perioperative analgesia has traditionally been provided by opioid analgesics. However, aggressive use of opioids can be associated with an increased incidence of postoperative nausea and vomiting, which may in turn contribute to a delayed discharge from the day-care facility. In order to minimize these opioid-related adverse effects, "balanced" analgesia (6) involving the use of opioid and non-opioid analgesic drugs [local anesthetics and non-steroidal anti-inflammatory drugs (NSAIDs)] is becoming increasingly popular.

In this article, the rationale for the perioperative use of local anesthetic drugs, NSAIDs and non-pharmacologic techniques will be reviewed.

Local Anesthetic Techniques

Peripheral nerve blocks and wound infiltration with local anesthetics are becoming increasingly popular adjuvants to general anesthesia because they can provide significant intraoperative and postoperative analgesia. These techniques can decrease the incidence of pain and reduce the requirements for opioid analgesics in the perioperative period. Pain relief in the early postoperative period from the residual block of the local anesthetic techniques provides for a rapid and smooth recovery, enabling earlier ambulation and discharge. Local anesthesia and effective postoperative pain control can decrease the incidence of nausea and vomiting, and thereby potentially lowering the incidence of unanticipated hospital admissions after ambulatory surgery. Struggling, crying, and restlessness can result in hematoma formation and thereby delay wound healing. Adequate pain control leads to decreased manipulation of the surgical site and thereby reduces swelling, hematoma formation, and infection (4).

Carefully controlled clinical studies are needed to identify the most efficient techniques and the most suitable local anesthetic and/or local anesthetic mixtures for peripheral blocks. Blockade of the ilioinguinal and iliohypogastric nerves with bupivacaine significantly decreases the anesthetic and analgesic requirements in children and adults undergoing inguinal herniorrhaphy (7-9). Infiltration of the ilioinguinal, iliohypogastric and genitofemoral nerves with 0.25% bupivacaine provided 6-8 hours of effective analgesia after inguinal herniorrhaphy (10). In addition, pain from a Pfannenstiel's incision can be treated with bilateral blockade of the ilioinguinal and iliohypogastric nerves (11). Although, this technique can be useful in providing analgesia from the skin and layers of the anterior abdominal wall, it does not block visceral pain.

Subcutaneous ring block of the penis with 0.25% bupivacaine effectively provides analgesia after circumcision (12). For postcircumcision pain, penile block with a mixture of 1% lidocaine and 0.25% bupivacaine is as effective as 0.25% bupivacaine alone, however, with significantly lower serum levels of bupivacaine (13). Similarly, infiltration of the mesosalpinx in the area of the Yoon ring placement, with 0.5% bupivacaine or 1% etidocaine, significantly decreases the postoperative pain and cramping after laparoscopic tubal ligation (14, 15). Pain after knee surgery has been successfully treated with femoral nerve blocks (16). However, complete anesthesia of the knee would require anesthetizing not only the femoral nerve but also the obturator, lateral femoral cutaneous, and sciatic nerves.

While subcutaneous infiltration of the operative site with local anesthetics remains a popular technique for decreasing the postoperative opioid analgesic requirement (17,18), other simplified local anesthetic delivery systems have been described in the anesthesia literature. Topical analgesia with lidocaine aerosol was found to be highly effective in decreasing pain, as well as the opioid analgesic requirement, after inguinal herniorrhaphy (19) (Figure 1). Instillation of 0.25% bupivacaine into the hernia wound provided similar postoperative pain relief as ilioinguinal/iliohypogastric nerve block in children (20). The simple application of topical lidocaine jelly, lidocaine ointment, or lidocaine spray has been shown to be as effective as nerve blocks and parenteral opioids in providing pain relief after outpatient circumcision (21,22) (Table 1). Although, pain relief was comparable with all topical techniques, children preferred lidocaine spray if repeated application was necessary. Intracavity and wound instillation of local anesthetics is another simple and effective technique for providing pain relief during the early postoperative period. Intraperitoneal administration of local anesthetics (80 ml, 0.5% lidocaine

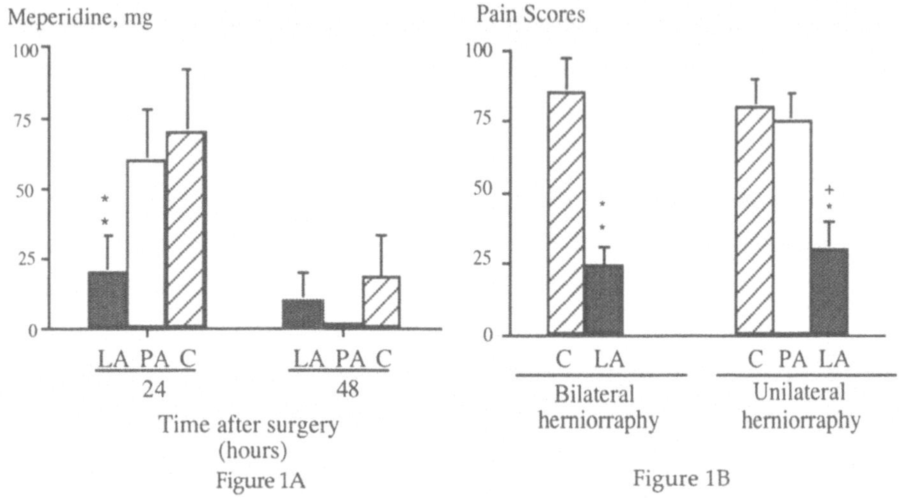

Figure 1A: Meperidine requirements in the first 24 hr after inguinal hernia repair were significantly reduced for patients treated with lidocaine aerosol (LA) in the wound, compared with patients treated with placebo aerosol (PA) or untreated control patients (C). Bars show mean requirement, whiskers demarcate SEM (**P < 0.01).

Figure 1B: 24 hr after surgery, pain scores on palpation of the herniorrhaphy wound were significantly less when treated with LA in the wound (left portion of panel). There was a significant reduction of pain scores with LA (**P<0.01). Seven patients having bilateral hernia repair (right portion of panel) were randomly assigned to treatment on one wide with LA or PA, while the other side was left untreated as a paired control. There was a significant response compared with control for LA (*P<0.05), and for LA versus PA (⁺P<0.05).

[Data from Sinclair et al. (19).]

Table 1. Comparative effects of parenteral morphine, bupivacaine nerve block, and topical lidocaine for postoperative pain relief after outpatient circumcision[a].

	Control	Morphine Sulfate (.2 mg/kg)	Nerve Block (1.0-1.5 ml)	Lidocaine Jelly (0.5-1.0 ml)
Age (yr)	5 ± 2	5±2	4±2	4 ± 2
Pain in postanesthesia care unit (%)	92	27	7[b]	5[b]
Pain-free period (h)	1.1 ± 1.0	4.8 ± 1.7[b]	5.2 ± 1.7[b]	5.3 ± 1.9[b]
Analgesic doses (n)				
0-24 h	1.9 ± 1.0	2.0±0.9	1.5 ± 1.1	1.7 ± 1.1
24-48 h	1.5 ± 1.3	0.7 ± 1.1	1.0 ± 1.1[b]	0.7 ± 1.2[b]

[a] Mean values ± SD

[b] Significant difference from the control group, p<0.05

[Data from Tree-Trakarn and Pirayavaraporn (21).]

and 0.125% bupivacaine with epinephrine) during laparoscopy was found to be an efficient method of reducing the intensity of postoperative scapular pain (23). Continuous (24,25) or intermittent perfusion (25-28) of the surgical wound with local anesthetic solutions is also an effective technique for pain control after superficial (non-cavitary) procedures. In contrast, several authors using various techniques of local anesthetic wound infiltration have failed to find significant differences in pain relief or opioid usage (29,30). The variable results may be due to differences in local anesthetic dose, timing, and concentration.

Local anesthetics are frequently injected into the knee joint to provide analgesia during arthroscopic surgery and to facilitate early recovery. Administration of bupivacaine, lidocaine, mepivacaine, or prilocaine either by single instillation or by controlled pressure-irrigation systems have been described (31-34). Although intraarticular bupivacaine, 25-40 ml, 0.25%, has been demonstrated to be a safe (35,36) and effective analgesic, the mean duration of analgesia is only 2 hours (37,38). In another study, intraarticular instillation of 30 ml of 0.5% bupivacaine reduced the opioid requirements and facilitated early mobilization after knee arthroscopy, but did not significantly decrease the patients' perception of pain (39). However, the results in the postarthroscopy model are inconsistent (40-42).

In recent years, increasing evidence has been obtained to suggest that intraarticular morphine, either alone or in combination with bupivacaine, can produce effective and long-lasting analgesia following knee arthroscopy (43-46). Combining intraarticular bupivacaine 0.5% and ketorolac 60 mg decreased pain on arrival in the PACU after arthroscopy compared to either the local anesthetic or NSAIDs alone. The combination, however, did not result in earlier discharge. Well-controlled studies are few and highly controversial (47-49).

Although local anesthetic supplementation usually decreases the severity of pain in the immediate (50) period, patients may still complain of significant pain after discharge due to difficulty in anticipating the degree of pain at the time the patient is allowed to go home (51). Thus, a limitation to a single dose of local anesthetic is duration. These situations may arise when a long-lasting local anesthetic like bupivacaine is used. Combination of local anesthetic techniques with NSAIDs may be used as a part of multimodal therapy to achieve a better pain control throughout the perioperative period. The concept of "balanced analgesia" consists of administration of agents affecting the various physiological processes involved in nociception in order to produce more effective analgesia with fewer side effects (52).

Another factor which has encouraged the increased use of local anesthetic techniques is the concept of preemptive analgesia (53,54). Prophylactic neural blockade prior to surgical incision (and other noxious perioperative stimuli) may prevent the nociceptive input from altering the excitability of the central nervous system. The application of preemptive analgesic techniques is alleged to reduce postoperative pain and skeletal muscle spasm. Preincisional infiltration of bupivacaine in combination with general anesthesia was reported to be superior to spinal anesthesia in relieving postoperative pain (55). These findings suggest that inhibition of peripheral sensitization may be important in prevention of postoperative pain. Similarly, infiltration of the tonsillar bed with bupivacaine prior to tonsillectomy is reported to decrease both constant pain and pain on swallowing for up to 5 days after surgery (56). However, only a few controlled studies have compared neural block administered before and after the surgical stimulus (57).

In conclusion, wound infiltration and peripheral nerve blocks are found to be simple, safe and effective. Availability of new local anesthetic drugs, with less toxicity and long duration, which selectively block sensory neural fibers may further increase advantages of these techniques. Increasing use of local anesthetic techniques in combination with NSAIDs and opioid analgesics can markedly enhance the safety and efficacy of analgesic drugs in the perioperative period. A multimodal approach can decrease morbidity and permit earlier ambulation and discharge after elective operations. More importantly, improved analgesic techniques will increase patient satisfaction and enhance their perception of ambulatory anesthesia and surgery.

Non-steroidal Anti-inflammatory Drugs

Oral non-steroidal anti-inflammatory drugs (NSAIDs) have long been used in medicine for their anti-inflammatory, antipyretic and analgesic properties. With the introduction of parenteral preparations of

NSAIDs, more widespread use of these drugs has been reported in the management of postoperative pain. NSAIDs block the synthesis of prostaglandins by inhibition of the enzyme cyclooxygenase (58). Prostaglandins mediate several components of the inflammatory response including fever, pain and vasodilation (59,60). In addition, NSAIDs also have prostaglandin-independent effects such as inhibition of neutrophil migration and lymphocyte responsiveness which contribute to their anti-inflammatory and analgesic properties (61).

Traditionally, the analgesic properties of NSAIDs have been attributed to their inhibitory effects on the synthesis of prostaglandins in the peripheral nerves. Inhibition of prostaglandin synthesis by NSAIDs decreases the tissue inflammatory response to surgical trauma and hence, reduces peripheral nociception and pain perception (62) (Figure 2). However, recent *in vivo* animal studies suggest that the central response to painful stimuli may also be modulated by NSAIDs inhibition of prostaglandin synthesis (63). Several recent observations support this central antinociceptor effect of the NSAIDs. Firstly, NSAIDs produce a dose-dependent depression of the rat thalamic response to peripheral nociceptor input. Secondly, they interfere with transmitters or modulators other than prostaglandins in the nociceptive system and the spinal cord (64).

Since the NSAIDs have analgesic properties comparable to opioid compounds (65-67) without opioid-related side effects (68,69), anesthesiologists often administer these drugs as adjuvants during and after surgery. When ketorolac and dezocine, a μ-receptor agonist-antagonist, were administered as adjuvants to propofol-N_2O anesthesia, both analgesic drugs were associated with improved postoperative analgesia and patient comfort when compared to fentanyl (70). However, ketorolac was associated with a lower incidence of nausea and vomiting, and patients tolerated oral fluids and were judged "fit for discharge" significantly earlier than those in the dezocine treatment group. Similarly, while ketorolac provided postoperative pain relief similar to that of fentanyl (71) it was associated with less nausea, somnolence, and an earlier return of bowel function when compared to fentanyl. Furthermore, the administration of ketorolac as an alternative to fentanyl for augmentation of local anesthesia during monitored anesthesia care resulted in significantly less

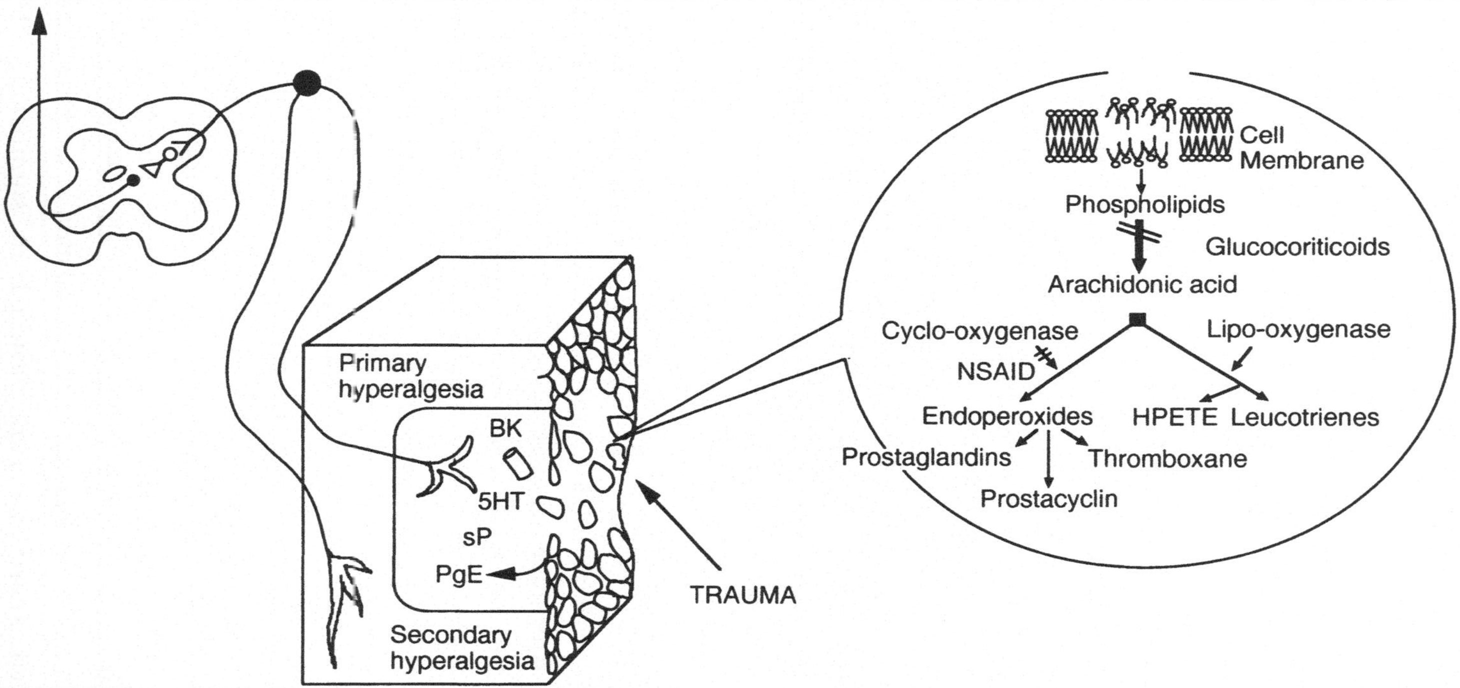

Figure 2. Tissue injury leads to release of substance P (sP) from nerve endings and release of algogenic substances (e.g., bradykinin (BK), serotonin (5HT), histamine and arachidonic cascade metabolites) resulting in vasodilatation, hyperalgesia). Secondary hyperalgesia results probably from functional changes in both the peripheral and central nervous system. Arachidonic acid can be metabolized to the prostaglandin endoperoxides (PgE) by the enzyme cyclooxygenase or to hydroperoxy derivatives (HPETE) and leucotriens by the lipoxygenase pathway. NSAIDs inhibit the biosynthesis of prostaglandins by means of an acetylation and consequent inactivation of cyclo-oxygenase.

postoperative pruritus, nausea or vomiting (72). However, when ketorolac was substituted for, or combined with fentanyl for minor gynecological procedures (73-75), it failed to significantly decrease intraoperative opioid requirements, shorten recovery times or decrease postoperative side effects. When ketorolac or saline were administered prior to induction, post-intubation, and in the Postanesthesia Care Unit (PACU) in patients undergoing laparoscopic cholecystectomy, ketorolac decreased immediate postoperative opioid requirements, but failed to influence either emetic sequelae or ventilatory function (76). These seemingly conflicting results can be explained by the timing and dose of ketorolac administered, as well as differences in surgical procedures.

Using shock wave lithotripsy to evaluate the effect of NSAIDs on visceral pain, diclofenac was administered as an adjuvant to a fentanyl-midazolam sedative technique. While diclofenac was associated with improved hemodynamic stability, only a marginal opioid-sparing effect could be demonstrated (77). Furthermore, when this drug was administered intravenously prior to outpatient arthroscopic surgery and compared to either fentanyl 1 mg/kg, IV, or placebo, diclofenac was associated with similar visual analog pain scores to fentanyl (78). However, following laparoscopic surgery, diclofenac had no effect on the recovery profile in the immediate postoperative period, but resulted in decreased pain and analgesic requirements 24 hours postoperatively (79).

Preoperative oral or rectal administration of NSAIDs is also effective in the management of postoperative pain. When oral naproxen was administered prior to laparoscopic surgery, postoperative pain scores, opioid requirements, and time to discharge were significantly shorter when compared to placebo (80). Furthermore, in the late recovery period and after discharge from the outpatient facility, oral ibuprofen (800 mg) or naproxen suppositories (500 mg), were associated with superior analgesia and less nausea compared to fentanyl, 75 μg, IV or placebo (81,82). Intraarticular injection of ketorolac produced no reduction in postoperative pain when compared to intraarticular bupivacaine (83). Similarly, there was no advantage in combining acetylsalicylic acid with local anesthetic during intravenous regional anesthesia (46).

At the extremes of age, opioid-related adverse effects may be of particular concern to the anesthesiologist. When diclofenac and acetaminophen were administered preoperatively to pediatric patients, both the preoperative incidence of restlessness and crying, as well as the postoperative meperidine requirements were lower in the diclofenac-treated patients (84). When oral ketorolac (0.9 mg/kg in juice) was compared to both acetaminophen and placebo for bilateral myringotomy procedures in children, the ketorolac-treated patients recorded lower pain scores and required less analgesia in the early postoperative period (85). Similarly, in pediatric patients, the intraoperative administration of ketorolac as an adjuvant to general anesthesia provided postoperative analgesia comparable to morphine (86). The ketorolac-treated patients experienced less postoperative nausea and vomiting. As expected, when either morphine or ketorolac were administered to pediatric patients for postoperative pain relief, ketorolac-induced analgesia developed more slowly but was more sustained than morphine (87).

In a study designed to assess postoperative pain in elderly patients following orthopedic procedures, no significant difference could be demonstrated between patients receiving intramuscular ketorolac or papaveretum followed by the oral administration of either ketorolac or a paracetamol-dextropropoxyphene combination (88).

Due to the weak analgesic properties of the NSAIDs they have limited use in the management of acute intraoperative pain. However, despite the seemingly conflicting reports in the literature, the NSAIDs are useful adjuvants in the management of postoperative pain in the ambulatory setting. Importantly, it appears that the clinical efficacy of this group of analgesic drugs depends upon the time, route of administration, as well as the surgical procedure. Finally, since the NSAIDs may be associated with less postoperative nausea, vomiting and respiratory depression when compared to the opioid analgesic drugs, their use in outpatient anesthesia will contribute not only a shorter postoperative recovery period, but may also lead to improved patient comfort and safety.

Non-pharmacologic Techniques

The use of transcutaneous electric nerve stimulation (TENS) or acupuncture-like transcutaneous electrical nerve stimulation (ALTENS) and percutaneous electrical nerve stimulation (electroacupuncture) have been described in the treatment of chronic pain. Given the inherent side effects produced by both opioid and non-opioid analgesics, as well as the local anesthetics, it is not surprising that the nonpharmacologic approaches to managing acute postoperative pain have been evaluated in the outpatient setting. The mechanisms by which TENS, ALTENS, and electroacupuncture may exert their analgesic action have not been completely elucidated. Possible mechanisms include: (i) an influence on descending pain inhibitory pathways, (ii) an inhibition of substance-P release in central nervous structures, (iii) and the release of endogenous opiate substances (89-92).

Transcutaneous electrical nerve stimulation has been reported to produce a 15-30% decrease in the postoperative opioid requirement (93). Pulmonary function was reportedly less depressed in TENS-treated patients than in a sham-treated group (94). In addition, Jensen et al. reported a more rapid recovery of joint mobility after outpatient arthroscopic surgery (95). Nevertheless, other investigative groups have reported no significant decrease in the requirement for opioid analgesic medication or improvement in the quality of postoperative pain control (96, 97). When used after superficial surgical procedures, proper application of the stimulating electrodes and proper patient instruction appear to be important factors in achieving success with TENS (98). A double-blind prospective study involving electroacupuncture and ALTENS combined with a standardized intubation general anesthesia technique for retroperitoneal lymph node resection showed a reduction of the need for opiates intraoperatively and in the early postoperative period (99). Transcutaneous electrical nerve stimulation (TENS) has been used as an adjuvant during and after minor outpatient surgical procedures. However, very few studies have documented the concomitant use of electroacupuncture and/or ALTENS with a conventional anesthetic or analgesic technique for pain relief during and after surgery. Clinical efficacy of this technique remains controversial because potential sources of bias and/or absence of blindness preclude conclusive findings. Other nonpharmacologic approaches (e.g., cryoanalgesia, ultrasound, and hypnosis) have also been evaluated as potentially useful adjuvants to opioid analgesics in the early postoperative period (100-102). For most of these modalities, clinical studies have yielded conflicting or inconclusive data (103).

SUMMARY

As more extensive and painful surgery procedures (e.g., laparoscopic cholecystectomy, laminectomy, knee reconstructions, hysterectomies) are being undertaken on an outpatient basis, availability of sophisticated postoperative analgesic regimens are necessary to optimize the benefits of day-care surgery for both the patient and the health care provider.

However, outcome studies are needed to evaluate the effect of these newer therapeutic approaches with respect to postoperative side effects, and other important recovery parameters. Recent studies suggest that factors other than pain *per se* must be controlled in order to reduce postoperative morbidity and facilitate the recovery process. Not surprisingly, the anesthetic technique can influence the analgesic requirement in the early postoperative period. Although opioid analgesics will continue to play an important role, the adjunctive use of both local anesthetic agents and non-steroidal anti-inflammatory analgesics will likely assume a greater role in the future. Use of drug combinations (e.g., opiates and local anesthetics, opiates and NSAIDs) may provide for improved analgesia with fewer opioid-induced side effects than opioid analgesics alone. Finally, safer and simpler analgesic delivery systems are needed to improve our future ability to provide cost-effective pain relief after day-care surgery.

In conclusion, as a result of our enhanced understanding of the mechanisms of acute pain and the physiologic basis of nociception, the provision of "stress free" anesthesia with minimal postoperative discomfort is now possible for most patients undergoing elective surgical procedures. The aim of an analgesic technique should not only be to lower the pain scores but also to facilitate earlier mobilization and to reduce perioperative complications. If future clinical studies clarify the issues which have been raised by experimental work in animals, clinicians may be able to effectively treat postoperative pain using combination of "balanced," "preemptive," and "peripheral" analgesia.

REFERENCES

1. Armitage EN: Postoperative pain-prevention or relief (editorial)? Br J Anaesth 63:136-138, 1989
2. White PF: Current and future trends in acute pain management. Clin J Pain 5:S51-S58, 1989
3. Wildsmith JA: Symposium on aspects of pain. Br J Anaesth 63:135, 1989
4. White P: Pain management after day-case surgery. Curr Opinion in Anesthesiol 1:70-75, 1988
5. Poler S, Zelcer J, White P: Postoperative pain management. Outpatient Anesthesia. Edited by White P. New York, Churchill-Livingstone, 1990, pp. 417-451
6. Code W: NSAIDs and balanced analgesia (editorial). Can J Anaesth 40:5,401-405, 1993
7. Cross GD, Barrett RF: Comparison of two regional techniques for postoperative analgesia in children following herniotomy and orchiopexy. Anaesthesia 42:845-849, 1987
8. Langer JC, Shandling B, Rosenberg M: Intraoperative bupivacaine during outpatient hernia repair in children: A randomized double-blind trial. J Ped Surg 22:267-270, 1987
9. Ding Y, White P: Outpatient herniorrhaphy: Use of ilioinguinal-hypogastric nerve block (IHNB) with 0.25% bupivacaine during MAC (abstract). Anesth Analg 76:S80, 1993
10. Hinkle RJ: Percutaneous inguinal blocks for the outpatient management of post-herniorrhaphy pain in children. Anesthesiology 67:411-413, 1987
11. Bunting P, McConachie I: Ilioinguinal nerve blockade for analgesia after caesarean section. Br J Anaesth 61:773-775, 1988
12. Elder P, Belman A, Hannallagh R, et al: Postcircumcision pain: A prospective evaluation of subcutaneous ring block of the penis. Reg Anesth 9:48-49, 1984
13. Sfez M, Le Mapihan Y, Mazoit X, Dreux-Boucard H: Local anesthetic serum concentrations after penile nerve block in children. Anesth Analg 71:423-426, 1990
14. Alexander CD, Wetchler BV, Thompson RE: Bupivacaine infiltration of the mesosalpinx in ambulatory surgical laparoscopic tubal sterilization. Can J Anaesth 34:362-365, 1987
15. Baram D, Smith C, Stinson S: Intraoperative etidocaine for reducing postoperative pain after laparoscopic tubal ligation. J Rep Med 35:407-410, 1990
16. Tierney E, Lewis G, Hurtig JB, et al: Femoral nerve block with bupivacaine 0.25% for postoperative analgesia after open knee surgery. Can J Anaesth 34:455-458, 1987
17. Owen H, Galloway DJ, Mitchell KG: Analgesia by wound infiltration after surgical excision of benign breast lumps. Ann R Coll Surg Engl 67:114-115, 1985

18. Moss G, Regal ME, Lichtig L: Reducing postoperative pain, narcotics, and length of hospitalization. Surgery 99:206-210, 1986
19. Sinclair R, Cassuto J, Högström S, et al: Topical anesthesia with lidocaine aerosol in the control of postoperative pain. Anesthesiology 68:895-901, 1988
20. Casey WF, Rice LJ, Hannallah RS, Broadman L, et al: A comparison between bupivacaine instillation versus ilioinguinal/iliohypogastric nerve block for postoperative analgesia following inguinal herniorrhaphy in children. Anesthesiology 72:637-639, 1990
21. Tree-Trakarn T, Pirayavaraporn S: Postoperative pain relief for circumcision in children: Comparison among morphine, nerve block, and topical analgesia. Anesthesiology 62:519-522, 1985
22. Tree-Trakarn T, Pirayavaraporn S, Lertakyamanee J: Topical analgesia for relief of post-circumcision pain. Anesthesiology 67:395-399, 1987
23. Narchi P, Benhamou D, Fernandez H: Intraperitoneal local anaesthetic for shoulder pain after day-case laparoscopy. Lancet 338:1569-1570, 1991
24. Thomas DF, Lambert WG, Williams KL: The direct perfusion of surgical wounds with local anaesthetic solution: An approach to postoperative pain? Ann R Coll Surg Engl 65:226-229, 1983
25. Gibbs P, Purushotam A, Auld C, Cuschieri RJ: Continuous wound perfusion with bupivacaine for postoperative wound pain. Br J Surg 75:923-924, 1988
26. Hashemi K, Middleton MD: Subcutaneous bupivacaine for postoperative analgesia after herniorrhaphy. Ann R Coll Surg Engl 65:38-39, 1983
27. Levack ID, Robertson GS: The direct perfusion of surgical wounds with local anaesthetic solution (letter). Ann R Coll Surg Engl 66:146, 1984
28. Levack ID, Holmes JD, Robertson GS: Abdominal wound perfusion for the relief of postoperative pain. Br J Anaesth 58:615-619, 1986
29. Cameron AE, Cross FW: Pain and mobility after inguinal herniorrhaphy: Ineffectiveness of subcutaneous bupivacaine. Br J Surg 72:68-69, 1985
30. Aull L, Woodward ER, Rout RW, Paulus DA: Analgesia and postoperative hypoxaemia after gastric partition with and without bupivacaine wound infiltration. Can J Anaesth 37:S53, 1990
31. Butterworth JF IV, Carnes RS III, Samuel MP, et al: Effect of adrenaline on plasma concentrations of bupivacaine following intra-articular injection of bupivacaine for knee arthroscopy. Br J Anaesth 65:537-539, 1990
32. Dahl MR, Dasta JF, Zuelzer W, McSweeney TD: Lidocaine local anesthesia for arthroscopic knee surgery. Anesth Analg 71:670-674, 1990
33. Hultin J, Hamberg P, Stenström A: Knee arthroscopy using local anesthesia. Arthroscopy 8:239-241, 1992

34. Wredmark T, Rolf L: Arthroscopy under local anaesthesia using controlled pressure-irrigation with prilocaine. J Bone Joint Surg: 64:583-585, 1982
35. Katz J, Kaeding CS, Hill JR, Henthorn TK: The pharmacokinetics of bupivacaine when injected intra-articularly after knee arthroscopy. Anesth Analg 67:872-875, 1988
36. Solanki DR, Enneking FK, Ivey FM, et al: Serum bupivacaine concentrations after intraarticular injection for pain relief after knee arthroscopy. Arthroscopy 8:44-47, 1992
37. Chirwa SS, MacLeod BA, Day B: Intraarticular bupivacaine (Marcaine) after arthroscopic meniscectomy: A randomized double-blind controlled study. Arthroscopy 5:33-35, 1989
38. Kaeding CC, Hill JA, Katz J, Benson L: Bupivacaine use after knee arthroscopy: Pharmacokinetics and pain control study. Arthroscopy 6:33-39, 1990
39. Smith I, Van Hemelrijck J, White P, Shively R: Effects of local anesthesia on recovery after outpatient arthroscopy. Anesth Analg 73:536-539, 1991
40. Milligan KA, Mowbray M, Mulrooney L, Standen P: Intra-articular bupivacaine for pain relief after arthroscopic surgery of the knee joint in daycase patients. Anaesthesia 43:563-564, 1988
41. Hughes DG: Intra-articular bupivacaine for pain relief in arthroscopic surgery (letter). Anaesthesia 40:821, 1985
42. Henderson RC, Campion ER, DeMasi RA, Taft TN: Postarthroscopy analgesia with bupivacaine. A prospective, randomized, blinded evaluation. Am J Sports Med 18:614-617, 1990
43. Joshi GP, McCarroll SM, Cooney CM, et al: Intra-articular morphine for pain relief after knee arthroscopy. J Bone Joint Surg 74:749-751, 1992
44. Stein C, Comisel K, Haimerl E, et al: Analgesic effect of intraarticular morphine after arthroscopic knee surgery. N Engl J Med 325:1123-1126, 1991
45. Khoury GF, Chen AC, Garland DE, Stein C: Intraarticular morphine, bupivacaine, and morphine/bupivacaine for pain control after knee videoarthroscopy. Anesthesiology 77:263-266, 1992
46. Corpataux J-B, Van Gessel E, Forster A, Gamulin Z: Does the addition of acetylsalicylic acid to local anesthetic during the Bier block improve postoperative analgesia? Anesthesiology 77:A811, 1992
47. Stein C: Peripheral mechanisms of opioid analgesia. Anesth Analg 76:182-191, 1993
48. Raja SN, Dickstein RE, Johnson CA: Comparison of postoperative analgesic effects of intraarticular bupivacaine and morphine following arthroscopic knee surgery. Anesthesiology 77:1143-1147, 1992
49. Heard SD, Edwards WT, Ferrari D, et al: Analgesic effect of intraarticular bupivacaine or morphine after arthroscopic knee

surgery: A randomized, prospective, double-blind study. Anesth Analg 74:822-826, 1992

50. Smith I, Shively RA, White PF: Effects of ketorolac and bupivacaine on recovery after outpatient arthroscopy. Anesth Analg 75:208-212, 1992
51. Meridy HW: Criteria for selection of ambulatory surgical patients and guidelines for anesthetic management: A retrospective study of 1553 cases. Anesth Analg 61:921-926, 1982
52. Dahl JB, Rosenberg J, Dirkes WE, et al: Prevention of postoperative pain by balanced analgesia. Br J Anaesth 64:518-520, 1990
53. Wall PD: The prevention of postoperative pain (editorial). Pain 33:289-290, 1988
54. Woolf CJ: Recent advances in the pathophysiology of acute pain. Br J Anaesth 63:139-146, 1989
55. Tverskoy M, Cozacov C, Ayache M, et al: Postoperative pain after inguinal herniorrhaphy with different types of anesthesia. Anesth Analg 70:29-35, 1990
56. Jebeles JA, Reilly JS, Gutierrez JF, et al: The effect of pre-incisional infiltration of tonsils with bupivacaine on the pain following tonsillectomy under general anesthesia. Pain 47:305-308, 1991
57. Dahl JB, Kehlet H: The value of pre-emptive analgesia in the treatment of postoperative pain. Br J Anaesth 70:434-439, 1993
58. Vane JR: Inhibition of prostaglandin synthesis as a mechanism of action for the aspirin-like drugs. Nature New Biol 231:232-236, 1971
59. Moncada S, Vane JR: Arachidonic acid metabolites and the interactions between platelets and blood-vessel walls. N Engl J Med 300:1142-1147, 1979
60. Trang LE: Prostaglandins and inflammation. Semin Arthritis Rheum 9:153-190, 1980
61. Abramson SB, Weissman G: The mechanisms of action of nonsteroidal anti-inflammatory drugs. Arthritis Rheum 32:1-9, 1989
62. Dahl J, Kehlet H: Non-steroidal antiinflammatory drugs: Rational for use in severe postoperative pain. Br J Anaesth 66:703-712, 1991
63. Malmberg AB, Yaksh TL: Hyperalgesia mediated by spinal glutamate or substance P receptor blocked by spinal cyclooxygenase inhibition. Science 257:1276-1278, 1992
64. Jurna I, Brune K: Central effect of the non-steroid anti-inflammatory agents, indomethacin, ibuprofen, and diclofenac, determined in C fibre-evoked activity in single neurons of the rat thalamus. Pain 41:71-80, 1990
65. Yee JP, Koshiver JE, Allbon C, et al: Comparison of intramuscular ketorolac tromethamine and morphine sulphate for analgesia of pain after major surgery. Pharmacotherapy 6:253-261, 1986
66. O'Hara DA, Fragen RJ, Kinzer MM et al: Ketorolac tromethamine as compared with morphine sulphate for the treatment of postoperative pain. Clin Pharm Ther 41:556-561, 1987

67. Powell H, Smallman JM, Morgan M: Comparison of intramuscular ketorolac and morphine in pain control after laparotomy. Anaesthesia 45:538-542, 1990
68. Murray AW, Brockway MS, Kenny GN: Comparison of the cardiorespiratory effects of ketorolac and alfentanil during propofol anesthesia. Br J Anaesth 63:601-603, 1989
69. Kenney G, Mcardle C, Aitkin H: Parenteral Ketorolac: Opiate-sparing effect and the lack of cardiorespiratory depression in the perioperative patient. Pharmacotherapy 10:127S-131S, 1990
70. Ding Y, White PF: Comparative effects of ketorolac, dezocine, and fentanyl as adjuvants during outpatient anesthesia. Anesth Analg 75:566-571, 1992
71. Wong HY, Carpenter RL, Kopacz DJ: A randomized double-blind evaluation of ketorolac tromethamine for postoperative analgesia in ambulatory surgery patients. Anesthesiology 78:6-14, 1993
72. Bosek BV, Smith DB, Cox C: Ketorolac or fentanyl to supplement local anesthesia? J Clin Anesth 4:480-483, 1992
73. Ding Y, White PF: Use of ketorolac and fentanyl during ambulatory surgery. Anesthesiology 77:A5, 1992
74. Ding Y, Fredman B, White P: Use of ketorolac and fentanyl during outpatient gynecological surgery. Anesth Analg (in press) 1993
75. Green C, Pandit S, Kothary S et al: No fentanyl sparing effect of intraoperative IV ketorolac after laparoscopic tubal ligation. Anesthesiology 77:A7, 1992
76. Liu J, Ding Y, White PF, et al: Effects of ketorolac on postoperative analgesia and ventilatory function after laparoscopic cholecystectomy. Anesth Analg 76:1061-1066, 1993
77. Fredman B, Jedeikin R, Olsfanger D, Aronheim M: The opioid-sparing effect of diclofenac sodium in outpatient extracorporeal shock wave lithotripsy (ESWL). J Clin Anesth 5:141-144, 1992
78. McLoughlin C, McKinney MS, Fee JP, et al: Diclofenac for day-care arthroscopy surgery: Comparison with a standard opioid therapy. Br J Anaesth 65:620-623, 1990
79. Gillberg LE, Harsten AS, Stahl LB: Preoperative diclofenac sodium reduces post-laparoscopy pain. Can J Anaesth 40:406-408, 1993
80. Comfort VK, Code WE, Rooney ME, Yip RW: Naproxen premedication reduces postoperative tubal ligation pain. Can J Anaesth 4:349-352, 1992
81. Rosenblum M, Weller RS, Conrad PL, et al: Ibuprofen provides longer lasting analgesia than fentanyl after laparoscopic surgery. Anesth Analg 73:255-259, 1991
82. Dueholm S, Forrest M, Hjortso E, et al: Pain relief following herniotomy: a double-blind randomized comparison between naproxen and placebo. Acta Anaesthesiol Scand 33:391-394, 1989
83. Monahan S, Johnson C, Downing J, et al: Post arthroscopy analgesia with intra-articular ketorolac. Anesthesiology 77:A854, 1992

84. Baer GA, Rorarius MG, Kolehmainen S, et al: The effect of paracetamol or diclofenac administered before operation on postoperative pain and behavior after adenoidectomy in small children. Anaesthesia 47:1078-1080, 1992
85. Watcha MF, Ramirez-Ruiz M, White PF, et al: Perioperative effects of oral ketorolac and acetaminophen in children undergoing bilateral myringotomy. Can J Anaesth 39:649-654, 1993
86. Watcha MF, Jones MB, Lagueruela RG, et al: Comparison of ketorolac and morphine as adjuvants during pediatric surgery. Anesthesiology 76:368-372, 1992
87. Maunaksela EL, Kokki H, Bullingham RE: Comparison of intravenous ketorolac with morphine for postoperative pain in children. Clin Pharmacol Ther 52:436-443, 1992
88. Smallman JM, Powell H, Ewart MC, et al: Ketorolac for postoperative analgesia in elderly patients. Anaesthesia 47:149-152, 1992
89. Takeshige C, Sato T, Mera T, et al: Descending pain inhibitory system involved in acupuncture analgesia. Brain Res Bull 29:617-634, 1992
90. Yonehara N, Sawada T, Matsuura H, Inoki R: Influence of electro-acupuncture on the release of substance P and the potential evoked by tooth pulp stimulation in the trigeminal nucleus caudalis of the rabbit. Neurosci Lett 142:53-56, 1992
91. Cheng RS, Pomeranz BH: Electroacupuncture analgesia is mediated by stereospecific opiate receptors and is reversed antagonists of type I receptors. Life Sci 26:631-638, 1980
92. Mayer D, Price D, Rafii A: Antagonism of acupuncture analgesia in man by narcotic antagonist naloxone. Brain Res 121:368-372, 1977
93. Tyler E, Caldwell C, Ghia JN: Transcutaneous electrical nerve stimulation: an alternative approach to the management of postoperative pain. Anesth Analg 61:449-456, 1982
94. Ali J, Yaffe CS, Serrette C: The effect of transcutaneous nerve stimulation on postoperative pain and pulmonary function. Surgery 89:507-512, 1981
95. Jensen JE, Conn RR, Hazelrigg G, Hewett JE: The use of transcutaneous neural stimulation and isokinetic testing in arthroscopic knee surgery. Am J Sports Med 13:27-35, 1985
96. McCallum MI, Glynn C, Moore RA, et al: Transcutaneous electrical nerve stimulation in the management of acute postoperative pain. Br J Anaesth 61:308-312, 1988
97. Smedley F, Taube M, Wastell C: Transcutaneous electrical nerve stimulation for pain relief following inguinal hernia repair: a controlled trial. Eur Surg Res 20:233, 1988
98. Cooperman AM, Hall B, Mikalacki K et al: Use of transcutaneous electrical stimulation in the control of postoperative pain. Am J Surg 133:185-187, 1977
99. Kho HG, van Egmond J, Zuang CF, et al: Acupuncture anaesthesia observations on its use for removal of thyroid adenomata and

influence on recovery and morbidity in a Chinese hospital. Anaesthesia 45:480-485, 1990

100. Khiroya RC, Davenport HT, Jones JG: Cryoanalgesia for pain after herniorrhaphy. Anaesthesia 41:73-76, 1986
101. Hashish I, Hai HK, Harvey W, et al: Reduction of postoperative pain and swelling by ultrasound treatment: A placebo effect. Pain 33:303-311, 1988
102. Houle M, McGrath PA, Moran G, Garrett OJ: The efficacy of hypnosis- and relaxation-induced analgesia on two dimensions of pain for cold pressor and electrical tooth pulp stimulation. Pain 33:241-251, 1988
103. Wood G, Lloyd JW, Bullingham RE, et al: Postoperative analgesia for day-case herniorrhaphy patients: A comparison of cryoanalgesia, paravertebral blockade and oral analgesia. Anaesthesia 36:603, 1981

EFFECT OF POSTOPERATIVE PAIN ON SURGICAL OUTCOME

H. Kehlet

Postoperative pain relief has two practical aims. The first is provision of subjective comfort, which is desirable for humanitarian reasons. The second is inhibition of trauma-induced nociceptive impulses to blunt autonomic and somatic reflex responses to pain, and to enhance subsequent restoration of function by allowing the patient to breathe, cough and move more easily. Subsequently, it has been assumed that these effects may reduce pulmonary, cardiovascular, thromboembolic and other complications and improve all-over postoperative outcome. However, the effects of nociceptive blockade and pain relief on postoperative morbidity are still debatable, despite the fact that pain relief with epidural or spinal local anesthetics has a pronounced inhibitory effect on the surgical stress response in lower body operations, but less so in upper body procedures (1-3).

Based upon the published randomized, controlled clinical trials, epidural or spinal anesthesia has been demonstrated to reduce intraoperative blood loss by about 30% in most lower body procedures (3,4). In addition, it has been shown to reduce thromboembolic complications by about 30-50% after hip and knee replacement and prostatectomy (3-5) and the risk of graft thrombosis after vascular surgery (6). Unfortunately, most thrombosis studies have included a control group not receiving appropriate antithrombotic prophylaxis; therefore, further studies are needed on this point.

It is well established that regional anesthesia with local anesthetics may improve postoperative pulmonary function. Cumulated data suggest a reduction in pulmonary infectious complications of about 40% in lower body procedures (3,4), but much less so in upper body procedures (3,4,6-9). The effect of pain relief and regional anesthesia on postoperative cardiac

T. H. Stanley and M. A. Ashburn (eds.), Anesthesiology and Pain Management, 171–175.

complications is debatable due to an insufficient amount of data. However, it is clear that a single dose of intraoperative epidural analgesia will have no positive effects on cardiac outcome after major procedures (7). Since continuous epidural analgesia with subsequent reduction of sympathetic cardiac stimulation and prevention of the increase in postoperative cardiac work should be beneficial, further studies are needed.

Regional anesthesia has no documented advantageous effects on postoperative mental dysfunction (3,4). In addition, there seems to be no documented evidence for positive effects on all-over postoperative changes in immune function and risk of infectious complications (3,4). Regional anesthesia with local anesthetics improves postoperative ileus (3,4), an advantageous effect which could be somewhat lost by combined treatment with epidural opioids. However, to date, limited studies suggest an improvement of postoperative ileus by combined epidural local anesthetic-opioid treatment (3,8,9).

The effect of spinal or epidural regimens on mortality has not been settled, but cumulated data from the high-risk group of patients undergoing acute surgery for hip fracture suggest a significant reduction in postoperative mortality (3,5), probably due to reduction of thromboembolic, pulmonary and cardiac complications.

Summarizing, the positive effects of neural blockade with local anesthetics have predominantly been observed in operations in the lower part of the body, where, incidentally, the technique is also the most effective to reduce the surgical stress response (1-3). In contrast, most controlled studies during upper abdominal and thoracic procedures have not been able to document similar important effects on all-over morbidity (3,4,6-16).

Postoperative pain relief by PCA opioid treatment has probably no major effect on postoperative outcome, based upon four randomized trials (17-20). In contrast, one study demonstrated improved outcome with high-dose opioid administered intra- and postoperatively in high risk neonates undergoing cardiac surgery (21).

Summarizing, and based upon the existing data from controlled trials, effective postoperative analgesia may not be followed by major improvements in postoperative outcome. The explanation hereto is most probably that the achieved pain relief has not been utilized to enhance mobilization and oral nutritional intake. Furthermore, most of the available studies have used suboptimal analgesic techniques and not taken advantage of the pronounced pain relief offered with multi-modal pain therapy (22).

Preliminary data from our group have demonstrated a major improvement in postoperative morbidity and reduction of hospital stay, following hip replacement (23) and after major colonic surgery (24), by a combined approach with enforced preoperative patient information, optimal pain relief with multi-modal pain therapy, enforced postoperative exercise and mobilization and early enteral nutrition. This combined approach incorporating team-work between the patient, the surgical nurse, the surgeon, and the anesthesiologist, represents an expansion of the conventional "acute pain service" in order to fully utilize the pain free state.

Our preliminary observations suggest such an approach, probably in the setting of a "postoperative rehabilitation unit," may lead to major improvements in all-over postoperative outcome (25).

REFERENCES

1. Kehlet H: Modification of responses to surgery by neural blockade: Clinical implications, Neural Blockade in Clinical Anesthesia and Management of Pain. Edited by Cousins MJ, Bridenbaugh PO. Philadelphia, J.B. Lippincott, 1988, pp. 145-190
2. Kehlet H: Surgical stress: The role of pain and analgesia. Br J Anaesth 63:189-195, 1989
3. Kehlet H: General vs. regional anesthesia, Principles and Practice of Anesthesiology. Edited by Rogers M, Tinker J, Covino B, Longnecker DE. St. Louis, C.V. Mosby, 1993, pp. 1218-1234
4. Scott NB, Kehlet H: Regional anaesthesia and surgical morbidity. Br J Surg 75:299-304, 1988
5. Sorenson RM, Pace NL: Anesthetic techniques during surgical repair of femoral neck fractures. A meta-analysis. Anesthesiology 77:1095-1104, 1992
6. Tuman KJ, McCarthy RJ, March RJ, et al: Effects of epidural anesthesia and analgesia on coagulation and outcome after major vascular surgery. Anesth Analg 73:696-704, 1991
7. Baron J-F, Bertrand M, Barré E, et al: Combined epidural and general anesthesia versus general anesthesia for abdominal aortic surgery. Anesthesiology 75:611-618, 1991

8. Seeling W, Bruckmooser K-P, Hüfner C, et al: Continuous thoracic epidural analgesia does not diminish postoperative complications after abdominal surgery in patients at risk. Anaesthesist 39:33-40, 1990
9. Jayr C, Thomas H, Rey A, et al: Postoperative pulmonary complications. Epidural analgesia using bupivacaine and opioids versus parenteral opioids. Anesthesiology 78:666-676, 1993
10. Rawal N, Sjöstrand U, Christofferson E, et al: Comparison of intramuscular and epidural morphine for postoperative analgesia in the grossly obese: Influence on postoperative ambulation and pulmonary function. Anesth Analg 63:583-592, 1984
11. Yeager MP, Glass DD, Neff RK, Brinck-Johnsen T: Epidural anesthesia and analgesia in high-risk surgical patients. Anesthesiology 66:729-736, 1987
12. Hjortsø N-C, Neumann P, Frøsig F, et al: A controlled study on the effect of epidural analgesia with local anaesthetics and morphine on morbidity after abdominal surgery. Acta Anaesthesiol Scand 29:790-796, 1985
13. Hendolin H, Lahtinen J, Lansimies E, et al: The effect of thoracic epidural analgesia on respiratory function after cholecystectomy. Acta Anaesthesiol Scand 31:645-651, 1987
14. Ryan P, Schweitzer SA, Woods RJ: Effect of epidural and general anesthesia compared with general anaesthesia alone in large bowel anastomoses. A prospective study. Eur J Surg 158:45-49, 1992
15. Jayr C, Mollié A, Bourgain JL, et al: Postoperative pulmonary complications: General anesthesia with postoperative parenteral morphine compared with epidural analgesia. Surgery 104:57-63, 1988
16. Bredtmann RD, Herden HN, Teichmann W, et al: Epidural analgesia in colonic surgery: Results of a randomized prospective study. Br J Surg 77:638-642, 1990
17. Egbert AM, Parks LH, Short LM, Burnett ML: Randomized trial of postoperative patient-controlled analgesia vs intramuscular narcotics in frail elderly men. Arch Intern Med 150:1897-1903, 1990
18. Jackson D: A study of pain management: Patient-controlled analgesia versus intramuscular analgesia. J Intraven Nurs 12:42-51, 1989
19. Kenady DE, Wilson JF, Schwartz RW, et al: A randomized comparison of patient-controlled versus standard analgesic requirements in patients undergoing cholecystectomy. Surg Gynecol Obstet 154:1495-1499, 1992
20. Wasylak TJ, Abbott FV, English MJ, Jeans M-E: Reduction of postoperative morbidity following patient-controlled morphine. Can J Anaesth 37:726-731, 1990
21. Anand KJ, Hickey PR: Halothane-morphine compared with high dose sufentanil for anesthesia and postoperative analgesia in neonatal cardiac surgery. N Engl J Med 326:1-9, 1992
22. Kehlet H, Dahl JB: The value of multi-modal or balanced analgesia in postoperative pain relief. Anesth Analg 1993 (in press)

23. Møiniche S, Hansen BL, Christensen S-E, et al: Activity of patients and duration of hospitalization following hip replacement with balanced treatment of pain and early mobilization. Ugeskr Læger 154:1495-1499, 1992
24. Møiniche S, Bülow S, Hesselfeldt P, et al: Convalescense and hospital stay after colonic surgery during balanced analgesia, enforced oral feeding and mobilization. Br J Surg (submitted)
25. Kehlet H: Postoperative pain relief—A look from the other side. Reg Anesth 1994 (in press)

POSTOPERATIVE PAIN MANAGEMENT IN CHILDREN

D. C. Tyler

Postoperative pain is perhaps the most common type of pain found in hospitalized children, and in the past, reports have shown that it has been poorly treated (1-3). The renewed interest in pain management in children in the past ten years has resulted in considerable attention to the problem of postoperative pain and the rapid development of organized postoperative pain services. One assumes that these changes have resulted in better pain management for children after surgery, although data to indicate conclusively that pain management is better are not available.

In discussing the topic of postoperative pain management, two aspects of the subject are particularly important. One is the organizational and educational component of a postoperative pain program and the second is the application of pharmacologic and other techniques to the treatment of pain. In this chapter I will review organizational aspects, discuss the applied pharmacology of postoperative pain management and conclude with some remarks about financial aspects.

Many steps need to occur before a child receives appropriate treatment of acute pain following surgery. Assuming that the physician has written appropriate orders for postoperative pain therapy, the nurse must evaluate the patient and determine whether or not pain is significant enough to warrant the risks of treatment. He or she must then carry out the procedure for obtaining the medication, deliver the treatment, and record the intervention. In this process nursing judgment about the patient's pain is a major component of ongoing postoperative pain management. When one considers that there are at least three shifts of nurses per day and that the patient may have a different nurse on each day in the hospital, one can begin to recognize the importance of nurse education. This education problem is significant even in those situations

T. H. Stanley and M. A. Ashburn (eds.), Anesthesiology and Pain Management, 177–187.

where standard parenteral opioid techniques are being used, and when a new technique, such as epidural opioids, is introduced, nurse education becomes even more important. No matter how good a job the physician does, if the therapy is not carried out continuously over a 24-hour period, the patient does not receive good pain relief.

One good way to ensure good nursing education is to have a nurse whose job it is to educate other nurses. Physicians and nurses are trained differently and as a result think differently. Nurses generally are taught to follow policies and procedures. If the physicians send a patient to the ward with a few terse instructions about a new technique and with orders for how to provide further therapy, the nurse may have no understanding of the goals of therapy, the principles behind it, or the problems associated with it. Having no policy and procedure, he or she has no framework on which to base further therapy. If a nurse is assigned to ensure pain education in the hospital, many of these problems can be obviated. He or she can develop policies and procedures and implement an educational program that will review the goals of therapy, the principles behind it and the problems associated with it. Armed with this information the nurse caring for the patient can do a much better job of providing of follow-up care.

Having this pain nurse make rounds with the Pain Service ensures that problems in communication are discovered and that appropriate follow-up can occur. The nurse can facilitate communications between the nurses on the floor and the doctors making rounds to clarify issues and to answer questions.

THE NATURE OF POSTOPERATIVE PAIN

Physiologic Issues

Acute pain may seem to be a fairly simple topic compared to the complex issues compared with chronic pain, but, when one begins to examine some of the issues involved with acute pain, the whole topic becomes more complex. Both physiologic and psychological factors contribute to perception of acute pain. Physiologically, postoperative pain is more complex than the ongoing nociception seen in the operating room, and hyperalgesia has been recognized as an important component. Hyperalgesia can be manifested as decreased pain threshold, increased pain for a given stimulus, and spread of pain to uninjured tissue. The cause of postoperative hyperalgesia is a subject of much research, and efforts are being made to modify the response as indicated in the section on prevention of postoperative pain discussed below. We believe that hyperalgesia develops in children as it does in adults, although this belief has not been clearly documented in very many places. Hyperalgesia has, however, been demonstrated in newborn infants (4). Presumably the same sorts of physiologic processes occur in the postoperative period in children.

Psychological Issues

The interaction of personality with pain and the psychological issues surrounding perception of pain in children are not very well understood. Reports in the literature indicate that emotional disturbances are common in children after surgery, particularly in young pre-verbal children (5). Some of the factors that contribute to these disturbances are pain, separation from parents, and fears arising from experiences within the hospital. These disturbances make pain more difficult to measure and leave the child less able to cope with pain.

PREVENTION OF POSTOPERATIVE PAIN

Prevention of postoperative pain involves both physiologic and psychological preparation and treatments.

Physiologic Measures

Preemptive analgesia has become a topic that is discussed considerably, although the number of studies that indicate preemptive analgesia is helpful are few. Data from the laboratory indicate that a sustained noxious input into the central nervous system changes the characteristics of the nervous system and leaves it in a hyperexcitable state (6-10). These data also suggest that if opioids are used before the noxious input, a small dose can prevent the hyperexcitability, but if the spinal cord does become hyperexcitable, higher doses of opioid are required to suppress the excitability (10).

Several studies have indicated that blocking the afferent input into the nervous system prior to surgical incision results in reduced pain postoperatively (11-13). In one study a group of patients had hernia repair under general anesthesia and a second group had local infiltration of lidocaine. Patients after the local anesthetic required less opioid, had less nausea and left the hospital sooner than after general anesthesia (11). In a second group of patients with hernia, those patients who had general anesthesia plus local infiltration had less pain in the postoperative period (12).

In a group of pediatric patients undergoing tonsillectomy, preoperative infiltration of the tonsillar bed with bupivacaine resulted in less pain over several days postoperatively when compared to postoperative infiltration with bupivacaine (13). Unfortunately, this study has not been repeated and questions remain about whether the numbness caused by the local infiltration is worse than the postoperative pain, considering that opioids can be used to treat the pain.

Another possible way of preventing postoperative pain is to administer an antiinflammatory agent prior to or during surgery (14-17). Studies with the new drug ketorolac indicate that this drug may provide some benefit in terms of sparing opioid use in the postoperative period.

Psychological Measures

One important factor in preemptive analgesia is preparation of the patient. Very little information is available, however, about what types of psychological techniques can be taught to children in the preoperative period to help them cope with postoperative pain. Generally, the belief among pediatric anesthesiologists is that children cope best with threatening experiences, including pain, when they can be with their parents, since parents can provide a major support. Attempts have been made recently to change hospital procedures to reduce the separation of child from parents as much as possible. With respect to preparation, the general recommendation is that the child should be prepared by receiving a simple explanation of what will happen and why (18,19). Viewing films or experiencing a type of surgical play can be helpful to children in preparing for surgery (20), and specific materials for preparation can be useful in reducing stress and anxiety (21-23).

TREATMENT OF POSTOPERATIVE PAIN IN CHILDREN

Little needs to be said about intramuscular injection (IM). Children do not like IM injections, and the absorption of the drug is such that IM injections do not work very well (24). It is my belief that this is a technique to be reserved for situations when nothing else is possible.

With intravenous administration of opioids, it is important to recognize that individual patients may require very different doses of opioid to achieve comfort. It is also important to recognize that bolus administration will result in fluctuations of blood level and variability in pain relief. In fact, what usually happens is that the patient's condition varies between somnolence from excess opioid to pain from inadequate amounts of opioid.

If intravenous opioids are to be used as a bolus, it is important that the patient leave the recovery room comfortable. The patient should receive a loading dose of opioid titrated to the point where the patient is comfortable. We do this in the recovery room by making the anesthesiologist responsible for ensuring that the patient is comfortable before leaving the recovery room. After the loading dose, patients receive small boluses relatively frequently, but certainly no more than every 2 to 3 hours for morphine.

A good way around the problems with bolus administration is to use continuous intravenous infusion. Here again, it is important that the patient receive a loading dose, a procedure that can be carried out in the recovery room. The patient is then begun on an infusion of 10 to 20 μg/kg/hr of morphine (25). While it is clear that if the patient has inadequate pain relief he or she should receive a bolus of morphine, the need for a bolus is frequently forgotten and the infusion rate is simply turned up. The result is that several hours pass until the patient achieves comfort.

It is important to have a reliable infusion pump, preferably locked so that the patient cannot alter the rate of infusion. It is also important to have good nursing observation to be able to detect patients who begin to receive excess opioid.

Patient controlled analgesia is an alternative to intravenous administration in patients who are old enough to understand the system. Our standard age criteria include patients 10 years of age and older who are able to communicate effectively at age level. Frequently patients as young as 5 or 6 years can also use PCA, particularly after some instruction. We feel that it is important that the patient is the one who pushes the button, otherwise the safety factor of the patient falling asleep when they begin to receive too much opioid is obviated.

We usually use morphine as the starting opioid, with a dose of 0.015 mg/kg, and a lockout of 8 minutes. If analgesia is inadequate with this dose, it is increased by 50%. Side effects are treated symptomatically. Occasionally, we see a patient who has significant side effects such as nausea and vomiting and itching and who does not have good pain relief. Often changing the opioid will improve pain relief and reduce side effects. In the past, we have changed to meperidine, but we have seen several patients who have had seizures associated with the use of meperidine. Consequently, we now use hydromorphone, in a dose of about 1/5 that of morphine.

When we began with the use of PCA, patients and their parents received extensive education in the use of the technique. With time, we have evolved to a brief discussion of PCA during the preanesthetic evaluation and education by the nurses as PCA is being started.

Problems that can result during the use of PCA usually occur because of programming errors or concomitant administration of other medications that can interfere with respiration or faults the set-up of the system.

Epidural administration of opioids has achieved popularity. Our own use of epidural opioids has diminished somewhat since we began using the technique in the mid-1980's, because of problems with side effects. Urinary retention, nausea and vomiting, and itching are frequent enough that epidural opioids do not seem indicated in patients who have brief or fairly minor pain. Previously, for instance, we used epidural opioids in patients following club foot repair, but we discovered that the side effects of the epidural opioids were keeping the patients in the hospital longer than they would have been had they had parenteral opioid administration.

Specifically, we now use epidural opioids for those patients who are having major surgery and who are expected to have moderate to severe pain in the postoperative period. This group would include patients who have thoracotomy, major intraabdominal or intrapelvic surgery, or orthopedic surgery involving hip osteotomy or other major procedures. Patients who have distal peripheral orthopedic procedures are generally treated with other techniques.

The choice between lumbar or sacral placement of the epidural catheter seems to vary according to geography and the training of the people in each individual hospital. Our preference is for caudal administration in patients under 8 or 9 years of age, because the caudal is a fairly easy approach, and, for residents who are not used to doing these procedures on smaller children, it is a less technically demanding procedure than a lumbar epidural. Some are concerned that use of the caudal route can lead to contamination of the catheter with fecal material because the catheter is placed so near the rectum. In several thousand cases, however, we have not had a problem with infection, although if a catheter is grossly soiled, we do remove it. This is an infrequent occurrence.

Generally the caudal catheter is placed at the time of surgery while the child is receiving general anesthesia. Bupivacaine, 1/4%, is used for analgesia during surgery. It is my preference that the block persist into the postoperative period to allow the anesthesiologist to ensure that local anesthetic block has been achieved. Some of the most difficult problems in postoperative pain management come from patients who begin to have pain 3 hours following surgery with an epidural catheter in place. The evaluator is able to determine whether the block was effective in the first place and generally will need to use local anesthetic to re-establish a block to ensure that the catheter is, in fact, in the right place.

We still continue to use bolus morphine in a dose of 30 to 40 μg/kg (26). This dose is relatively small, but for most patients it will be effective.

If the duration of analgesia is shorter than 6 hours we will increase the dose of morphine by approximately 50%.

To try to reduce side effects we are making some use of continuous infusions of bupivacaine and fentanyl. There are no good data, however, to indicate that this technique provides better analgesia or fewer side effects than bolus morphine. We make up a solution or 1/8 or 1/16% bupivacaine with 2 μg/cc of fentanyl. This infusion is run at a rate of 0.13 cc/kg/hr, with a maximum bupivacaine infusion of 0.4 mg/kg/hr (27). We fairly religiously hold to the maximum infusion of bupivacaine based on the data presented by Berde. If an infusion of bupivacaine and fentanyl is used, it seems necessary to have the catheter near the appropriate dermatomes. Some have tried to advance a caudal catheter cephalad to try to get to the correct dermatomes, based on the experience of Bosenberg (28). This technique is unreliable, however, and I feel that a lumbar epidural approach or the use of morphine is preferable.

Monitoring of patients in the postoperative period depends on the technique used for postoperative analgesia. For patients with intravenous techniques or PCA, monitoring is by nursing observation alone. We do, however, use a pulse oximeter to monitor patients who receive epidural opioids, mainly because we are not sure if respiratory depression will occur. Our experience indicates that it is quite rare, but we continue to use the pulse oximeter as a safety factor.

ECONOMIC ASPECTS

The economic aspects of postoperative pain management depend to a large extent on the hospital and the way in which its costs are passed along to the patient, however, every hospital is different. One of the factors to be considered is the unit cost of a bolus dose of morphine. If this is high enough, then PCA becomes relatively economical for the patient. With PCA the issues are whether the patient is charged for the PCA pump and/or tubing, the cost of the opioid used, and the cost of any administration or set-up fees that are involved.

Another issue with PCA is the physician's charge. Medicare is beginning to take issue with a separate charge for PCA, feeling that this charge should be bundled in with the surgeon's fee. This problem has not yet been an issue with the PCA in children, but it may be a problem in the future. We have made the argument in our institution that it is important for one service to be responsible for all PCA's to ensure quality control and to ensure that ongoing nursing education occurs. This may be an easier argument to make in a pediatric hospital as compared to an adult hospital. I believe that there are some specific issues related to the use of PCA in children that warrant special attention.

Issues regarding finances of epidural opioids come down to charges for medication and any administration charges, depending on who does the repeat injections. For bolus administrations, we have our nurses on the floor trained to make repeat injections, so the charge for this service is lumped in with the overall nursing charge. For epidural infusions, a pump will be required and this adds to the expense, depending on the type of pump and the expenses for mixing and formulating the drugs that will be infused.

These expenses need to be weighed against the time in the hospital, and if it can be demonstrated that time in the hospital is reduced by effective pain management then the overall economic gain for the medical system is positive. These data on outcome, however, are lacking in pediatric patients and, therefore, this question cannot be answered at this time.

REFERENCES

1. Beyer JE, DeGood DE, Ashley LC, Russell GA: Patterns of postoperative analgesic use with adults and children following cardiac surgery. Pain 17:71-81, 1983
2. Mather L, Mackie J: The incidence of postoperative pain in children. Pain 15:271-282, 1983
3. Schechter NL, Allen DA, Hanson K: Status of pediatric pain control: A comparison of hospital analgesic usage in children and adults. Pediatrics 77:11-15, 1986
4. Fitzgerald M, Millard C, MacIntosh N: Hyperalgesia in premature infants (letter). Lancet 1(8580):292, 1988
5. Levy DM: Psychic trauma of operations in children. Am J Dis Child 69:7-25, 1945
6. Wall PD: The prevention of postoperative pain (editorial). Pain 33:289-290, 1988
7. Wall PD, Woolf CJ: Muscle but not cutaneous C-afferent input produces prolonged increases in the excitability of the flexion reflex in the rat. J Physiol (Lond) 356:443-458, 1984

8. Wall PD, Woolf CJ: The brief and the prolonged facilitatory effects of unmyelinated afferent input on the rat spinal cord are independently influenced by peripheral nerve section. Neuroscience 17:1199-1205, 1986
9. Woolf CJ: Evidence for a central component of post-injury pain hypersensitivity. Nature 306:686-688, 1983
10. Woolf CJ, Wall PD: Morphine-sensitive and morphine-insensitive actions of C-fibre input on the rat spinal cord. Neurosci Lett 64:221-225, 1986
11. Makuria T, Alexander-Williams J, Keighley MR: Comparison between general and local anaesthesia for repair of groin hernias. Ann R Coll Surg Engl 61:291-294, 1979
12. Tverskoy M, Cozacov C, Ayache M, et al: Postoperative pain after inguinal herniorrhaphy with different types of anesthesia. Anesth Analg 70:29-35, 1990
13. Jebeles JA, Reilly JS, Gutierrez JF, et al: The effect of pre-incisional infiltration of tonsils with bupivacaine on the pain following tonsillectomy under general anesthesia. Pain 47:305-308, 1991
14. Hiller A, Pitkänen M, Tuominen M, Rosenberg PH: Intravenous indomethacin prevents venipuncture inflammatory sequelae. Acta Anaesthesiol Scand 32:27-29, 1988
15. Pavy T, Medley C, Murphy DF: Effect of indomethacin on pain relief after thoracotomy. Br J Anaesth 65:624-627, 1990
16. Tigerstedt I, Tammisto T, Neuvonen PJ: The efficacy of intravenous indomethacin in prevention of postoperative pain. Acta Anaesthesiol Scand 35:535-540, 1991
17. Maunuksela E-L, Olkkola KT, Korpela R: Does prophylactic intravenous infusion of indomethacin improve the management of postoperative pain in children? Can J Anaesth 35:123-127, 1988
18. Jackson K: Psychologic preparation as a method of reducing the emotional trauma of anesthesia in children. Anesthesiology 12:293-300, 1951
19. Vaughan GF: Children in hospital. Lancet 1:1117-1120, 1957
20. Melamed BG, Siegel LJ: Reduction of anxiety in children facing hospitalization and surgery by use of filmed modeling. J Consult Clin Psychol 43:511-521, 1975
21. Ferguson BF: Preparing young children for hospitalization: A comparison of two methods. Pediatrics 64:656-664, 1979
22. Visintainer MA, Wolfer JA: Psychological preparation for surgical pediatric patients: The effect on children's and parents' stress responses and adjustment. Pediatrics 56:187-202, 1975
23. Wolfer JA, Visintainer MA: Prehospital psychological preparation for tonsillectomy patients: Effects of children's and parents' adjustment. Pediatrics 64:646-655, 1979
24. Austin KL, Stapleton JV, Mather LE: Multiple intramuscular injections: A major source of variability in analgesic response to meperidine. Pain 8:47-62, 1980

25. Lynn AM, Opheim KE, Tyler DC: Morphine infusion after pediatric cardiac surgery. Crit Care Med 12:863-866, 1984
26. Krane EJ, Tyler DC, Jacobson LE: The dose response of caudal morphine in children. Anesthesiology 71:48-52, 1989
27. Berde CB: Convulsions associated with pediatric regional anesthesia (editorial). Anesth Analg 75:164-166, 1992
28. Bösenberg AT, Bland BA, Schulte-Steinberg O, Downing JW: Thoracic epidural anesthesia via caudal route in infants. Anesthesiology 69:265-269, 1988

PREEMPTIVE ANALGESIA

H. Kehlet and J. B. Dahl

Experimental studies in animals have demonstrated tissue injury or noxious stimulation results in long-term functional changes in the central nervous system, with expansion of receptive fields, facilitation of flexor motor neuronal responses and decrease in the threshold of dorsal horn neurons (1-4). Experience from clinical studies following capsaicin stimulation (5,6), thermal injury (7,8), or gynecological laparotomy (9) suggests similar post-injury changes to take place in humans. Consequently, it has been suggested that surgery may lead to spinal cord hyperexcitability, which may amplify and/or prolong postoperative pain (10).

Simultaneously, most but not all experimental studies have shown the hyperexcitability of dorsal horn neurons to be eliminated or reduced if *pre*-injury (preemptive) neural blockade with local anaesthetics or opioids were administered (1,4,12,13), while similar techniques applied postinjury had less or no effect (1,4,11-13). Intrathecal NSAID reduced excitability both when applied *pre*- or *post*-injury (14).

Consequently, the importance of "preemptive analgesia" or "timing" of analgesic regimens has been suggested to be of major importance in the treatment of postoperative pain (1,10). Unfortunately, the clinical documentation of the value of "preemptive analgesia" versus the same treatment applied later in the postoperative course has been hindered by lack of well-designed studies (15,16).

So far, 11 double-blind controlled studies comparing the same analgesic treatment applied pre- versus postoperatively are available. These studies evaluated neural blockade with local anesthetics (17-22), systemic (23) or epidural opioids (24), or NSAIDs (25-27).

Overall, the results of these studies have not documented preemptive analgesia or timing of analgesic treatment to be of *major*

T. H. Stanley and M. A. Ashburn (eds.), Anesthesiology and Pain Management, 189–194.

importance in the treatment and duration of postoperative pain. However, differences in the design of these studies require a further analysis of the data.

Two studies have investigated the effect of pre- versus postoperative administration of systemic (23) or epidural opioid (24) on postoperative pain scores and opioid requirements. In both these studies, no other analgesic treatment was given. In both studies, pain scores at almost all assessments were similar between pre- and postinjury opioid treatment groups at rest (23,24), or function (23), but opioid requirements were significantly reduced by preoperative systemic opioid administration with 10 mg of morphine IV (23). The other study only showed a decrease in opioid requirements at one of several periods of assessments, without any important overall reduction of opioid requirements following preemptive epidural fentanyl treatment (24). Interestingly, preinjury systemic opioid treatment also reduced postoperative secondary hyperalgesia assessed by von Frey hair stimulation (23). In contrast, all (17,18,20-22) but one study (19) comparing pre- versus postoperative neural blockade with local anesthetic wound infiltration or epidural analgesia have not been able to demonstrate preemptive analgesia or timing of treatment to be of clinical importance. In the only positive study (19), preemptive incisional infiltration did not change postoperative pain scores, but delayed first request for additional postoperative analgesics. Since preoperative opioid administration to some degree may reduce postoperative opioid requirements (23,24), it has been argued that the studies comparing pre- versus postoperative neural blockade, but with simultaneous pre- and/or intraoperative use of opioid (17,18,20,22), are difficult to interpret because of the use of opioids. However, in one of the negative preemptive neural blockade studies (21) no additional opioid was given pre- or intraoperatively. To some extent we think this is a hypothetical discussion, since it is common clinical practice to use small pre- or intraoperative doses of opioids, and this has not in any study resulted in sufficient low pain scores during rest and movement.

Taking all the neural *pre-* versus *post*emptive studies together, timing of neural blockade apparently has no important effect on postoperative pain scores and opioid requirements, whether perioperative opioids were administered or not. The explanation for this negative finding compared to the experimental neural blockade studies may be that the applied neural blockades do not provide sufficient "preemptive analgesia". Thus, it is well documented from studies using evoked potentials that such blockades do not provide total afferent blockade (28).

The three published studies comparing pre- versus postoperative administration of NSAID (25-27) have not documented preemptive use of NSAID to be more effective than the same dose given postoperatively. This is in accordance with experimental studies (14).

Summarizing, the results of these studies, in our opinion, demonstrate that the use of preemptive analgesia in its present form has not made a major contribution to the effectiveness of postoperative pain treatment.

This conclusion is further supported by the lack of prolonged antinociceptive effects of a preburn neural blockade with lidocaine infiltration versus a postburn neural blockade in volunteers (29). The explanation to the discrepancy between most of the experimental studies and the clinical studies may be due to the difference in extent of trauma, i.e., tissue injury, since several of the experimental studies have used a minor and very transient injury (pinch, capsaicin, etc.) where the afferent input and, thereby, central sensitization disappear rapidly. In contrast, a surgical operation is characterized by continuous wound inflammation and afferent input. Thus, in a human burn model, the time course of primary and secondary hyperalgesia was parallel, suggesting that secondary hyperalgesia needs an afferent input from the periphery, and that it does not outlast the duration of the primary hyperalgesia (inflammatory) response (8). Therefore, a short-lasting preemptive analgesic regimen, by whatever technique, may not have prolonged analgesic effects due to the upcoming afferent input and subsequent neuroplastic response in the spinal cord. Interestingly, the study demonstrating significant reduction of opioid requirements within the first 24-hour postoperative period in patients given 10 mg morphine IV preoperatively, found significantly higher pain scores during movement in the preemptive group versus the postemptive group at 48 hours postoperatively (23).

The literature also contains several studies comparing pre-operative neural blockade versus no blockade (4,15,16), and most of these studies suggest improved and prolonged pain relief by the neural blockade.

Although some of these results are interesting and positive, they need to be confirmed by others, and it shall be emphasized that these studies do not document the clinical value of "preemptive analgesia" compared with the same postinjury treatment (15,16).

Summarizing, post-injury central neuroplasticity is a fascinating research area, but so far its role for decreasing the magnitude and duration of postoperative pain has not been determined. Furthermore, the hypothesis of "prevention of pain by preemptive analgesia" is interesting and fruitful for future research; but a major breakthrough with improvement of postoperative pain treatment will probably merely come from a combination of "preemptive analgesia" and multi-modal pain therapy (30) and a duration of analgesic treatment as long as an increased afferent input from the surgical wound persists during function (mobilization).

REFERENCES

1. Woolf CJ: Central mechanisms of acute pain, Proceedings of the 6th World Congress of Pain. Edited by Bond MR, Charlton JE, Woolf CJ. Amsterdam, Elsevier, 1991, pp. 25-34
2. Dubner R, Ruda MA: Activity dependent neuronal plasticity following tissue injury and inflammation. Trends Neurosci 15:96-103, 1992
3. Treede R-D, Meyer RA, Raja SN, Campbell JN. Peripheral and central mechanisms of cutaneous hyperalgesia. Prog Neurobiol 38:397-421, 1992
4. Coderre TJ, Katz J, Vaccarino AL, Melzack R: Contribution of central neuroplasticity to pathological pain: Review of clinical and experimental evidence. Pain 52:259-285, 1993
5. LaMotte RH, Shain CN, Simone DA, Tsai EF: Neurogenic hyperalgesia: Psychophysical studies of underlying mechanisms. J Neurophysiol 66:190-211, 1991
6. Kolzenburg M, Lundberg LE, Torebjork HE: Dynamic and static components of mechanical hyperalgesia in human hairy skin. Pain 51:207-219, 1992
7. Raja SN, Meyer RA, Campbell JN: Peripheral mechanisms of somatic pain. Anesthesiology 68:571-590, 1988
8. Møiniche S, Dahl JB, Kehlet H: Time course of primary and secondary hyperalgesia after heat injury to the skin. Br J Anaesth 1993 (in press)
9. Dahl JB, Erichsen CJ, Fuglsang-Frederiksen A, Kehlet H: Pain sensation and nociceptive reflex excitability in surgical patients and human volunteers. Br J Anaesth 69:117-121, 1992

10. Wall PD: The prevention of postoperative pain (editorial). Pain 33:289-290, 1988
11. Coderre TJ, Vaccarino AL, Melzack R: Central nervous system plasticity of the tonic pain response to subcutaneous formalin injection. Brain Res 535:155-158, 1990
12. Dickenson AH, Sullivan AF: Subcutaneous formalin-induced activity of dorsal horn neurones in the rat: Differential response to an intrathecal opiate administrated pre or post formalin. Pain 30:349-360, 1987
13. Katz J, Vaccarino AL, Coderre TJ, Melzack R: Injury prior to neurectomy alters the pattern of autonomy in rats. Behavioral evidence of central neural plasticity. Anesthesiology 75:876-883, 1991
14. Malmberg AB, Yaksh TL: Hyperalgesia mediated by spinal glutamate or substance P receptor blocked by spinal cyclooxygenase inhibition. Science 257:1276-1279, 1992
15. McQuay HJ: Pre-emptive analgesia. Br J Anaesth 69:1-3, 1992
16. Dahl JB, Kehlet H: The value of pre-emptive analgesia in the treatment of postoperative pain. A critical analysis. Br J Anaesth 70:434-439, 1993
17. Dahl JB, Hansen BL, Hjortsø NC, et al: Influence of timing on the effect of continuous extradural analgesia with bupivacaine and morphine after major abdominal surgery. Br J Anaesth 69:4-8, 1992
18. Dierking GW, Dahl JB, Kanstrup J, et al: The effect of pre- versus postoperative inguinal field block on postoperative pain after herniorrhaphy. Br J Anaesth 68:344-348, 1992
19. Ejlersen E, Andersen HB, Eliasen K, Mogensen T: A comparison between preincisional and postincisional lidocaine infiltration and postoperative pain. Anesth Analg 74:495-498, 1992
20. Pryle BJ, Vanner RG, Enriquez N, Reynolds F: Can pre-emptive lumbar epidural blockade reduce postoperative pain following lower abdominal surgery? Anaesthesia 48:120-123, 1993
21. Rice LJ, Pudimat MA, Hannallah RS: Timing of caudal block placement in relation to surgery does not affect duration of postoperative analgesia in paediatric ambulatory patients. Can J Anaesth 37:429-431, 1990
22. Dahl JB, Daugaard JJ, Rasmussen B, et al: The effect of preemptive epidural analgesia with morphine and bupivacaine on pain at rest and during mobilization following total knee arthroplasty. Acta Anaesthesiol Scand 1993 (in press)
23. Richmond CE, Bromley LM, Woolf CJ: Preoperative morphine pre-empts postoperative pain. Lancet 342(8863):73-76, 1993
24. Katz J, Kavanagh BP, Sandler AN, et al: Preemptive analgesia. Clinical evidence of neuroplasticity contributing to postoperative pain. Anesthesiology 77:739-746, 1992
25. Gustafsson I, Nystrom E, Quiding H: Effect of preoperative paracetamol on pain after oral surgery. Eur J Clin Pharmacol 24:63-65, 1983

26. Sisk AL, Mosley RO, Martin RP: Comparison of preoperative and postoperative diflunisal for suppression of postoperative pain. J Oral Maxillofac Surg 47:464-468, 1989
27. Murphy DF, Medley C: Preoperative indomethacin for pain relief after thoracotomy: Comparison with postoperative indomethacin. Br J Anaesth 70:298-300, 1993
28. Dahl JB, Brennum J, Arendt-Nielsen L, et al: The effect of pre- versus postinjury infiltration with lidocaine on thermal and mechanical hyperalgesia after heat injury to the skin. Pain 53:43-51, 1993
29. Lund C: Somatosensory evoked potentials in the assessment of neural blockade. Dan Med Bull 40:266-272

THE SPINAL ROUTE OF ANALGESIA: OPIOIDS AND FUTURE OPTIONS

M. J. Cousins, L. E. Mather, N. Smart, and D. White

The demonstration by Yaksh and Rudy (1) that intrathecal morphine in rats produced long-lasting, dose-dependent, and naloxone-reversible analgesia led to the first use of spinal opioids in humans by Wang et al. (2) in 1979. Within months after the publication of this study of intrathecal morphine in cancer patients, Behar et al. (3) reported the epidural use of morphine in 10 patients and Cousins et al. (4) reported epidural use of meperidine. In the latter study, it was found that the time course of analgesia correlated with that of CSF rather than plasma meperidine concentrations, thus indicating a spinal site of action.

These first reports on spinal opioids generated much enthusiasm because long-lasting analgesia was seen to be produced without effect on motor or sympathetic neuronal systems and the term "selective spinal analgesia" was coined (4). A plethora of publications supporting their clinical efficacy rapidly followed, numbering over 100 in 1981.

However, in current use, neither epidural nor subarachnoid opioids provide the panacea which early reports appeared to promise. Respiratory depression, fortunately recognized at an early stage (5-7), and other side effects, including sedation, pruritus, nausea and vomiting, and urinary retention (4,5,8-12), have limited both their safety and clinical usefulness. In the treatment of cancer pain, high doses of morphine administered epidurally or intrathecally may produce toxic side effects such as hyperalgesia and localized "convulsions," e.g., in the legs.

Spinal opioid analgesia is still in the process of clinical development and recent advances in the neurobiological and pathophysiological understanding of acute pain give insight into how the spinal route of analgesia might best be used. Non-opioid analgesic receptor mechanisms modulating pain transmission in the dorsal horn

T. H. Stanley and M. A. Ashburn (eds.), Anesthesiology and Pain Management, 195–226.

have also been demonstrated and might be expected to play an important role in prevention as well as treatment of postoperative pain in the future (Table 1).

Table 1. Receptors at the common synapse: types, locations and actions.

Receptor Site	Receptor Type	Action	Mechanism
NK Dendritic spine	δ	inhibits NK transmission	hyperpolarization (↑ K^+ efflux)
	adenosine	inhibitory	hyperpolarization (↑ K^+ efflux)
	$5HT_{IB}$	inhibitory	hyperpolarization (↑ K^+ efflux)
	$GABA_B$	inhibitory	hyperpolarization (↑ K^+ efflux)
	α_2	inhibitory	hyperpolarization (↑ K^+ efflux)
NMDA Dendritic spine	μ	inhibitory	promotes K^+ efflux
	$GABA_A$	inhibitory	promotes Cl^- influx
	adenosine	inhibitory	promotes K^+ efflux
AMPA Dendritic spine	δ	inhibitory	promotes K^+ influx
	$GABA_A$	inhibitory	promotes Cl^- influx
Presynaptic	α_2	inhibitory	↓ SP release
	K	inhibitory	
	$GABA_B$	inhibitory	
	δ	inhibitory	↓ SP release
	$5HT_3$	inhibitory	
	NK-1	excitatory	↑ EAA release
	$5HT_2$	excitatory	

Abbreviations: see text

CLINICAL FACTORS INFLUENCING EPIDURAL OPIOID ADMINISTRATION

The clinical factors influencing opioid administration are summarized in Table 2.

Table 2. Epidural opioids: Clinical factors affecting use.

Factor	Effect
1. Drug	
High hydrophilicity e.g. morphine	Slow onset Long duration Extensive dermatomal spread Late onset respiratory depression
High lipid solubility, moderate receptor affinity e.g. fentanyl, sufentanil	Rapid onset Duration only slightly longer than im No late onset respiratory depression
High lipid solubility, high receptor affinity e.g. buprenorphine, lofentanil	Rapid onset Medium to long duration No late onset respiratory depression
2. Dose	
Correlates with efficacy up to a plateau Large interindividual differences Increasing dose hastens onset, prolongs duration but increases risk of complications Suggested initial doses of morphine by lumbar epidural catheter below: Thoracic, upper abdominal surgery <65 yrs 2-5 mg >65 yrs 2-4 mg Lower abdominal, hip surgery <65 yrs 2-5 mg >65 yrs 1-3 mg Lower limb surgery <65 yrs 2 mg >65 yrs 1-2 mg Dose reduced with thoracic catheter for thoracic and upper abdominal surgery	
3. Mode Drug Delivery	
Bolus versus infusion	For morphine, infusion low dose requirements effective analgesia few side effects but no rigorous controlled study of bolus v. infusion For fentanyl no benefits demonstrated

(Continued)

Table 2. Epidural opioids: Clinical factors affecting use. (Cont.)

Factor	**Effect**
4. Volume of Injectate	Prolongs duration of Morphine, Fentanyl, Sufentanil, Quickens onset (fentanyl) no effect on quality of analgesia
5. Effect of Adrenaline	Morphine + Adr: no effect Fentanyl + Adr: below fentanyl concentrations of: 10 μg/ml, ↑ analgesia 100 μg + 1 in 400,000 Adr: no effect on 1st dose but prolonged effect of subsequent dose Sufentanil + Adr: no effect Meperidine + Adr: no effect Diamorphine + Adr: prolonged duration
6. Site of Injection	Lipophilic drugs predicted to produce more sharply segmental analgesia than morphine. No controlled study has confirmed this.
7. **Timing of Injection**	Administration prior to surgery may i ncrease efficacy

Efficacy

The administration of spinal opioids requires technical skill and is not without serious complications. Simpler techniques for postoperative pain relief exist and adequate analgesia can be produced via the traditional systemic routes.

Postoperative Pain

Ultimately, the value of spinal opioids in acute pain management will depend on proving their greater benefit over alternative methods with safety equal to or better than that for existing and recently developed dose-optimization techniques (e.g., patient controlled analgesia). Spinal opioids are capable of relieving both visceral pain, such as after abdominal or thoracic surgery (13-15), and somatic pain, such as after orthopedic surgery (16-18). Comparison of efficacy with other techniques has yielded results with outcomes which range from a finding of no difference when compared to standard parenteral analgesics, to a finding of complete pain relief in all subjects. As many of the early studies on which these results are based had no randomization or blinding and often haphazard selections of dose, their conclusions must be questioned.

Criteria for evaluating the influence of study design on the outcome of trials of spinal opioids in acute and chronic pain have been published separately (19). It is not unreasonable to conclude that the failure to demonstrate analgesic efficacy may be due to problems in study design (19). Analgesia is usually determined by a verbal report or visual analogue scale (VAS). The reliability of VAS has been documented (20), although not specifically for postoperative pain. Comparisons for clinical analgesia should, in addition, utilize outcome criteria, including patient preference, patient expectations and satisfaction, patient performance (e.g., mobilization), and pulmonary function tests.

Double-blind designs should include "crossover" and also the use of "double dummy," e.g., simultaneous epidural and IV or IM routes so that the patient always receives treatment by both routes and is unaware which route is active (21). Recent studies by Ellis et al. and Loper et al. have employed this method (22,23).

Another significant problem with study designs is the lack of data on dosage equivalence between routes. The key to comparative studies is the use of "optimally effective" regimen for the alternative routes (19). The margin of safety between the minimum effective analgesic dose and the dose associated with toxic effects requires clear definition before spinal opioids can be compared with other routes of administration. For example, there are currently no clear data about the incidence and severity of adverse respiratory effects associated with intramuscular opioids.

Spinal Opioids in Labor

When used alone, epidural opioids have been shown to produce poorer obstetric quality analgesia than local anesthetics (24). Analgesia is not achieved reliably and is of limited duration. There is also a high incidence of side effects (24).

In doses of 2 and 5 mg, epidural morphine is ineffective (25). However, 7.5 mg is often effective in the first stage of labor but not in the second stage (26). In comparison, epidural bupivacaine 0.5% was found to be effective in all patients in stages one and two (26), and 0.25% bupivacaine fully effective (27). Fentanyl (28) and meperidine (29) have been found to provide good analgesia, but it is of short duration and is inadequate for the second stage of labor (30). Epidural fentanyl 150-200 μg produced pain relief until late first stage, but severe pain was experienced thereafter (28). This is a high dose epidurally and the effects were probably produced partly by systemic action. Epidural meperidine 100 mg provides reasonable but relatively brief analgesia (160 ± 90 min) (31), while lower doses are ineffective (29,32). Again, the dose is large and there is probably additional systemic action. It would seem that the actions of meperidine do not lead to sympathetic nerve blockade and consequent hypotension. Sufentanil is reported to be effective in first stage labor in doses as low as 2.5 μg.

The combination of low-dose epidural opioid and local anesthetic can produce better analgesia in labor than either similar doses of local anesthetic or opioid used alone. There is little or no motor blockade and the parturient retains the urge to bear down at delivery. In one prospective, randomized, double-blind trial in which saline placebo infusion was compared to a continuous infusion of 0.0625% bupivacaine plus fentanyl 2 μg/ml for second stage labor pain, it was demonstrated that the local anesthetic/opioid combination produced good to excellent analgesia in 76% of mothers without increasing the rate of instrumental delivery or cesarean section (33). Another study showed a very low incidence of urinary retention requiring bladder catheterization after epidural meperidine/bupivacaine analgesia: the frequency of catheterization is known to rise with increasingly dense degrees of neural block (34).

Epidural local anesthetic/opioid combinations appear to have no unexpected adverse effects on neonatal outcome (24).

Intrathecal use of opioids in labor may be valuable in patients with cardiovascular compromise. However, in some settings this technique is used as the method of choice over epidural opioids. A small dose of morphine (0.25 mg) may be added to the subarachnoid anesthetic for cesarean section, to produce long-lasting postoperative analgesia.

Complications

Nausea and Vomiting

Nausea and vomiting are well documented side effects of spinal opioids and appear to be more common after intrathecal injection, although formal study of this point is lacking. There is a wide range of reported incidence (8-75%) after epidural administration. Stenseth et al. (35) reported that epidural morphine 4-6 mg was associated with nausea or vomiting in 34% of patients, while a similar figure (40%) was reported by Fuller et al. (36) in a retrospective study of epidural morphine for analgesia in 4800 patients after cesarean section.

It should be remembered that a 30% incidence of nausea and vomiting accompanies routine parenteral use of opioids in postoperative patients (37), and several studies have demonstrated an equal (38-40) or lower (41-43) incidence with spinal opioids as compared to systemic opioids. Lipid soluble agents such as meperidine, fentanyl and sufentanil appear to be associated with a lower incidence of vomiting than morphine (21,44,45); however, controlled data are not available.

Transdermal scopolamine 1.5 mg, IV metoclopramide, IV droperidol, and IV naloxone have all been recommended for treatment. Naloxone, 5 μg/kg/hr IV, antagonizes nausea and vomiting without diminishing analgesia (46). Ondansetron is reported to reduce the incidence of nausea and vomiting by up to 50% and may become a valuable agent for prevention and treatment of nausea and vomiting. Further studies are required to determine the severity and frequency of nausea and vomiting in comparison to other pain relief techniques and for different opioid drugs administered spinally.

Pruritus

Pruritus may be a rudimentary itch reflex with an afferent spinal arc and may be enkephalin mediated (47). Pruritus need not be confined to the segmental area of action of the opioid but also occurs around the head and neck (48). In the reported clinical series, the incidence of pruritus with epidural morphine varies from 1-100% (13,33).

Lipid soluble opioid mu-agonists such as meperidine, fentanyl and diamorphine all produce pruritus, but few comparative data are available. When meperidine, 50 mg, was used for post-cesarean section pain, Brownridge reported that 505 of 2000 patients admitted to pruritus, but only on direct questioning and in only one patient was it troublesome (49).

Urinary Retention

Urinary retention is a troublesome complication of spinal opioids and is viewed as a contraindication to their use by some surgeons in procedures such as hip replacement where bladder catheterization may result in infection. The reported incidence varies widely. In a study of morphine (6 mg), Torda and Pybus (14) found that only 1 patient of 24 required bladder catheterization while 39% of postoperative patients required bladder catheterization in another series (38). An incidence of 90% or more has been quoted in young males receiving epidural morphine (50).

Spinal morphine reduces volume-evoked micturition reflex, detrusor muscle tone and bladder capacity while urethral sphincter tone is increased. It is proposed, but not definitively proven, that these effects are due to vesicosphincter dysynergia, possibly by inhibition at a spinal level of post ganglionic nerves to the urinary bladder (37,46).

Current evidence suggests that the urodynamic effects of epidural morphine are not dose related (46). Anecdotal reports suggest that the incidence is lower following lipid soluble opioids (e.g., methadone, sufentanil, fentanyl) (51,52), but this has not undergone rigorous clinical evaluation. Treatment consists of naloxone, 0.1 mg IV, followed by in and out bladder catheterization if naloxone is ineffective (53).

CNS Effects

Dysphoria has been reported in volunteer studies (54,55) and sedation has been observed in clinical studies (50,53). Sedation is reported to be less troublesome with low doses of morphine (56), meperidine (21), or fentanyl (57). Sufentanil has a high incidence of sedation shortly after epidural administration and this has again been shown to be reduced by decreasing the dose from 75 μg to 50 μg (44).

Respiratory Depression

Respiratory depression is the "most feared" complication associated with the use of spinal opioids and has undeniably limited their clinical use (37). Although opioid administration by any route can produce respiratory depression, spinal administration of morphine poses a special problem because the onset may be delayed several hours and may not be entirely predictable.

There are two mechanisms by which opioids can be delivered to the respiratory center. Systemic uptake into the circulation and subsequent delivery to the CNS produces early respiratory depression occurring with 2 hours of drug administration. Cephalad spread of morphine in the CSF is responsible for late respiratory depression occurring beyond 6 hours. Several pharmacokinetic studies have shown hydrophilic opioids such as morphine persist in the CSF for the greatest time and undergo the greatest cephalad spread (58-61). Thus morphine is the drug most likely to be associated with late onset respiratory depression.

Incidence

The true incidence of clinically significant respiratory depression is unknown but is thought to be low (62). Several extensive studies with data on large numbers of patients are frequently cited and are summarized in Table 3. There is a large difference in the incidence of respiratory depression between various studies ranging from 0.083% to 3.1%.

The studies have made possible the identification of certain factors which predispose to respiratory depression (35,37,63,64). Elderly or debilitated patients, co-existing respiratory disease, intrathecal or thoracic epidural administration, lack of previous exposure to opioids and raised intrathoracic pressure all increase the likelihood of respiratory depression. Hydrophilic drugs (e.g., morphine), large or repeated doses, or concomitant administration of parenteral opioids have also been shown to predispose to respiratory depression.

Low risk groups may also exist. The physiological changes of pregnancy that include increased alveolar ventilation and enhanced sensitivity to CO_2 may confer some protection against respiratory depression in the obstetric population (36,64,65). Life threatening delayed respiratory depression, however, can occur in the absence of any risk factors. Jyu and Lamb (66) reported severe respiratory depression in a healthy 49-year-old male 5 hours after 2.5 mg epidural morphine while Reiz and Westberg (12) documented severe respiratory depression 4 hours after a second dose of 2 mg epidural morphine in a fit patient.

Monitoring

Clearly, the safe use of spinal opioids requires that measures be taken to detect at the earliest opportunity the appearance of respiratory depression so that appropriate treatment can be implemented promptly. Ideally, monitoring should be continuous, (to detect transient hypoxemia, hypoventilation or apnea), non-invasive and comfortable.

Respiratory depression may be indicated by a slowing of the rate of ventilation. However, intermittent monitoring of respiratory rate is a very poor indicator of hypoventilation and is an insufficient monitor on its own. Transient events occur relatively frequently and may be missed: normal rates do not exclude respiratory depression. Ready et al. (53) described a patient with a $PaCO_2$ of 95 mmHg despite a rate of 12. Similarly, Rawal and Wattwil (67) found that patients given epidural morphine after cholecystectomy had respiratory rates greater than control despite the presence of significant respiratory depression.

Ready et al. (53) have suggested the frequent recording of level of consciousness in addition to respiratory rate. Changes in respiratory pattern, reduced respiratory effort, airway obstruction, the presence of other severe side effects (e.g., vomiting) and increasing sedation are other indicators of impending severe respiratory depression. Their detection requires close surveillance by nursing staff and a sufficient number of nurses trained to detect these signs; also staff able to administer naloxone must be available. In a retrospective study of 4,800 patients who received epidural morphine for post-cesarean section pain, hourly nursing observations of respiratory rate detected respiratory depression episodes with on other respiratory sequelae in 12 patients (36).

Ready et al. have suggested criteria for determining when to use a respiratory monitor and these are based on known risk factors (52). The most effective monitor in these circumstances is probably the pulse oximeter which is simple to use and provides a constant monitor of hemoglobin saturation. Some authors assert the safe use of spinal opioids in all patients outside the obstetric environment requires pulse oximetry and apnea monitors (64). Respiratory depression occurs progressively and

Table 3. Incidence of respiratory depression following epidural morphine: large scale epidemiological studies.

Author	Sample no.	Dose (mg)	Incidence	Comments	Ref. no.
Gustafsson	6-9000	2-4	0.25-0.4%	Retrospective	16
Stenseth	1085	4-6	0.9%	Found respiratory depression more frequent after thoracic epidural In 90%, diagnosis of resp. depression on basis of bradypnea	35
Ready	623	4-5	0.6%	75% had intra-operative narcotics Poor correlation between resp. rate and degree of hypoventilation	53
Rawal	11000	4	0.09%	Retrospective	63
Reiz and Westberg	1200	2	0.083%	Small dose	12
Fuller	4880	2-5	0.25%	Obstetric population Retrospective	36
Writer	128	5	3.1%	Prospective, continual observations of respiratory rate only	65

sudden apnea is not seen. Monitoring should be directed at identifying worsening respiratory depression rather than at its end point, apnea. Nevertheless, it seems prudent that at risk patients should be nursed in a medium or critical care area (68).

Comparative Risk of Respiratory Depression with Other Routes of Administration

Stimulated by fear of respiratory arrest in patients receiving spinal opioids, respiratory depression has been vigorously investigated and widely documented. Spinal opioids have thereby earned somewhat of a reputation for respiratory depression. In contrast, IM, IV, and PCA administration is perceived as low risk and patients often have respiration monitored infrequently and intermittently. However, with the possible exception of morphine and its risk of late onset respiratory depression, spinal administration of opioids may be no more likely to produce respiratory depression than opioids administered IM, IV or by PCA.

Non-Opioid Spinal Analgesics

The spinal administration of opioids blocks synaptic transmission between nociceptive afferents and dorsal horn neurones, and segmental analgesia is produced without impairment of motor, sympathetic, or other sensory functions. These benefits must be balanced against side effects of which respiratory depression is the most worrisome.

The identification of other, non-opioid analgesic receptor systems at this site suggests that new types of analgesic drugs can be developed. Used either alone or in combination with opioids, these may be able to produce similar or superior benefits to opioids without the drawbacks. The site of action of the non-opioid drugs discussed below is shown in Table 1.

Adrenoreceptor Agents

The most extensively studied drug to date has been clonidine, an α_2 agonist which is also effective at α_1 adrenoreceptors in higher doses. Epidural clonidine has been shown to produce analgesia in animal studies (69-71) and in humans (72-75). The mechanism is postulated to be by activation of presynaptic and postsynaptic α_2 receptors which inhibit substance P release (76) and reduce dorsal horn neurone firing (77).

Conflicting reports exist as to the efficacy of clonidine in the treatment of postoperative pain. In one double-blind, placebo-controlled study, for example, epidural clonidine, 3 μg/kg, failed to show any analgesic effects in post-thoracotomy pain (78). It seems probable that lack of effect in this and some other studies was due to inadequate dosing. At doses less than 400 μg (73-75,78), clonidine appears relatively ineffective, whereas doses greater than 600 μg have been shown to be efficacious (79,80). The onset and duration of analgesia are similar to fentanyl although there is one report of prolonged analgesia (18-24 hr) (72).

Like spinal opioids, clonidine produces side effects. These include hypotension (81-83), bradycardia (84), hyperglycemia (85), reduced serum cortisol (80), and sedation (86). Hypotension is the main side effect and is probably caused by inhibition of preganglionic sympathetic nerve activity in the spinal cord. Rostral spread of clonidine in the CSF to the brain stem could conceivably produce late onset hypotension similar to late onset respiratory depression resulting from the rostral spread of opioids although this has been observed neither in animals nor humans.

Clonidine may have a "ceiling" effect at high dose limiting its action. This has been demonstrated in intravenous use and may be due to α_1 effects. Dexmedetomidine is a new α_2 adrenoreceptor agonist 10-100 times more selective for the α_2 adrenoreceptor agonist than clonidine (87). Although it has not been used spinally as yet, phase II studies are currently underway for IV use. Epidural and intrathecal use may show advantages over clonidine, particularly because of lack of α_1 effects but no clinical trials have been carried out to verify this.

Several reports show that by combining clonidine with opioids, greater analgesia can be produced than when either is used alone. $Alpha_2$ agonists significantly shift the opioid dose-response curve when they are administered intrathecally (88-91). Electrophysiological, behavioral and clinical studies have all demonstrated potentiation of opioid analgesia by clonidine. The interaction appears to occur mainly at a spinal cord level (92-95), although there are reports of central mechanisms as well. Whether such effects are additive or synergistic remains unclear. Plummer et al. (96) reported synergic effects in rats, but only in a narrow dose range of morphine and clonidine.

By acting on different receptor mechanisms which mediate the same effect (i.e., analgesia), the total dose of each drug can be reduced thereby or preventing side effects.

The optimal dose of clonidine, the preferred route of administration (bolus or infusion), and whether it should be used alone or in combination with other agents remains unanswered. At present, clonidine's clinical usefulness appears to be limited by its short duration of action and hemodynamic depression.

GABA - Receptor Agents

Midazolam inhibits EAA transmission by interacting with a receptor complex that includes a $GABA_A$ recognition site, a benzodiazepine binding site, and a chloride channel. In rats (97) and humans (98), intrathecal midazolam has produced segmental analgesia in a dose dependent manner blocked by the benzodiazepine antagonist flumazenil. Goodchild has shown that analgesia in rats is produced by an action on spinal cord benzodiazepine receptors (97). Midazolam has been used epidurally and is effective in relieving somatic but not visceral pain. Used intrathecally, small doses of midazolam have been shown to markedly potentiate the effects of morphine (99).

Baclofen

Baclofen is a $GABA_B$ agonist and produces antinociception in rats (100-103) and primates (104). $GABA_B$ receptors are present on primary afferent terminals in laminae I-IV of the dorsal horn (105) and presynaptic inhibition may account for the antinociceptive effects of baclofen (106-111).

There is also evidence for postsynaptic $GABA_B$ receptors (112) which may be coupled to potassium conductance via a G-protein (113-115), but these appear to be less important as regards baclofen's antinociceptive activity. In mice baclofen appears to inhibit SP mediated behavior but not EAA mediated behavior (116,117).

Adenosine - Receptor Agents

Several studies have demonstrated the antinociceptive effects of adenosine agonists following intrathecal administration to animals (118-

123). Adenosine receptors are classified into A1 and A2 receptors (124) and both are present in the spinal cord of rats (125). The antinociceptive effects of A1 and A2 receptor agonists can be revered with adenosine antagonists (methylxanthines) suggesting an action at adenosine receptors. Adenosine receptors are widespread in the dorsal horn and, like opioids, inhibit both EAA and SP mediated nociception. Adenosine antagonists administered spinally might therefore be expected to be powerful analgesics. One animal study suggested that selective A1 agonists, e.g., R-phenylisopropyl-adenosine (R-PIA) are potentially more useful as candidates for the future treatment of pain in humans as they produce antinociception without motor impairment, a side effect of less selective agents such as N-ethylcarboxamide-adenosine (NECA) (126).

Excitatory Amino Acid (EAA) Receptors

Ketamine is a non-competitive antagonist of the NMDA operated channel (127) and has been shown to block nociceptive excitation of dorsal horn neurones (128). NMDA transmission is central in the development of hyperalgesia, and NMDA antagonists prevent wind up, and changes in gene expression. The development of new competitive or non-competitive NMDA antagonists for spinal administration is likely to become a key issue in pain relief. Ketamine itself exerts a multiplicity of actions (129) and clinically a racemate is used. Exploration of the pharmacology of its enantiomers is indicated. Its clinical efficacy in enhancing bupivacaine when administered caudally in children has been reported (130).

Clinical studies have been done using the NMDA receptor antagonist, 3- (2-carboxypiperazin-4-yl)propyl-1-phosphonic acid (CPP), which has been shown to prevent "wind-up" in experimental animals (131,132). Intrathecal administration of CPP in a patient with neuropathic pain attenuated the pain radiating beyond the territory of the damaged nerve, however, the pain and allodynia persisted within this region of innervation (133). Like Ketamine, however, psychomimetic side effects may limit the use of CPP.

Recent animal studies have shown that activation of the metabotropic glutamate agonists, NMDA, AMPA and kainic acid, on rat dorsal horn neurons, may potentiate the excitatory actions of EAA in nociception (134,135). Although intrathecal administration of the selective antagonist for the metabotropic receptor, 2-amino-3-phosphopropionic acid, had no effect on formalin-induced pain in rat behavioral studies (136), further experimentation in animals models of clinically relevant pain states is warranted.

Opioid - Receptor Agents

It is unlikely that any of the present generation of kappa agonists will be useful in man because of limitations in analgesic effects and a high incidence of dysphoric side effects (137,138).

Damgo is a selective mu opioid agonist and blocks NMDA transmission (91).

Serotonin Receptor Agents

Ketanserin is a $5HT_2$ antagonist which blocks SP-like behavior in mice (90).

2 methyl serotonin is a selective $5HT_3$ agonist that blocks scratching and biting behavior induced by centrally administered SP and NMDA in mice (139).

Other Agents

Somatostatin exists in the CNS (140), is found in high concentrations in the dorsal horn of the spinal cord (141), and has been reported to be anti-nociceptive (142). It has been shown to produce segmental analgesia to pinprick (143) but there are major concerns about neurotoxicity. Somatostatin 1-14 administered intrathecally in animals may be neurotoxic at doses less than those which produce analgesia (144-148). The relevance of these studies to humans is unclear, but until the mechanisms of toxicity are elucidated, and the potential for neurotoxicity in humans has been excluded, somatostatin is not a candidate for spinal administration. It should be remembered that all new drugs which seek to exploit non-opioid receptor mechanisms in the dorsal horn of the spinal cord are potentially neurotoxic. Extensive and thorough studies must be undertaken in animals before application to the epidural or intrathecal space in humans.

Combination Therapy

The co-administration of two or more drugs which provide analgesia at distinct and separate sites of action potentially has many benefits and offers the prospect of a major advance in postoperative pain management. The drugs may have additive or synergistic effects resulting in improved analgesia and smaller doses of each agent can be administered so that dose related side effects are reduced.

For example, Schulze et al. (149) randomized cholecystectomy patients to receive either intermittent nicomorphine and acetaminophen on request or the combination of epidural bupivacaine and morphine plus systemic indomethacin. The latter regimen contains agents which act at three distinct sites: peripherally on cyclo-oxygenase, on the sensory axon, and in the dorsal horn. Postoperative pain at rest and during coughing as assessed by VAS was virtually abolished in this group, which contrasted with the high pain scores in the other group receiving "conventional analgesia."

In clinical practice, the most commonly used epidural combination to date is an opioid plus a local anesthetic. Local anesthetic blocks afferent input to the spinal cord and thus prevent the development of hyperexcitability. Recent evidence suggests that opioids cannot do this as effectively and are not able completely to block afferent input into the neuraxis (150).

Hypotension, high block, systemic toxicity and motor block all limit the clinical usefulness of local anesthetics for postoperative pain management but these unwanted side effects can be minimized if dilute solutions are used in low dose. Good analgesia can still be produced by the addition of opioids. Also used in low dose, the toxic effects of the mixture are less than when either agent is used alone and in higher dose.

Several investigators have reported an additive effect of epidural opioids and local anesthetics (151-155), particularly fentanyl and bupivacaine. Fentanyl, 50-150 μg, combined with bupivacaine, 0.125%, 0.25% or 0.5%, provided better analgesia than the local anesthetic alone (156-159). Even subanalgesic doses of dilute bupivacaine, 0.068%, when combined with fentanyl gave similar analgesia to 0.25% (30). Onset time to surgical anesthesia may be reduced (151,160) and the duration of analgesia prolonged (151). There may be an increase in the degree of motor block (30,161), although some investigators have not found this.

In obstetric practice, the addition of fentanyl (50-100 μg), sufentanil (20-30 μg), morphine (2 mg), alfentanil (10 μg/kg), butorphanol (2-3 mg) to bupivacaine has been found to potentiate intraoperative analgesia (162,163) with no adverse maternal or neonatal effects (163-166). One study found that the further inclusion of epinephrine produced further potentiation (167). The incidence of nausea and vomiting during surgical manipulation of the uterus is actually reduced.

In other types of surgery, low-dose opioid-dilute local anesthetic combinations have been used successfully; diamorphine (168), sufentanil (169), fentanyl (151), and morphine (170) have provided analgesia with minimal side effects related either to opioid or local anesthetic agent. For example, the use of local anesthetic/opioid combinations results in a more rapid return of bowel function than when opioid alone is used (171). This may facilitate the recovery process and perhaps contribute to a shorter hospital stay. Thus, local anesthetic/opioid combinations are clearly promising and after major surgery, continuous central nerve block with such combinations is becoming the standard by which other methods are judged. Opioids themselves have been combined to improve analgesia. Taiwo et al. (172) administered intrathecally in rats a selective delta agonist DPDPE and a selective kappa agonist U50 488H. A degree of analgesic synergy was demonstrated. In postoperative dental patients, the analgesia produced by pentazocine, a kappa agonist, but not that by morphine, a mu agonist, was potentiated by naloxone (172). This unusual effect was mediated at a site with characteristics of the delta opioid receptor. Butorphanol, a partial agonist, when combined with fentanyl has a dose-dependent effect on antinociception (173). At low doses of butorphanol (1 mg), the analgesic effect of fentanyl/50 μg was reversed. This is due to butorphanol-mediated mu receptor antagonism. At higher doses (2-3 mg) the kappa agonist effect of butorphanol predominates and analgesia is produced. Determining the most effective dose of each agent in any combination may be complex as this example demonstrates. Clearly the identification of optimal regimen for the treatment of postoperative pain will require numerous, extensive, controlled, comparative trials.

CONCLUSION

The spinal administration of opioid analgesic drugs produces powerful analgesia without motor or autonomic block. In addition, patient outcome may be improved and morbidity and mortality may be decreased when compared with other methods of pain relief.

Major regional and systemic pharmacokinetic differences between hydrophilic and lipophilic drugs result in different pharmacodynamic effects.

Fear of respiratory depression has limited the clinical use of spinal opioids but it is important to realize that administration of the same drugs by other, perhaps less effective routes, is not without hazard. Respiratory depression is related to the dose of spinal opioids (174). Adequate surveillance remains the mainstay of safe use and requires the provision of monitoring equipment and a sufficient number of nurses able reliably to identify and if necessary treat respiratory depression. Pulse oximetry is currently the best monitoring device (174). Effective liaison between physicians, nursing staff and administrators is necessary to ensure adequate training, administrative arrangements and medical backup. Nursing care protocols can improve safety by defining clearly patient management and include monitoring instructions, prescription orders and orders for the treatment of side effects. The development of continuous, non-invasive monitoring able to detect hypoxemia, severe hypoventilation and apnea remains a priority.

Recent advances in understanding of the pathophysiology of pain and the neurobiology of the synapse between primary afferent fibers and second order neurones in the dorsal horn have profound implications for the management of all types of pain.

Mu receptors are widely distributed pre- and postsynaptically and mu agonists (e.g., morphine) inhibit both EAA-NMDA and SP mediated transmission to produce analgesia. NMDA receptors are important in the development of hyperexcitability which begins with sustained activity in C-fiber afferents. Wind up, LTP and gene expression have all been shown to be modified by NMDA antagonists. Opioids too can block the effects of NMDA activation, but are known to be less effective once these changes have occurred. It now seems important not merely to interrupt nociceptive transmission at the common synapse but to prevent the development of hyperexcitability in other areas of the spinal cord. Clearly, spinal opioids should be administered early and preferably prior to noxious stimulation to maximize their effects and improve the choices of effective analgesia. Numerous other non-opioid analgesic receptor mechanisms have been identified and these offer new opportunities for pharmacological manipulation of nociceptive transmission. New drugs active at these sites await investigation and development. Used either alone or in combination with opioids, such drugs hold out the prospect of improved analgesia with fewer or no side effects. They may also be able to abolish established hyperexcitability, a property which would be very useful in the treatment of cancer pain and chronic pain. The most thoroughly investigated to date is clonidine. Other new agents, however, must not be introduced into large scale clinical trials without undergoing rigorous investigation to exclude neurotoxicity. Somatostatin 1-14, for example, has recently been withdrawn from clinical investigation for this reason.

The combination of two or more drugs with the same effect but acting at different sites looks likely to provide a major advance in the treatment of severe pain. Effects may be additive or synergistic so that the dose of each drug in the combination can be reduced to minimize side effects while analgesia is preserved or increased. Opioid-local anesthetic combinations are already in widespread use and have been shown to be of benefit. Combination therapy is however in its infancy and identification of effective regimens will require extensive clinical trials.

FUTURE DIRECTIONS

Calcium Channel Blockers

In general, the release of neuropeptides and classical transmitters involved in pain transmission requires the influx of Ca^{2+}. The route of calcium influx, however, varies depending on transmitter and stimulus (175). In many cases, the influx is via voltage dependent Ca^{2+} channels. There have been four voltage dependent Ca^{2+} channels described, termed T, N, L and P-type channels (176,177). Pharmacological agents known to block these channels are ω-conotoxin, which blocks the N- and L-type channels; dihydropyridines, which block L-type channel; and ω-agatoxin, which blocks the P-type channel. The release of substance P induced by electrical stimulation, for example, requires an influx via the N-type voltage dependent Ca^{2+} channel, since it is blocked by w-conotoxin but not by dihydropyridines (178). Recent evidence examining the release of glutamate from rat synaptosomes prepared from the frontal cortex, show that the release is ω-agatoxin-sensitive, but ω-conotoxin-insensitive (179). P-type Ca^{2+} channels are also found in DRG cells and spinal neurons where they may also be involved in transmitter release (176). Further studies are required to obtain selective, non-toxic Ca^{2+} channel blockers that can be used clinically.

Veratridine

Veratridine applied locally to the rabbit vagus nerve, preferentially inhibits electrically-evoked impulses in C- and A δ-fibers propagating centrally, with no effect on Aβ-fibers (180). Presumably, the inhibitory effect is similar to the collision phenomenon described by Iggo (1958) (181), which only occurs when there is simultaneous spontaneous or evoked activity. If this is the case, the veratridine-induced depolarization would, in turn, be inhibited by the simultaneous spontaneous or evoked activity. Therefore, in the absence of spontaneous or evoked activity, veratridine may, itself, induce pain by activating nociceptors. More work is required before this technique could be considered an effective treatment.

REFERENCES

1. Yaksh TL, Rudy TA: Analgesia mediated by a direct spinal action of narcotics. Science 192:1357-1358, 1976
2. Wang JK, Nauss LA, Thomas JE: Pain relief by intrathecally applied morphine in man. Anesthesiology 50:149-151, 1979
3. Behar M, Magora F, Olshwang D, Davidson JT: Epidural morphine in treatment of pain. Lancet 1(8115):527-529, 1979
4. Cousins MJ, Mather LE, Glynn CJ, et al: Selective spinal analgesia (letter). Lancet 1(8126):1141-1142, 1979
5. Glynn CJ, Mather LE, Cousins MJ, et al: Spinal narcotics and respiratory depression (letter). Lancet 2(8138):356-357, 1979
6. Liolios A, Andersen FH: Selective spinal analgesia (letter). Lancet 2(8138):357, 1979
7. Scott DB, McClure J: Selective epidural analgesia (letter). Lancet 1(8131):1410-1411, 1979

8. Boas RA: Hazards of epidural morphine. Anaesth Intensive Care 8:377-378, 1980
9. Cousins MJ, Glynn CJ, Wilson PR, et al: Aspects of epidural morphine (letter). Lancet 2(8142):584, 1979
10. Cousins MJ, Glynn CJ, Wilson PR, et al: Epidural morphine (letter). Anaesth Intensive Care 8:217-219, 1980
11. Davies GK, Tolhurst-Cleaver CL, James TL: Respiratory depression after intrathecal narcotics. Anaesthesia 35:1080-1083, 1980
12. Reiz S, Westberg M: Side effects of epidural morphine (letter). Lancet 2(8187):203-204, 1980
13. Bromage PR, Camporesi E, Chestnut D: Epidural narcotics for postoperative analgesia. Anesth Analg 59:473-480, 1980
14. Torda TA, Pybus DA: Extradural administration of morphine and bupivacaine. A controlled comparison. Br J Anaesth 56:141-146, 1984
15. Glynn CJ, Mather LE, Cousins MJ, et al: Peridural meperidine in humans: Analgesic response, pharmacokinetics and transmission into CSF. Anesthesiology 55:520-526, 1981
16. Gustafsson LL, Schildt B, Jacobsen K: Adverse effects of extradural and intrathecal opiates: Report of a nationwide survey in Sweden. Br J Anaesth 54:479-486, 1982
17. Ebert J, Varner PD: The effective use of epidural morphine sulfate for postoperative orthopedic pain. Anesthesiology 53:257-258, 1980
18. Barron DW, Strong JE: Postoperative analgesia in major orthopaedic surgery. Epidural and intrathecal opiates. Anaesthesia 36:937-941, 1981
19. Cousins MJ, Plummer JP: Spinal opioids in acute and chronic pain, The design of analgesic clinical trials. Advances in Pain Research and Therapy. Edited by Max M, Portenoy R, Laska E. New York, Raven Press, 1991, pp. 457-479
20. Revill SI, Robinson JO, Rosen M, Hogg MI: The reliability of a linear analogue scale for evaluating pain. Anaesthesia 31:1191-1198, 1976
21. Brownridge P, Frewin DB: A comparative study of techniques of postoperative analgesia following caesarean section and lower abdominal surgery. Anaesth Intensive Care 13:123-130, 1985
22. Ellis DJ, Millar WL, Reisner LS: A randomized double-blind comparision of epidural versus intravenous fentanyl infusion of analgesia after cesarean section. Anesthesiology 72:981-986, 1990
23. Loper KA, Ready LB, Downey M, et al: Epidural and intravenous fentanyl infusions are clinically equivalent after knee surgery. Anesth Analg 70:72-75, 1990
24. Brownridge P, Cohen SE: Neural blockade for obstetrics and gynecology surgery, Neural Blockade in Clinical Anesthesia and Management of Pain. Edited by Cousins MJ, Bridenbaugh PO. Philadelphia, J.B. Lippincott, 1988, pp. 593-634
25. Booker PD, Wilkes RG, Bryson JHL, Beddard J: Obstetric pain relief using epidural morphine. Anaesthesia 35:377-379, 1980

26. Hughes SC, Rosen MA, Shnider SM, et al: Maternal and neonatal effects of epidural morphine for labor and delivery. Anesth Analg 63:319-324, 1984
27. Writer WDR: Epidural morphine for post-caesarean analgesia (editorial). Can J Anaesth 37:608-612, 1990
28. Currie LES, O'Sullivan GM, Seegobin R: Epidural fentanyl in labour. Anaesthesia 36:965-969, 1981
29. Perriss BW: Epidural pethidine in labour. A study of dose requirements. Anaesthesia 35:380-382, 1980
30. Cohen SE, Tan S, Albright GA, Halpern J: Epidural fentanyl/bupivacaine mixtures for obstetric analgesia. Anesthesiology 67:403-407, 1987
31. Baraka A, Maktabi M, Noueihid R: Epidural meperidine-bupivacaine for obstetric analgesia. Anesth Analg 61:652-656, 1982
32. Hammonds W, Bramwell RS, Hug CC, et al: A comparison of epidural meperidine and bupivacaine for relief of labor pain. Anesth Analg 61:187-188, 1982
33. Chestnut DH, Pollack KL, Laszewski LJ, et al: Continuous epidural infusion of bupivacaine-fentanyl during the second stage of labour (abstract). Anesthesiology 71:A841, 1989
34. Brownridge P: Epidural bupivacaine-pethidine mixture: Clinical experience using a low-dose combination in labour. Aust N Z J Obstet Gynaecol 28:17-24, 1988
35. Stenseth R, Sellevold O, Breivik H: Epidural morphine for postoperative pain: Experience with 1085 patients. Acta Anaesthesiol Scand 29:148-156, 1985
36. Fuller JG, McMorland GH, Douglas MJ, Palmer L: Epidural morphine for analgesia after caesarean section: A report of 4,880 patients. Can J Anaesth 37:636-640, 1990
37. Cousins MJ, Mather LE: Intrathecal and epidural administration of opioids. Anesthesiology 61:276-310, 1984
38. Lanz E, Theiss D, Riess W, Sommer U: Epidural morphine for postoperative analgesia: A double-blind study. Anesth Analg 61:236-240, 1982
39. Harrison DM, Sinatra R, Morgese L, Chung JH: Epidural narcotic and patient-controlled analgesia for post-cesarean section pain relief. Anesthesiology 68:454-457, 1988
40. Klinck JR, Lindop MJ: Epidural morphine in the elderly. A controlled trial after upper abdominal surgery. Anaesthesia 37:907-912, 1982
41. Camann WR, Loferski BL, Fanciullo GJ, et al: Does epidural administration of butorphanol offer any clinical advantage over the intravenous route? A double-blind, placebo-controlled trial. Anesthesiology 76:216-220, 1992
42. Eisenach JC, Grice SC, Dewan DM: Patient-controlled analgesia following cesarean section: A comparison with epidural and intramuscular narcotics. Anesthesiology 68:444-448, 1988

43. Reiz S, Ahlin J, Ahrenfeld B, et al: Epidural morphine for postoperative pain relief. Acta Anaesthesiol Scand 25:111-114, 1981
44. Donadoni R, Rolly G, Noorduin H, et al: Epidural sufentanil for postoperative pain relief. Anaesthesia 40:634-638, 1985
45. Wells DG, Davies G: Profound central nervous system depression from epidural fentanyl for extracorporeal shock wave lithotripsy. Anesthesiology 67:991-992, 1987
46. Rawal N, Möllefors K, Axelsson K, et al: An experimental study of urodynamic effects of epidural morphine and of naloxone reversal. Anesth Analg 62:641-647, 1983
47. Yaksh TL, Elde RP: Factors governing release of methionine enkephalin-like immunoreactivity from mesencephalon and spinal cord of the cat *in vivo*. J Neurophysiol 46:1056-1075, 1981
48. Ballantyne JC, Loach AB, Carr DB: Itching after epidural and spinal opiates. Pain 33:149-160, 1988
49. Brownridge P: Epidural and intrathecal opiates for postoperative pain relief (letter). Anaesthesia 38:74-76, 1983
50. Bromage PR: The price of intraspinal narcotic analgesia: Basic constraints. Anesth Analg 60:461-463, 1981
51. Naulty JS, Johnson M, Burger GA, et al: Epidural fentanyl for post-cesarean delivery pain management. Anesthesiology 59:A415, 1983
52. Evron S, Samueloff A, Simon A, et al: Urinary function during epidural analgesia with methadone and morphine in post-cesarean section patients. Pain 23:135-144, 1985
53. Ready LB, Oden R, Chadwick HS, et al: Development of an anesthesiology-based postoperative pain management service. Anesthesiology 68:100-106, 1988
54. Bromage PR, Camporesi EM, Durant PA, Neilsen CH: Non-respiratory side effects of epidural morphine. Anesth Analg 61:490-495, 1982
55. Knill RL, Clement JL, Thompson WR: Epidural morphine causes delayed and prolonged ventilatory depression. Can Anaesth Soc J 28:537-543, 1981
56. Lanz E, Kehrberger E, Theiss D: Epidural morphine: A clinical double-blind study of dosage. Anesth Analg 64:786-791, 1985
57. Ahuja BR, Strunin L: Respiratory effects of epidural fentanyl. Changes in end-tidal CO_2 and respiratory rate following single doses and continuous infusions of epidural fentanyl. Anaesthesia 40:949-955, 1985
58. Gourlay GK, Cherry DA, Cousins MJ: Cephalad migration of morphine in CSF following lumbar epidural administration in patients with cancer pain. Pain 23:317-326, 1985
59. Gourlay GK, Cherry DA, Plummer JL, et al: The influence of drug polarity on the absorption of opioid drugs into CSF and subsequent cephalad migration following lumbar epidural administration: Application to morphine and pethidine. Pain 31:297-305, 1987

60. Gourlay GK, Murphy TM, Plummer JL, et al: Pharmacokinetics of fentanyl in lumbar and cervical CSF following lumbar epidural and intravenous administration. Pain 38:253-259, 1989
61. Sjostrom S, Tamsen A, Persson MP, Hartvig P: Pharmacokinetics of intrathecal morphine and meperidine in humans. Anesthesiology 67:889-895, 1987
62. Sandler AN: Epidural opiate analgesia for acute pain relief. Can J Anaesth 37:533-534, 1990
63. Rawal N, Arnér S, Gustafsson LL, Allvin R: Present state of extradural and intrathecal opioid analgesia in Sweden. Br J Anaesth 59:791-799, 1987
64. Etches RC, Sandler AN, Daley MD: Respiratory depression and spinal opioids. Can J Anaesth 36:165-185, 1989
65. Writer WDR, Hurtig JB, Evans D, et al: Epidural morphine prophylaxis of postoperative pain: Report of a double blind multicentre study. Can Anaesth Soc J 32:330-338, 1985
66. Jyu C, Lamb JD: Respiratory depression following epidural morphine. Can Anaesth J 32:99-100, 1982
67. Rawal N, Wattwil M: Respiratory depression after epidural morphine—An experimental and clinical study. Anesth Analg 63:8-14, 1984
68. Cousins MJ, Cherry DA, Gourlay GK: Acute and chronic pain: Use of spinal opioids, Neural Blockade in Clinical Anesthesia and Management of Pain. Edited by Cousins MJ, Bridenbaugh PO. Philadelphia, J.B. Lippincott, 1988, pp. 955-1029
69. Eisenach JC, Dewan DM, Rose JC, Angelo JM: Epidural clonidine produces antinociception, but not hypotension, in sheep. Anesthesiology 66:496-501, 1987
70. Bentley GA, Copeland IW, Starr J: The actions of some alpha adrenoceptor agonists and antagonists in antinociceptive test in mice. Clin Exp Pharmacol Physiol 4:405-419, 1977
71. Yaksh TL: Spinal opiate analgesia: Characteristics and principles of action. Pain 11:293-346, 1981
72. Kalia PK, Madan R, Batra RK, et al: Clinical study on epidural clonidine for postoperative analgesia. Indian J Med Res 83:550-552, 1986
73. Boico O, Bonnet F, Rostaing S, et al: Epidural clonidine produces postoperative analgesia (abstract). Anesthesiology 69:A388, 1988
74. Mok MS, Wang JJ, Chan JH, et al: Analgesia effect of epidural clonidine and nalbuphine in combined use (abstract). Anesthesiology 69:A398, 1988
75. Bonnet F, Boico O, Rostaing S, et al: Clonidine for postoperative analgesia: Epidural versus IM study (abstract). Anesthesiology 69:A395, 1988
76. Kuraishi Y, Hirota N, Sato Y, et al: Noradrenergic inhibition of the release of substance P from the primary afferents in the rabbit spinal dorsal horn. Brain Res 359:177-182, 1985

77. Fleetwood-Walker SM, Mitchell R, Hope PJ, et al: An alpha-2 receptor mediates the selective inhibition by noradrenaline of nociceptive responses of identified dorsal horn neurones. Brain Res 334:243-254, 1985
78. Gordh T Jr: Epidural clonidine for treatment of postoperative pain after thoracotomy. A double-blind, placebo-controlled study. Acta Anaesthesiol Scand 32:702-709, 1988
79. Germain IT, Neron A, Lamssy A: Analgesic effect of epidural clonidine, Proceedings of the VIth World Congress on Pain. Edited by Dubner R, Gebhart GF, Bond MR. New York, Elsevier Science Publishers, 1988, pp. 472-476
80. Eisenach JC, Lysak SZ, Viscomi CM: Epidural clonidine analgesia following surgery: Phase I. Anesthesiology 71:640-646, 1989
81. Coombs DW, Saunders RL, LaChance D, et al: Intrathecal morphine tolerance: Use of intrathecal clonidine, DADLE, and intraventricular morphine. Anesthesiology 62:357-363, 1985
82. Coombs DW, Saunders RL, Fratkin JD, et al: Continuous intrathecal hydromorphone and clonodine for intractable cancer pain. J Neurosurg 64:890-894, 1986
83. Glynn CJ, Teddy PJ, Moore RA, et al: Role of spinal noradrenergic spinal system in transmission of pain in patients with spinal cord injury. Lancet 2(8518):1249-1250, 1986
84. Byrd BF III, Collins HW, Primm RK: Risk factors for severe bradycardia during oral clonidine therapy for hypertension. Arch Intern Med 148:729-733, 1988
85. Metz SA, Halter JB, Robertson RP: Induction of defective insulin secretion and impaired glucose tolerance by clonidine. Selective stimulation of metabolic alpha-adrenergic pathways. Diabetes 27:554-562, 1978
86. Bonnet F, Boico O, Rostaing S, et al: Clonidine-induced analgesia in postoperative patients: Epidural versus intramuscular administration. Anesthesiology 72:423-427, 1990
87. Maze M, Segal IS, Bloor BC: Clonidine and other alpha-2 adrenergic agonists: Strategies for the rational use of these novel anesthetic agents. J Clin Anesth 1:146-157, 1988
88. Watkins JC, Krogsgaard-Larsen P, Honore T: Structure-activity relationships in the development of excitatory amino acid receptor agonists and competitive antagonists. Trends Pharmacol Sci 11:25-33, 1990
89. Yaksh TL: Pharmacology of spinal adrenergic systems which modulate spinal nociceptive processing. Pharmacol Biochem Behav 22:845-858, 1985
90. Hylden JL, Wilcox GL: Pharmacological characterization of substance P-induced nociception in mice: Modulation by opioid and noradrenergic agonists at the spinal level. J Pharmacol Exp Ther 226:398-404, 1983

91. Wilcox GL: Excitatory neurotransmitters and pain, Proceedings of VIth World Congress on Pain. Edited by Bond MR, Charlton JE, Woolf CJ. Amsterdam, Elsevier Science Publishers, 1991, pp. 97-118
92. Spaulding TC, Venafro JJ, Ma MG, Fielding S: The dissociation of the antinociceptive effect of clonidine from supraspinal structures. Neuropharmacology 18:103-105, 1979
93. Howe JR, Wang JY, Yaksh TL: Selective antagonism of the antinociceptive effect of intrathecally applied alpha adrenergic agonists by intrathecal prazosin and intrathecal yohimbine. J Pharmacol Exp Ther 224:552-558, 1983
94. Terenius L: Stereospecific interaction between narcotic analgesics and a synaptic plasma membrane fraction of rat cerebral cortex. Acta Pharmacol Toxicol 32:317-320, 1973
95. Sullivan AF, Dashwood MR, Dickenson AH: Alpha-2 adrenoreceptor modulation of nociception in rat spinal cord: Location, effects and interactions with morphine. Eur J Pharmacol 138:169-177, 1987
96. Plummer JL, Cmielewski PL, Reynolds GD, et al: Influence of polarity on dose-response relationships of intrathecal opioids in rats. Pain 40:339-347, 1990
97. Goodchild CS, Serrao JM: Intrathecal midazolam in the rat: evidence for spinally-mediated analgesia. Br J Anaesth 59:1563-1570, 1987
98. Goodchild CS, Noble J: The effects of intrathecal midazolam on sympathetic nervous system reflexes in man—A pilot study. Br J Clin Pharmacol 23:279-285, 1987
99. Yanez A, Sabbe MB, Stevens CW, Yaksh TL: Interaction of midazolam and morphine in the spinal cord of the rat. Neuropharmacology 29:359-364, 1990
100. Wilson PR, Yaksh TL: Baclofen is antinociceptive in the spinal intrathecal space of animals. Eur J Pharmacol 51:323-330, 1978
101. Smith DF: Stereoselectivity of spinal neurotransmission: Effects of baclofen enantiomer on tail-flick reflex in rats. J Neural Transm 60:63-67, 1984
102. Hammond DL, Drower EJ: Effects of intrathecally administered THIP, baclofen and muscimol on nociceptive threshold. Eur J Pharmacol 103:121-125, 1984
103. Sawynok J: Baclofen activates two distinct receptors in the rat spinal cord and guinea pig ileum. Neuropharmacology 25:795-798, 1986
104. Yaksh TL, Reddy SVR: Studies in the primate on the analgesic effects associated with intrathecal actions of opiates, alpha-adrenergic agonists and baclofen. Anesthesiology 54:451-467, 1981
105. Price GW, Wilkin GP, Turnbull MJ, Bowery NG: Are baclofen sensitive GABAB receptors present on primary afferent terminals of the spinal cord? Nature 307:71-74, 1984
106. Davidoff RA, Sears ES: The effects of Lioresal on synaptic activity in the isolated spinal cord. Neurology 24:957-963, 1974

107. Henry JL, Ben-Ari Y: Actions of the p-chlorophenyl derivative of GABA, Lioresal, on nociceptive and non-nociceptive units in the spinal cord of the cat. Bran Res 117:540-544, 1976
108. Fox S, Krnjevic K, Morris ME, et al: Action of baclofen on mammalian synaptic transmission. Neuroscience 3:495-515, 1978
109. Henry JL: Effects of intravenously administered enantiomers of baclofen on functionally identified units in lumbar dorsal horn of the spinal cat. Neuropharmacology 21:1073-1083, 1982
110. Henry JL: Pharmacological studies on the prolonged depressant effects of baclofen on lumbar dorsal horn units in the cat. Neuropharmacology 21:1085-1093, 1982
111. Kangrga I, Randic M, Jeftinija S: Adenosine and (-) baclofen have a neuromodulatory role in the rat spinal dorsal horn. Soc Neurosci Abstr 13:1134-1136, 1987
112. Sawynok J, Moochhala SM, Pillay DJ: Substance P, injected intrathecally, antagonizes the spinal antinociceptive effect of morphine, baclofen and noradrenaline. Neuropharmacology 23:741-747, 1984
113. Crunelli V, Haby M, Jassik-Gerschenfeld D, et al: Cl^- and K^+ dependent inhibitory postsynaptic potentials evoked by interneurones of the rat lateral geniculate neurones. J Physiol (Lond) 399:153-176, 1988
114. Dolphin AC, Scott RH: Calcium channel currents and their inhibition by (-) baclofen in rat sensory neurones: Modulation by guanine nucleotides. J Physiol (Lond) 386:1-17, 1988
115. Soltesz I, Haby M, Leresche N, Crunelli V: The GABAB antagonist phaclofen inhibits the late K^+ dependent IPSP in cat and rat thalamic and hippocampal neurones. Brain Res 448:351-354, 1988
116. Aanonsen LM, Wilcox GL: Muscimol, gamma-aminobutyric acid receptors and excitatory amino acids in the mouse spinal cord. J Pharmacol Exp Ther 248:1034-1038, 1989
117. Huang AS, Wilcox GL: Baclofen, gamma aminobutyric acid B receptors and substance P in the mouse spinal cord. J Pharmacol Exp Ther 248:1026-1033, 1989
118. Holmgren M, Hedner J, Mellstrand T, et al: Evidence for a spinal antinociceptive effect of adenosine in the rat. Pain 2:S157, 1984
119. Post C: Antinociceptive effects in mice after intrathecal injection of 5-N-ethylcarboxamide adenosine. Neurosci Lett 51:325-330, 1984
120. Sawynok J, Sweeney MI, White TD: Classification of adenosine receptors mediating antinociception in the rat spinal cord. Br J Pharmacol 88:923-930, 1986
121. Sawynok J, Sweeney MI: The role of purines in nociception. Neuroscience 32:557-569, 1989
122. DeLander GE, Hopkins CJ: Involvement of A2 adenosine receptors in spinal mechanisms of antinociception. Eur J Pharmacol 139:215-223, 1987

123. Fastbom J, Post C, Fredholm BB: Antinociceptive effects and spinal distribution of two adenosine receptor agonists after intrathecal administration. Pharmacol Toxicol 66:69-72, 1990
124. van Calker D, Muller M, Hamprecht B: Adenosine regulates via two different types of receptors, the accumulation of cyclic AMP in cultured brain cells. J Neurochem 33:999-1005, 1979
125. Choca JI, Proudfit HK, Green RD: Characterisation of adenosine receptors in the rat spinal cord. Soc Neurosci Abstr 11:573-577, 1985
126. Karlsten R, Gordh T Jr, Hartvig P, Post C: Effects of intrathecal injection of the adenosine receptor agonists R-phenylisopropyl-adenosine and N-ethylcarboxamide-adenosine on nociception and motor function in the rat. Anesth Analg 71:60-64, 1990
127. Anis NA, Berry SC, Burton NR, Lodge D: The dissociative anaesthetics, ketamine and phencyclidine, selectively reduce excitation of central mammalian neurones by N-methyl-aspartate. Br J Pharmacol 79:565-575, 1983
128. Kitahata LM, Taub A, Kosada Y: Lamina-specific suppression of dorsal-horn unit activity by ketamine hydrochloride. Anesthesiology 38:4-11, 1973
129. Baumeister A, Advokat C: Evidence for a supraspinal mechanism in the opioid-mediated antinociceptive effect of ketamine. Brain Res 556:351-353, 1991
130. Naguib M, Sharif AM, Seraj M, et al: Ketamine for caudal analgesia in children: Comparison with caudal bupivacaine. Br J Anaesth 67:559-564, 1991
131. Davies J, Evans RH, Herrling PL, et al: CPP, a new potent and selective NMDA antagonist. Depression of central neurons responses, affinity for [3H] D-AP5 binding sites on brain membranes and anticonvulsant activity. Brain Res 382:169-173, 1986
132. Woolf CJ, Thompson SW: The induction and maintenance of central sensitization is dependent on N-methyl-D-aspartic acid receptor activation: Implications for the treatment of post-injury pain hypersensitivity states. Pain 44:293-299, 1991
133. Kristensen JD, Svensson B, Gordh T Jr: The NMDA-receptor antagonist CPP abolishes neurogenic 'wind-up pain' after intrathecal administration in humans. Pain 51:249-253, 1992
134. Bleakman D, Rusin KI, Chard PS, et al: Metabotropic glutamate receptors potentiate inotropic glutamate responses in the rat dorsal horn. Mol Pharmacol 42:192-196, 1992
135. Cerne R, Randic M: Modulation of AMPA and NMDA response in rat spinal dorsal horn neurons by trans-1-aminocyclopentane-1, 3-dicarboxylic acid. Neurosci Lett 144:180-184, 1992
136. Coderre TJ, Melzack R: The contribution of excitatory amino acids to central sensitization and persistent nociception after formalin-induced tissue injury. J Neurosci 12:3665-3670, 1992
137. Millan MJ: K-opioid receptors and analgesia. Trends Pharmacol Sci 11:70-76, 1990

138. Millan MJ, Czlonkowski A, Lipkowski A, Herz A: Kappa opioid receptor mediated antinociception in the rat. II. Supraspinal in addition to spinal sites of action. J Pharmacol Exp Ther 251:342-350, 1989
139. Lei S, Wilcox GL: Effects of excitatory amino acids and mu opioid agonists on nociceptive projection neurones in rat. Pain (Suppl) 5:S124, 1990
140. Patel Y, Rao K, Reichlin S: Somatostatin in human cerebrospinal fluid. N Engl J Med 296:529-533, 1977
141. Massari VJ, Tizabi Y, Park CH, et al: Distribution and origin of bombesin, substance P and somatostatin in cat spinal cord. Peptides 4:673-681, 1983
142. Morton CR, Hutchison WD, Hendry IA, Duggan AW: Somatostatin: Evidence for a role in thermal nociception. Brain Res 488:89-96, 1989
143. Carli P, Ecoffey C, Chrubasik J, et al: Spread of analgesia and ventilatory response to CO_2 following epidural somatostatin. Anesthesiology 65 (Suppl) 216, 1986
144. Ackerman E, Chrubasik J, Weinstock M, Wunsch E: Effect of intrathecal somatostatin on pain threshold in rats. Schermz Pain Doleur 2:41-42, 1985
145. Gaumann DM, Yaksh TL, Post C, et al: Intrathecal somatostatin in cat and mouse studies on pain, motor behaviour, and histopathology. Anesth Analg 68:623-632, 1989
146. Gaumann DM, Yaksh TL: Intrathecal somatostatin in rats: Antinociception only in presence of toxic effects. Anesthesiology 68:733-742, 1988
147. Long JB, Martinez-Arizala A, Kraimer JM, Haladay JW: Intrathecal somatostatin causes handlimb paralysis and reduces spinal cord blood flow in rats. Soc Neurosci 13:1309-1313, 1987
148. Mollenholt P, Post C, Rawal N, et al: Antinociceptive and 'neurotoxic' actions of somatostatin in rat spinal cord after intrathecal administration. Pain 32:95-105, 1988
149. Schulze S, Roikjaer O, Hasselstrom L, et al: Epidural bupivacaine and morphine plus systemic indomethacin eliminates pain but not systemic response and convalescence after cholecystectomy. Surgery 103:321-327, 1988
150. Tverskoy M, Cozacov C, Ayache M, et al: Postoperative pain after inguinal herniorrhaphy with different types of anesthesia. Anesth Analg 70:29-35, 1990
151. Tewes PA, Vella LM, Thomas S, Goll HM: Epidural fentanyl and bupivacaine combinations in patients undergoing pelvic surgery. Anesthesiology 69:3A406, 1988
152. Rucci FS, Cardamone M, Migliori P: Fentanyl and bupivacaine mixtures for extradural blockade. Br J Anaesth 57:275-284, 1985
153. Phillips G: Continuous infusion epidural analgesia in labor: The effect of adding sufentanil to 0.125% bupivacaine. Anesth Analg 67:462-465, 1988

154. Vandermeulen E, Vertommen J, Van Aken H, et al: Epidural bupivacaine with sufentanil in labour. Anesthesiology 71:A844, 1989
155. Chestnut DH, Laszewski LJ, Pollack KL, et al: Continuous epidural infusion of 0.0625% bupivacaine-0.0002% fentanyl during the second stage of labour. Anesthesiology 72:613-618, 1990
156. Justins DM, Knott C, Luthman J, Reynolds F: Epidural versus intramuscular fentanyl. Analgesia and pharmacokinetics in labour. Anaesthesia 38:937-942, 1983
157. Vella LM, Willatts DG, Knott C, et al: Epidural fentanyl in labour. An evaluation of the systemic contribution to analgesia. Anaesthesia 40:741-747, 1985
158. Skerman JH, Thompson BA, Goldstein M, et al: Combined continuous epidural fentanyl and bupivacaine in labor: A randomised study. Anesthesiology 63:A450, 1985
159. Youngstrom R, Eastwood D, Patel H, et al: Epidural fentanyl and bupivacaine in labor: Double blind study. Anesthesiology 61:A414, 1984
160. Milon D, Bentue Ferrer D, Noury D: Anesthesie peridurale pour cesarienne par association bupivacaine fentanyl. Ann Fr Anesth Reanim 2:273-279, 1983
161. Bromage PR, Kapiwal G, Tamilarasan A, et al: Influence of epinephrine and fentanyl as adjuvants on the quality of epidural blockade with 0.5% bupivacaine (abstract). Reg Anesth 13:252, 1988
162. King MJ, Bowden MI, Cooper GM: Epidural fentanyl and 0.5% bupivacaine for elective caesarean section. Anaesthesia 45:285-288, 1990
163. Naulty JS, Datta S, Ostheimer GW, et al: Epidural fentanyl for post-cesarean delivery pain management. Anesthesiology 63:694-698, 1985
164. Ackerman WE, Juneja MM, Colclough GW, Kaczorowski DM: Epidural fentanyl significantly decreases nausea and vomiting during uterine manipulation in awake patients undergoing caesarean section. Anesthesiology 69:A679, 1988
165. Gaffud MP, Bansal P, Lawton C, et al: Surgical analgesia for cesarean delivery with epidural bupivacaine and fentanyl. Anesthesiology 65:331-334, 1986
166. Paech MJ, Westmore MD, Speirs HM: A double blind comparison of epidural bupivacaine and bupivacaine-fentanyl for caesarean section. Anaesth Intensive Care 18:22-30, 1990
167. Noble DW, Morrison LM, Brockway MS, McClure JH: Adrenaline, fentanyl or adrenaline and fentanyl as adjuncts to bupivacaine for extradural anaesthesia in elective caesarean section. Br J Anaesth 66:645-650, 1991
168. Lee A, Simpson D, Whitefield A, Scott DB: Postoperative analgesia by continuous extradural infusion of bupivacaine and diamorphine. Br J Anaesth 60:845-850, 1988
169. Zwarts SJ, Hasenbos MAMW, Gielen MJM, Kho HG: The effect of continuous epidural analgesia with sufentanil and bupivacaine

during and after thoracic surgery on the plasma cortisol concentration and pain relief. Reg Anesth 14:183-188, 1989

170. Gregg RV, Denson DD, Knarr DC, Stueburg RC: Continuous epidural infusions of bupivacaine and morphine versus systemic narcotic analgesics for postoperative pain relief. Anesthesiology 69:A384, 1988
171. Scheinin B, Asantila R, Orko R: Effect of bupivacaine and morphine on pain and bowel function after colonic surgery. Acta Anaesthesiol Scand 31:161-164, 1987
172. Taiwo YO, Miaskowski C, Levine JD: Interactions of kappa and delta opioids in the production of analgesia in animals and humans. Pain (Suppl) 5:S265, 1990
173. Naulty JS, La Bove P, Datta S, et al: Epidural butorphanol/fentanyl for post-cesarean delivery analgesia. Anesthesiology 67:A463, 1987
174. Bailey PL, Rhondeau S, Schafer PG, et al: Dose-response pharmacology of intrathecal morphine in human volunteers. Anesthesiology 79:49-59, 1993
175. Miller RJ: Multiple calcium channels and neuronal function. Science 235:46-52, 1987
176. Mintz IM, Adams ME, Bean BP: P-type calcium channels in rat central and peripheral neurons. Neuron 9:85-95, 1992
177. Tsien RW, Lipscombe D, Madison DV, et al: Multiple types of neuronal calcium channels and their selective modulation. Trends Neurosci 11:431-438, 1988
178. Holt GG IV, Dunlap K, Kream RM: Characterization of the electrically evoke release of substance P from dorsal root ganglion neurons: methods and dihydropyridine sensitivity. J Neurosci 8:463-471, 1988
179. Turner TJ, Adams ME, Dunlap K: Calcium channels coupled to glutamate release identified by omega-Aga-IVA. Science 258:310-313, 1992
180. Schneider M, Datta S, Strichartz G: A preferential inhibition of impulses in C-fibers of the rabbit vagus nerve by veratridine, an activator of sodium channels. Anesthesiology 74:270-280, 1991
181. Iggo A: The electrophysiological identification of single nerve fibres, with particular reference to the slowest-conducting vagal afferent fibres in the cat. J Physiol (Lond) 142:110-126, 1958

PROBLEMS OF PAIN MEASUREMENT IN CHILDREN

D. C. Tyler

One of the major problems in managing pain in children is the difficulty of measurement of pain intensity. In order to treat pain effectively, one needs to know whether a child is in pain and whether the intensity of the pain is significant enough to warrant subjecting the child to the risks involved in treatment of pain. In addition to making judgments about the appropriate forms of pain therapy, there is another important reason for measurement of pain in children. Regular use of these measurement techniques by nurses will help raise awareness of staff about the need for appropriate pain therapy. We have attempted to have pain measured on all children in the postoperative period as a way of ensuring that children are treated appropriately. If a measurement is made and a number is charted on the patient's notes, then it is more likely that the child will be treated than if no attempt is made to measure pain at all. It is our belief that systematic attempts at pain measurement are important to the overall success of a pain program in a hospital.

Quantifying a subjective perception such as pain is hard enough in adults, but the problem becomes much more difficult in younger children, and quantification may be impossible in the smallest children. The clinical problem is this: When faced with a crying two-year-old, how can one tell whether the child is in pain, or is suffering from separation anxiety, hunger, cold, or any number of other feelings, all of which result in distress and crying. Partly as a result of this problem of measurement, treatment of pain in children lags behind what is currently available for adults.

Fortunately some techniques are being developed which can be used in a clinical setting to estimate pain intensity. For children over 7 or 8 years of age, the use of techniques such as a visual analog scale allows measurement in a useful way, and, for younger children, behavioral observation techniques are becoming more sophisticated. In this paper I

T. H. Stanley and M. A. Ashburn (eds.), Anesthesiology and Pain Management, 227–236.

will review some of the techniques available for pain measurement and then make suggestions about the best techniques that are available for specific ages of children. I will be dealing with pain measurement, that is quantification of pain intensity, not the complicated issue of pain assessment, which involves understanding other dimensions of the child's pain, including the physiologic, psychological, and social factors that contribute to pain and the effects of pain on the child's functioning within his or her family, in school, and in society.

TYPES OF MEASUREMENT TOOLS

In general there are three different strategies for measuring pain: physiologic measurements, behavioral observation, and patient report. While physiologic measures, such as changes in pulse and blood pressure, would be convenient ways to measure pain because they are easily quantified, there is no indication that any measurable physiologic variable correlates with pain perception. Even using sophisticated electrophysiologic techniques, pain cannot be quantified in a physiologic manner.

Behavioral observation is frequently used in young children who are not able to report their pain in a meaningful way. This type of measurement technique is particularly useful in pre-verbal children. In using behavioral observation, one selects a group of behaviors that are assumed to correlate with pain, scores those behaviors in a systematic way, and develops an overall score, the magnitude of which is felt to indicate the child's pain.

Patient report is the gold standard of measurement of pain in adults and for children who are beginning to be verbal, that is, above age four or five patient reports can be useful. Children above age seven or eight have sufficient understanding of numerical systems that they can use a visual analog scale in a reasonably accurate way. I will now discuss these techniques in more detail.

SPECIFIC TECHNIQUES OF PAIN MEASUREMENT

Physiologic Changes

Heart rate and blood pressure. It is a common belief among physicians and nurses in many hospitals that an increase in heart rate and blood pressure are indicative of pain, and most anesthesiologists believe that increased pulse and blood pressure are indicative of pain in an anesthetized patient. In babies, after a short, sharp stimulus, such as skin lancing, heart rate increases, although the response is variable (1-7). When a large number of babies are examined, however, these techniques are not reliable (2,4). More importantly, in a setting of sustained pain, such as in a postoperative situation, no data are available to indicate that there is any correlation of physiologic variables with intensity of pain. Too many other variables interfere with the patient's pulse rate and blood pressure to make them a meaningful measurement of pain.

Palmar sweating. Palmar sweating occurs with emotional arousal and by 37 weeks of gestation, babies will respond to emotional arousal with palmar sweating (8,9). There is also an increase in palmar sweating in response to a short, sharp stimulus (8,10), but the use of palmar sweating to estimate the intensity of sustained or prolonged pain, as in the postoperative situation, has not been examined.

Metabolic changes. Numerous studies have evaluated the changes in stress hormones that occur with pain. During and following surgery there is an increase in blood levels of stress hormones and this increase in stress hormone output can be attenuated with intraoperative anesthesia or with effective postoperative pain management (11–14). Unfortunately, however, many other factors besides pain result in a stress response and, consequently, the stress response is not a very precise measure of pain. In addition, the studies take time to be performed, and, therefore, measurement of hormones is not a clinically useful way of indicating whether or not a patient is having pain.

pO_2 changes. In babies subjected to circumcision without anesthesia it has been shown that pO_2 is lower than in patients who have circumcision after administration of a local anesthetic (6). Unfortunately, pO_2 is a very imprecise technique to use because other factors may influence the patient's pO_2, particularly in the immediate postoperative period.

Behavioral Scoring Systems

Characteristic of cry. One behavioral characteristic that has been examined in an attempt to measure pain in pre-verbal children is the type of cry. Recent reports suggest that babies make specific types of cry associated with pain (2,4,6,7,12,15-19). Unfortunately there is a good bit of overlap with nonpainful types of cries, and complicated spectrographic equipment is necessary in order to measure cry accurately. Consequently, cry is not a clinically useful method currently, although it shows some promise in the future.

Facial expressions. Another behavioral approach to measure pain is by examination of changes in facial expression. Human beings develop unique facial expressions in response to certain emotional situations (20), and there is, in fact, a facial expression associated with pain. Babies also develop unique facial expressions that are felt to be characteristic of pain, since these facial expressions occur in response to a painful stimulus (2,16,17,21). A coding system has been developed to try to evaluate facial expressions as a measure of pain, but as yet, facial expression is not a clinically useful tool.

Attia infant pain score. This scoring system was developed to attempt to measure pain in infants. The observer scores certain behaviors, including sleep during the preceding hour, facial expression, quality of cries, spontaneous motor activity, response to stimulation, flexion of fingers and toes, sucking, tone, consolability and sociability. Intuitive variations of this scoring system are probably used by experienced neonatal nurses in telling whether or not infants have pain. The Attia system has been published, but only limited work has been done to validate this scoring system (22).

CHEOPS

This is a behavioral scoring system developed at the Children's Hospital of Eastern Ontario (23). With this tool, the observer evaluates six aspects of behavior, including cry, facial expression, verbal output, movements of torso, touching of wound, and movement of legs. Each of these six categories is scored within a defined range and the total score added up. The scores range from 4 to 13, with 4 indicating no pain and 13 indicating intense pain. Some validation of this scoring system has been done in the immediate postoperative period in the recovery room (23), and in the latter postoperative period (24). There has been some suggestion recently that the CHEOPS scale might not be a valid measure of postoperative pain after the patient leaves the recovery room (25,26).

Observer pain scale. Another scoring system is based on a fairly simple 1 to 5 scale (27): 1-laughing, euphoric, 2-happy, content, playful, 3-calm or asleep, 4-mild to moderate pain, crying, grimacing, restlessness, can distract with toy, food, parent, 5-severe pain, crying, screaming, inconsolable. Some validation has been done with this scoring system (24) and it provides some benefit with patients in the postoperative period in that it involves an evaluation similar to that used on busy hospital wards.

Objective pain scale. The objective pain scale is a five-point, behavioral observation scale that examines blood pressure, crying, moving, agitation and verbalization or body language. Some validation has been done of this scale (28-30).

Patient Report. The best method to measure pain is by patient report. If the child is mature enough to use a numerical system, adult-based techniques can generally be used.

Visual analog scales. Visual analog scales are felt to be a valid method of measuring pain in adults. Several studies have examined visual analog scales in children and found them to be reliable in children above age 7 or 8 (31-33). At around this age, children are beginning to understand the number system and learn that one quantity is bigger than another, and using these concepts, they can quantitate pain with a visual analog scale.

Numerical scales. In many children's hospitals numerical scales are sometimes used in place of visual analog scales because they require no equipment. The child is asked to choose a number between 0 and 10 indicating their pain intensity. The pain thermometer is a variation of a numerical scale. A picture of a thermometer marked between 0 and 100 or 1 and 10 is presented, and the child is asked to indicate on the thermometer the intensity of pain.

Poker chip. This tool is a measure of pain intensity in which the child is asked to conceive of pain as "pieces of hurt" and to select from four poker chips the number that indicates pain intensity. There has been some initial validation with this tool, but it has not been thoroughly investigated (34,35).

Faces scales. There are a number of variations of faces scales. A series of cartoons, pictures, or actual photographs of faces with different expressions on them are presented to the child. The expressions range from a child who is sad and crying, to one who is happy and smiling. The child is asked to indicate the intensity of his or her pain by selecting the face that indicates how he or she feels. Children are able to use these scales to rate affect and to rate pain intensity (24,33,36-38), although in the postoperative situation a frightened child with pain may not cooperate with these scales.

Oucher scale. The Oucher scale is a variation of a faces scale in which a series of photographs of children are positioned next to a numerical scale. The photographs depict children in graded variations of distress. The child uses either the numerical or the faces scale to indicate pain intensity. This tool has undergone fairly extensive validation (39-41).

MEASUREMENT OF PAIN IN DIFFERENT AGE GROUPS

In deciding which scale to use, it is important evaluate the purpose of the scale. If it is being used for research purposes, one must ensure that adequate validation has been performed to ensure that the data obtained are reliable and valid. If on the other hand the pain scale is used in the clinical setting for measurement of pain in a child who needs treatment, then the clinical situation requires that the clinician use whatever scale is currently available and validation is not an issue except as a long-term measure to improve pain management in any given hospital or other clinical setting.

Infants (0-6 Months)

Infants are the most difficult age group to measure pain. Subtle clues may be all that are available to make an estimate of pain intensity. In the postoperative situation one should make use of all clues such as whether the patient had a recent painful event and when the last pain medication was given and then observe the infant's behavior, noting such things as movement, crying, facial expression and response to handling and soothing. If pain therapy is used, the infant's response to therapy should also be used as part of the evaluation.

Pre-verbal Children (6 Months to 3 Years)

In this group of children, behavioral observation is the only technique that will be of any use, as patient report is not reliable. We have found that the CHEOPS is a useful method of quantifying pain, although it has certain limitations, particularly in the postoperative period.

Preschool Children (3 Years to 6 Years)

In this age group patient report may be helpful at times. We would recommend using a faces scale or the Oucher scale in those patients who can cooperate, or the CHEOPS scale in those who cannot. Discussion with parents can sometimes be very helpful in indicating whether or not they feel the patient has pain, as the patient may discuss it with the parent but not with a doctor or nurse.

School Age Children and Adolescents (6 Years to Adult)

For most patients in this age group, patient report can be used. We would recommend either a visual analog scale or a numerical scale.

In conclusion pain measurement is difficult, but not impossible in infants and children. Systematic measurement and recording of pain intensity should become part of routine postoperative care.

REFERENCES

1. Möltner A, Hölzl R, Strian F: Heart rate changes as an autonomic component of the pain response. Pain 43:81-89, 1990
2. Johnston CC, Strada ME: Acute pain response in infants: A multidimensional description. Pain 24:373-382, 1986
3. Fisichelli VR, Karelitz S, Fisichelli RM, Cooper J: The course of induced crying activity in the first year of life. Pediatr Res 8:921-928, 1974

4. Field T, Goldson E: Pacifying effects of nonnutritive sucking on term and preterm neonates during heelstick procedures. Pediatrics 74:1012-1015, 1984
5. Dixon S, Snyder J, Holve R, Bromberger P: Behavioral effects of circumcision with and without anesthesia. J Dev Behav Pediatr 5:246-250, 1984
6. Williamson PS, Williamson ML: Physiologic stress reduction by a local anesthetic during newborn circumcision. Pediatrics 71:36-40, 1983
7. Owens ME, Todt EH: Pain in infancy: Neonatal reaction to a heel lance. Pain 20:77-86, 1984
8. Harpin VA, Rutter N: Development of emotional sweating in the newborn infant. Arch Dis Child 57:691-695, 1982
9. Verbov J, Baxter J: Onset of palmar sweating in newborn infants. Br J Dermatol 90:269-276, 1974
10. Harpin VA, Rutter N: Making heel pricks less painful. Arch Dis Child 58:226-228, 1983
11. Anand KJS, Sippell WG, Aynsley-Green A: Randomised trial of fentanyl anaesthesia in preterm babies undergoing surgery: Effects on the stress response. Lancet 1(8524):62-66, 1987
12. Kirya C, Werthmann MW Jr: Neonatal circumcision and penile dorsal nerve block—A painless procedure. J Pediatr 92:998-1000, 1978
13. Stang HJ, Gunnar MR, Snellman L, Condon LM: Local anesthesia for neonatal circumcision. Effect on distress and cortisol response. JAMA 259:1507-1511, 1988
14. Williamson PS, Evans ND: Neonatal cortisol response to circumcision with anesthesia. Clin Pediatr (Phila) 25:412-415, 1986
15. Wasz-Höckert O, Lind J, Vourenkoski V, et al: The infant cry. A spectrographic and auditory analysis. Clin Devel Med 29:8-42, 1968
16. Grunau RV, Craig KD: Pain expression in neonates: Facial action and cry. Pain 28:395-410, 1987
17. Grunau RV, Johnston CC, Craig KD: Neonatal facial and cry responses to invasive and non-invasive procedures. Pain 42:295-305, 1990
18. Porter FL, Miller RH, Marshall RE: Neonatal pain cries: Effect of circumcision on acoustic features and perceived urgency. Child Dev 57:790-802, 1986
19. Wolff PH: The natural history of crying and other vocalizations in early infancy, Determinants of Infant Behaviour IV. Edited by Foss BM. London, Methuen & Co Ltd, 1969, pp. 81-109
20. Ekman P, Øster H: Facial expressions of emotion. Ann R Psych 30:527-554, 1979
21. Izard CE, Hembree EA, Dougherty LM, Spizzirri CC: Changes in facial expressions of 2- to 19-month-old infants following acute pain. Devel Psych 19:418-426, 1983

22. Barrier G, Attia J, Mayer MN, et al: Measurement of post-operative pain and narcotic administration in infants using a new clinical scoring system. Intensive Care Med (Suppl 1) 15:S37-S39, 1989.
23. McGrath PJ, Johnson G, Goodman JT, et al: CHEOPS: A behavioral scale for rating postoperative pain in children, Advances in Pain Research and Therapy. Edited by Fields HL, Dubner R and Cervero F. New York, Raven Press, 1985, pp. 395-402
24. Tyler DC, Tu A, Douthit J, Chapman CR: Toward validation of pain measurement tools for children: A pilot study. Pain 52:301-309, 1993.
25. Büttner W, Breitkopf L, Finke W, Schwanitz M: Critical aspects of an outside evaluation of postoperative pain in infants. Anaesthesist 39:151-157, 1990
26. Beyer JE, McGrath PJ, Berde CB: Discordance between self-report and behavioral pain measures in children aged 3-7 years after surgery. J Pain Symptom Manage 5:350-356, 1990
27. Krane EJ, Jacobson LE, Lynn AM, et al: Caudal morphine for post-operative analgesia in children: A comparison with caudal bupivacaine and intravenous morphine. Anesth Analg 66:647-653, 1987
28. Broadman LM, Hannallah RS, Belman AB, et al: Post-circumcision analgesia—a prospective evaluation of subcutaneous ring block of the penis. Anesthesiology 67:399-402, 1987
29. Broadman LM, Rice LJ, Hannallah RS: Testing the validity of an objective pain scale for infants and children (abstract). Anesthesiology 69:A770, 1988
30. Hannallah RS, Broadman LM, Belman AB, et al: Comparison of caudal and ilioinguinal/iliohypogastric nerve blocks for control of post-orchiopexy pain in pediatric ambulatory surgery. Anesthesiology 66:832-834, 1987
31. Abu-Saad H, Holzemer WL: Measuring children's self-assessment of pain. Issues Compr Pediatr Nurs 5:337-349, 1981
32. Scott PJ, Ansell BM, Huskisson EC: Measurement of pain in juvenile chronic polyarthritis. Ann Rheum Dis 36:186-187, 1977
33. McGrath PA, de Veber LL, Hearn MT: Multidimensional pain assessment in children, Advances in Pain Research and Therapy. Edited by Fields HL, Dubner R and Cervero F. New York, Raven Press, 1985, pp. 387-393
34. Hester NK: The preoperational child's reaction to immunization. Nurs Res 28:250-255, 1979
35. Hester NO, Foster R, Kristensen K: Measurement of pain in children: Generalizability and validity of the pain ladder and the poker chip tool, Advances in Pain Research and Therapy. Edited by Fields HL, Dubner R and Cervero F. New York, Raven Press, 1990, pp. 79-84
36. Bieri D, Reeve RA, Champion GD, et al: The Faces Pain Scale for the self-assessment of the severity of pain experienced by children: Development, initial validation, and preliminary investigation for ratio scale properties. Pain 41:139-150, 1990

37. Maunuksela E-L, Olkkola KT, Korpela R: Measurement of pain in children with self-reporting and behavioral assessment. Clin Pharmacol Ther 42:137-141, 1987
38. Pothmann R: Comparison of the Visual Analog Scale (VAS) and a Smiley Analog Scale (SAS) for the evaluation of pain in children, Advances in Pain Research and Therapy. Edited by Tyler DC and Krane EJ. New York, Raven Press, 1990, pp. 95-99
39. Beyer JE: "The Oucher: A user's manual and technical report." The Hospital Play Equipment Co. Evanston, IL, USA, 1984
40. Beyer JE, Aradine CR: Content validity of an instrument to measure young children's perceptions of the intensity of their pain. J Pediatr Nurs 1:386-395, 1986
41. Beyer JE, Aradine CR: Patterns of pediatric pain intensity: A methodological investigation of a self-report scale. Clin J Pain 3:130-141, 1987

POST SPINAL CORD INJURY PAIN: MECHANISMS AND TREATMENT OPTIONS

P. J. Siddall and M. J. Cousins

INTRODUCTION

Pain is a frequent and debilitating accompaniment of spinal cord injury (SCI) (1). SCI pain, like other forms of deafferentation pain where there is loss or modification of normal afferent sensory inputs, is notoriously resistant to currently available modes of treatment and highlights our lack of understanding of basic pain mechanisms.

A recent review of ten publications over the past four decades revealed that an average of 69% of SCI patients reported experiencing pain and in nearly one third the pain was severe (2). Although loss of function is considered the most significant consequence of SCI, pain itself has a direct bearing on the ability or otherwise of the spinally injured person to regain their optimal level of activity. Bonica (2) reports that 36% of a population of 885 SCI outpatients were unemployed and stated that it was the severity of their pain rather than the loss of motor function that was preventing their return to employment. The impact of pain following SCI is also demonstrated by a study that reported that 37% of higher level SCI patients with pain and 23% of lower level SCI patients would, if they had the chance, trade pain relief for loss of bladder, bowel or sexual function.

The epidemiological factors that are involved in the development of SCI pain are unclear. It has been suggested on the basis of observation that pain is more common following cervical injuries (3). On the other hand Davis and Martin (4) reported from their experience during the World War II that there was a higher incidence of pain following thoracic and lumbosacral injuries. Yet again it has been stated that the conus and cauda equina injuries are more likely to be associated with pain (5).

T. H. Stanley and M. A. Ashburn (eds.), Anesthesiology and Pain Management, 237–251.

The type of injury may also be a factor in the development of pain. It has been suggested that injuries that result in severe damage to the cord, such as gunshot wounds, are more likely to result in pain (5). Similarly, it is not clear whether completeness of the lesion is more or less likely to result in pain. Evidence from autopsy studies of spinal cord injured patients suggests that pain is more likely to be associated with incompleteness (6).

CLINICAL PRESENTATION

Types of Pain

Pain following spinal cord injury presents in several ways and various authors have proposed categories in an attempt to classify different types of pain. These include:

Musculoskeletal pain. Musculoskeletal pain arises from damage to structures such as the bones, ligaments, intervertebral discs and facet joints. It is usually situated close to the level of injury and is described as either a sharp or dull and aching pain which is localized to the site of injury. Chronic musculoskeletal pain is generally due to overuse or overcompensation of muscle groups associated with mobility and transfer.

Radicular pain. Radicular pain occurs at or immediately above the level of injury and radiates in a dermatomal pattern corresponding to the nerve roots affected. This pain is due to direct damage to dorsal nerve roots at or near the site of injury.

Segmental pain. Segmental, transitional zone pain, or girdle pain occurs at or above the level of sensory loss and usually covers one to three segments in width. It is described as a burning, aching or sharp, shooting pain and is associated with hyperalgesia of the affected dermatomes. Although similar to radicular pain, it is probably due to functional changes in neurons within the spinal cord at or above the level of injury.

Syringomyelia must always be considered in the patient who has delayed onset of segmental pain especially where there is a rising level of sensory loss. Nashold (5) reports that 65% of their group of paraplegics who had a delayed onset of pain exhibited a syringomyelia with the average onset being six years following the initial spinal injury.

Visceral pain. Pain which is visceral in nature is often seen following spinal cord injury, more commonly in quadriplegics. Although intra-abdominal pathology may be demonstrated, in many patients no pathology can be found that provides an explanation for a nociceptive basis to this type of pain despite multiple investigations. It is often poorly localized, although attributed to the lower abdomen and pelvic region, and often related to disturbances of bladder or bowel function.

Dysesthetic pain. This type of pain, which is also referred to as central or deafferentation pain, presents as a spontaneous and/or evoked dysesthesia, usually diffuse pain caudad to the level of spinal cord injury. It is characterized by sensations of burning, aching, stabbing or electric shocks with hyperalgesia and often develops some time after the initial injury. Although it is difficult in many studies to allocate pain types to specific categories, it appears that of all the groups the diffuse dysesthetic type of pain is the most common (2).

Although not included in the list of pain types, the contribution of psychological and environmental components to these pains must be considered and it has been suggested that psychogenic pain should also be included as a type of pain following spinal cord injury (7,8). However psychological factors should probably be considered as a contribution to any of these pains rather than being considered an entity in its own right.

As well as these main categories, there are several other pain presentations. These include reflex sympathetic dystrophy (9) and limb pain associated with compressive mononeuropathies (10). The other disturbance of sensory function following spinal cord injury is phantom sensations. Although often not painful, they are sometimes distressing to the patient and often underreported. Bors (11) found that the incidence was as high as 100%.

Pain Features

Pain and hyperalgesia are often, but not always, seen immediately following SCI. Syringomyelia may result in the expression of pain some time following the initial injury. Patients with SCI pain also demonstrate abnormalities of sensory and autonomic function. The dysesthetic component of the pain can be triggered by normally innocuous stimuli such as light touch or vibration and even emotional changes such as anxiety or anger. Increased sweating is often found cephalad to the lesion. These different types of pain and other features have been consistently reported in patients with SCI. However, a comprehensive description of the pain and its pathophysiology or underlying mechanisms remains to be provided. How is it that a patient that has a clinically complete spinal lesion can have evoked pain or hyperalgesia from an area whose sensory input is caudad to the lesion? How is it that patients experience visceral pain when the spinal lesion is above the currently understood neural inputs from visceral pathways? Similarly, what is the basis of the diffuse, burning, "dysesthetic" or phantom pains experienced by patients with spinal cord lesions. It has been suggested that such dysesthetic sensations are a result of intact residual fibers within the damaged cord; however this type of pain has been observed even in those people in which an entire segment of the cord has been removed and, therefore, there is no possibility of afferent transmission by the spinal route (12).

These questions highlight the complexity and lack of knowledge about SCI pain. Despite this situation, no rigorous and systematic attempt has been made to examine and document the contribution made by nociceptive, neuropathic, psychologic and environmental factors to SCI pain. Furthermore, there are few reports of controlled studies that determine the efficacy of pharmacologic and other treatment modalities in this condition. If treatment is to be effective, the mechanisms and the level at which they occur need to be identified clearly.

MECHANISMS

Possible mechanisms for SCI pain include (13-15):

Peripheral Mechanisms

SCI results in extensive damage to bones, joints, discs, ligaments and muscles at the site of injury (16). All of these structures are potential sources of nociceptive pain via peripheral mechanisms. The peripheral nervous system (PNS) may also contribute to neuropathic pain following SCI since it is known that normally innocuous sensory stimuli can induce severe pain in patients with spinal cord lesions. Although little is known about the mechanisms of pain resulting from central nervous system (CNS) lesions, there is extensive data on neuropathic pain following peripheral nerve injury. Pain and hyperalgesia resulting from CNS or PNS lesions share similar characteristics and therefore may share common mechanisms. Possible peripheral mechanisms of neuropathic pain are: sprouting of undamaged sensory neurons into denervated tissue; sensitization of primary afferent neurons; and sympathetic activation or sensitization of primary afferents. Often patients with SCI will feel pain in areas below the level of the lesion. A possible reason for this is sprouting of intact primary afferent neurons into the denervated region. It has been shown, in experimental animals, that when a peripheral nerve is cut, nerves that supply the adjacent skin area sends sprouts into the denervated area (17). Furthermore, the area now innervated by the sprouting nerve becomes hyperresponsive to mildly noxious stimuli (17). Sensitization of primary afferent neurons may contribute to the exaggerated responses induced by normally innocuous stimuli. Sensitization is characterized by a decrease in threshold, increased firing frequency and spontaneous firing. The mechanism underlying sensitization is not entirely understood, but recent evidence suggests that it is partially mediated by humoral factors such as metabolites of arachidonic acid. Products of both the cyclooxygenase (for example, PGI2) and lipoxygenase (for example, 8R, 15S diHETE) pathways of arachidonic acid metabolism have been shown to increase the excitability of sprouting nerve terminals of the sciatic nerve (18). The sympathetic nervous system may also contribute to the sensitization of primary afferent neurons. Indeed, sympathetic block can, in some cases, relieve pain associated with CNS lesions (19). Activation of postganglionic sympathetic neurons increases the excitability of sprouting primary afferent neurons (20). Sympathetic sensitization is thought to be mediated by the release of noradrenaline which then acts via the $alpha_2$-adrenergic receptor (20).

Local Irritation At the Site of Injury

It may be that following SCI local trauma results in scar tissue and irritation of cells and fibers of sensory pathways and nuclei. This "irritated focus" may then become responsive to incoming signals which under normal conditions would not elicit a response. There is evidence at least in peripheral nerves that damaged fibers following injury become hypersensitive, generate new receptors and give rise to afterdischarges (21). It is possible that spinal neurons behave in the same way resulting in ongoing pain. Clinical evidence suggests that pain originates in the spinal cord just rostral to the level of injury as cordectomy, which removes the spinal cord 2 to 3 cm above the level of injury, has been reported to result in pain relief.

Activation of Alternative Pathways Outside the Spinal Cord

Recent demonstration of "plasticity" of the nervous system raises the possibility of the development of alternative sensory pathways (Figure 1). This may occur through regrowth of visceral nociceptive afferents which then join the spinal cord at a higher level, through activation of otherwise silent vagal afferents or through activation of a general systemic response following a locally generated neurohumoral reaction. The involvement of the sympathetic nervous system is also suggested by the vasomotor and other autonomic changes seen in cases of SCI (19).

Activation of Alternative Pathways Within the Spinal Cord

In patients who have incomplete lesions, pain may also be a result of conduction in alternative pathways within the spinal cord. The dorsal column pathway, spinocervicothalamic, spinoparabrachial, spinohypothalamic tracts and multisynaptic ascending system are all suggested as candidates for this pathway (22) for review. These normally subsidiary or latent pathways may become activated with lesions of the lateral spinothalamic pathway.

Abnormal Firing and/or Anatomical Reorganization of Spinal and Supraspinal Deafferented Neurons

There is abundant evidence that several changes take place at synapses which lose their normal afferent input. These changes include

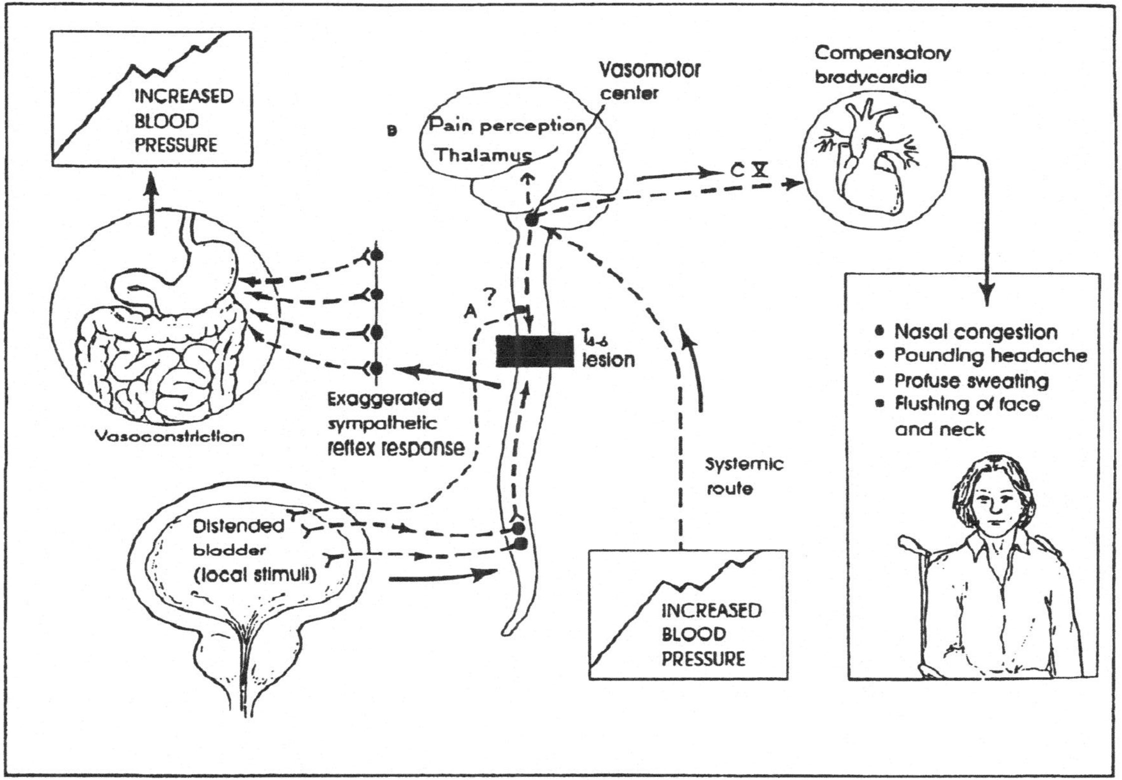

Figure 1 . Two possible mechanisms of pain following spinal cord injury. (A) Visceral afferents may rejoin at a higher level of the cord and bypass the site of lesion or (B) a general systemic response, as occurs with autonomic dysreflexia, may activate higher pathways following a peripheral stimulus. (Adapted from Zejdlik CP: Management of Spinal Cord Injury, 2nd Ed. Boston, Jones and Bartlett Publishers, 1992, p322.)

reinnervation by other axons, substitution of excitatory synapses for inhibitory ones, and activation of previously ineffective synapses (23,24). It has been demonstrated that the central terminals of deafferented primary myelinated afferent neurons undergo structural reorganization, with sprouting into lamina II of the dorsal horn (25). Nociceptive input may result in the expression of certain genes within cells which may then be associated with delayed and long-lasting changes in cell responsivity (26,27). It has been demonstrated that both spinal (28) and thalamic (29,30) neurons show abnormal firing patterns following spinal cord injury. Therefore it may be that sensory neurons in the higher central nervous system show these changes following spinal cord injury and act as a spontaneous pain generating mechanism.

Loss of Inhibitory Mechanisms

Pain may be a result of the loss of normally active inhibitory mechanisms (27). It is well known that inhibition of nociceptive transmission occurs at various levels of the neuraxis. Several lines of evidence indicate that posterior column fibers exert an inhibitory influence on pain afferents in lateral pathways and clinical evidence suggests that the integrity of this pathway is important in the expression of hyperalgesia (15,31). Therefore, it is possible that this balance is destroyed with spinal cord lesions, and this mechanism alone or in combination with the one described above results in ongoing pain.

The last two mechanisms above provide a plausible explanation for spontaneous dysesthesia in areas below the level of the spinal lesion even when the lesion is complete. However, they fail to provide an explanation for evoked pain or hyperalgesia localized to a specific area below the level of a complete lesion. It may be that some patients reported in the literature as having complete lesions in the absence of neurophysiological testing, in fact, do have some residual spinal function.

Clearly there are a variety of mechanisms that have been suggested in an attempt to explain SCI pain. The precise mechanisms responsible, however, are unknown. Therefore, while there are a variety of treatment approaches that have been used, the reason for their effectiveness or lack of it is unknown.

MANAGEMENT

As with other deafferentation pain syndromes, treatment is often ineffectual and unsatisfying for both patient and practitioner. Various approaches have been utilized with varying degrees of success and there is a general lack of controlled studies.

Simple Analgesics

Simple analgesics are helpful for musculoskeletal pain but because of their predominantly peripheral action are largely ineffective in the management of SCI deafferentation pain.

Anticonvulsants

Anticonvulsants such as carbamazepine, are more effective in the management of radicular or segmental pain, particularly where there is a sharp, shooting component (32). Other anticonvulsants such as sodium valproate and clonazepam are also used although evidence of their effectiveness is limited. Their effect is probably due to suppression of aberrant nerve activity at a spinal or higher level.

Antidepressants

It has been reported that tricyclic antidepressants are most effective in the management of dysesthetic pain (1). The presumed mechanism of action is thought to be their ability to inhibit the reuptake of serotonin and noradrenaline and therefore increase pain inhibitory mechanisms. There is also evidence from a case report that the use of an anticonvulsant (carbamazepine) in addition to a tricyclic antidepressant (amitriptyline) is more effective than the use of these agents by themselves (33).

Local Anesthetics

Lidocaine administered intravenously (34) and oral mexiletine have both been used with success in the management of SCI pain. They probably act in a similar manner to anticonvulsants by dampening central aberrant neuronal activity.

Alpha-adrenergic Agonists

Clonidine has been administered to patients with SCI pain by the epidural route and has been found to be more effective than morphine for pain relief (35) suggesting that alpha-adrenergic agonists may have a useful role in this problem. Evidence from our own experience (Siddall et al., submitted to *Pain*) has also demonstrated the effectiveness of clonidine combined with morphine administered intrathecally for dysesthetic SCI pain while intrathecal morphine alone was ineffective.

Opioids

The long term use of opioids may be necessary in the patient with SCI pain who is unable to achieve pain relief with other methods. However, the dysesthetic type of pain, which is the most common type of chronic pain problem, is often unresponsive to even high doses of opioid agents.

Anesthetic Blockade

Anesthetic blockade at several levels may be useful in reducing pain following SCI. This may include the use of sympathetic, epidural or spinal blockade.

Stimulation Techniques

Dorsal column stimulation. This technique has been reported to be successful in the management of other types of neuropathic pain such as arachnoiditis. However, it is generally not successful in the management of SCI pain although there are reports that it may be useful if the spinal cord lesion is incomplete (36).

Transcutaneous electrical nerve stimulation (TENS). TENS has been used for the treatment of SCI pain but with limited success (37). It appears to be more effective in those patients that have incomplete lesions.

Surgical Procedures

DREZ lesions. Dorsal root entry zone (DREZ) lesions that involve two to three spinal segments have been proposed as being effective in the management of SCI pain. However, evidence from studies in which this procedure has been used indicates that good outcome is dependent to a large extent on the nature of their pain (38). Those who have radicular pain are more likely to have a favorable outcome while those who have the diffuse, distal or burning pain are less likely to do well. The procedure also carries the risk of cerebrospinal fluid leaks, as well as changes in sensory level or motor function.

Cordotomy. The largest study of this procedure indicates that up to 56% of paraplegics obtain relief following a high spinal cordotomy (39). However, in a number of patients the pain recurred and consideration must be given to the consequences of raising the level of sensory loss in the already compromised patient.

Cordectomy. The use of cordectomy as a pain relieving measure is controversial. Early studies (4) found that cordectomy was unsuccessful in producing long term relief and more recently cases are described in which pain was felt even after verified total spinal transection (12). However, more recent studies have indicated a better success rate with removal of the cord at least two to three segments above the level of injury (5). This success is presumably due to removal of the focus of aberrant neuronal activity in the spinal cord described previously in this article. Despite these reports of pain relief many spinally injured patients are understandably reluctant to consider removal of sections of their spinal cord.

Other surgical procedures that have been used with varying results in the management of SCI pain include commissurotomy, dorsal rhizotomy and surgical sympathectomy.

Psychological Treatment

The patient with SCI undergoes a huge adjustment in relationships, lifestyle, vocation and self-image that need to be addressed. Pain report may be an expression of difficulty in adjustment and, therefore, psychological approaches that attempt to deal with these issues may be helpful in reducing the experience of pain.

Physical Treatment

Physical treatment is important in the management of SCI pain particularly in the case of musculoskeletal pain. Changes in posture, exercises, adjustments to wheelchairs and other forms of physical treatment modalities may be helpful in treating pain that is arising from a mechanical source.

FUTURE DIRECTIONS

There are many questions that remain unanswered about SCI pain. We are still unclear as to the mechanisms that underlie this pain, and there is a dearth of controlled studies which examine the effectiveness of treatment. Therefore, there exists at both a basic and a clinical level a need for studies which elucidate SCI pain mechanisms and which present a rational approach to its management.

REFERENCES

1. Donovan WH, Dimitrijevic MR, Dahm L, Dimitrijevic M: Neurophysiological approaches to chronic pain following spinal cord injury. Paraplegia 20:135-146, 1982
2. Bonica JJ: Introduction: Semantic, epidemiologic, and educational issues. Pain and Central Nervous System Disease, The Central Pain Syndromes. Edited by Casey KL. New York, Raven Press, 1991, pp. 13-29
3. Holmes G: Pain of central origin. Contributions to Medical and Biological Research, Vol. 1. New York, PB Hoeber, 1919, pp. 235-246
4. Davis L, Martin J: Studies upon spinal cord injuries. J Neurosurg 4:483-491, 1947
5. Nashold BS: Paraplegia and pain. Deafferentation Pain Syndromes: Pathophysiology and Treatment. Edited by Nashold BS, Ovelmen-Levitt J. New York, Raven Press, 1991, pp. 301-319
6. Kakulas BA, Smith E, Gaekwad U, et al: The neuropathology of pain and abnormal sensations in human spinal cord injury derived from the clincopathological data base at the Royal Perth Hospital. Recent Achievements in Restorative Neurology, Vol. 3, Altered Sensation

and Pain. Edited by Dimitrijevic MR, Wall PD, Lindblom U. Basel, Karger, 1990, pp. 37-41

7. Summers JD, Rapoff MA, Varghese G, et al: Psychosocial factors in chronic spinal cord injury pain. Pain 47:183-189, 1991
8. Davidoff G, Roth EJ: Clinical characteristics of central (dysesthetic) pain in spinal cord injury patients. Pain and Central Nervous System Disease: The Central Pain Syndromes. Edited by Casey KL. New York, Raven Press, 1991, pp. 77-83
9. Cremer S, Maynard F, Davidoff G: The reflex sympathetic dystrophy syndrome associated with traumatic myelopathy: Report of 5 cases. Pain 37:187-192, 1989
10. Davidoff G, Werner RA, Waring WP: Compression mononeuropathies of the upper extremities in chronic paraplegia. Paraplegia 29:17-24, 1991
11. Bors E: Phantom limbs of patients with spinal cord injury. Arch Neurol Psychol 66:610-631, 1951
12. Melzack R, Loeser JD: Phantom body pain in paraplegics: Evidence for a central "pattern generating mechanism" for pain. Pain 4:195-210, 1978
13. Pagni CA: Central pain due to spinal cord and brain stem damage, Textbook of Pain. Edited by Wall PD, Melzack R. London, Churchill Livingstone, 1989, pp. 634-655
14. Tasker RR, Dostrovsky JO: Deafferentation and central pain, Textbook of Pain. Edited by Wall PD, Melzack R. London, Churchill Livingstone, 1989, pp. 154-180
15. Tasker RR, de Carvalho G, Dostrovsky JO: The history of central pain syndromes, with observations concerning pathophysiology and treatment, Pain and Central Nervous System Disease: The Central Pain Syndromes. Edited by Casey KL. New York, Raven Press, 1991, pp. 31-58
16. Kakulas BA, Taylor JR: Pathology of injuries of the vertebral column and spinal cord. Elsevier Science, 21-51, 1992
17. Nixon BJ, Doucette R, Jackson PC, Diamond J: Impulse activity evokes precocious sprouting of nociceptive nerves into denervated skin. Somatosensory Research 2:97-126, 1984
18. Devor M, White D, Goetzl E, Levine J: Eicosanoids increase spontaneous activity of C-fiber nerve endings in rat sciatic nerve neuroma. Neuroreport 3:21-24, 1992
19. Loh L, Nathan PW, Schott GD: Pain due to lesions of central nervous system removed by sympathetic block. Br Med J 282:1026-1028, 1981
20. Sato J, Perl ER: Adrenergic excitation of cutaneous pain receptors induced by peripheral nerve injury. Science 251:1608-1610, 1991
21. Dubner R: Neuronal plasticity and pain following peripheral tissue inflammation or nerve injury, Pain Research and Clinical Management, Vol. 4, Proceedings of the VIth World Congress on Pain. Edited by Bond M, Charlton E, Woolf CJ. Amsterdam, Elsevier, 1991, pp. 263-276

22. Craig AD: Supraspinal pathways and mechanisms relevant to central pain, Pain and Central Nervous System Disease: The Central Pain Syndromes. Edited by Casey KL. New York, Raven Press, 1991, pp. 157-170
23. Dubner R: Neuronal plasticity in the spinal and medullary dorsal horns: A possible role in central pain mechanisms, Pain and Central Nervous System Disease: The Central Pain Syndromes. Edited by Casey KL. New York, Raven Press, 1991, pp. 143-155
24. Loeser JD: Definition, aetiology and neurological assessment of pain originating in the nervous system following deafferentation. Pain Suppl:S81-S80, 1981
25. Woolf CJ, Shortland P, Coggeshall RE: Peripheral nerve injury triggers central sprouting of myelinated afferents. Nature 355:75-78, 1992
26. Hunt SP, Pini A, Evan G: Induction of c-fos-like protein in spinal cord neurons following sensory stimulation. Nature 328:632-634, 1987
27. Zimmerman M: Central nervous mechanisms modulating pain-related information: Do they become deficient after lesions of the peripheral or central nervous system? Pain and Central Nervous System Disease: The Central Pain Syndromes. Edited by Casey KL. New York, Raven Press, 1991, pp. 183-199
28. Loeser JD, Ward AA, White LE: Chronic deafferentation of human spinal cord neurons. J Neurosurg 29:48-50, 1968
29. Lenz FA, Kwan HC, Dostrovsky JO, Tasker RR: Characteristics of the bursting pattern of action potentials that occurs in the thalamus of patients with central pain. Brain Res 496:357-360, 1989
30. Lenz FA: The thalamus and central pain syndromes: Human and animal studies, Pain and Central Nervous System Disease: The Central Pain Syndromes. Edited by Casey KL. New York, Raven Press, 1991, pp. 171-182
31. Beric A, Dimitrijevic MR, Lindblom U: Central dysesthesia syndrome in spinal cord injury patients. Pain 34:109-116, 1988
32. Farkash AE, Portenoy RK: The pharmacological management of chronic pain in the paraplegic patient. J Am Paraplegia Soc 9:41-50, 1986
33. Sandford PR, Lindblom LB, Haddox JD: Amitriptyline and carbamazepine in the treatment of dysesthetic pain in spinal cord injury. Arch Phys Med Rehabil 73:300-301, 1992
34. Backonja M, Gombar KA: Response of central pain syndromes to intravenous lidocaine. J Pain Symptom Manage 7:172-178, 1992
35. Glynn CJ, Jamous MA, Teddy PJ, et al: Role of spinal noradrenergic system in transmission of pain in patients with spinal cord injury. Lancet ii:1249-1250, 1986
36. Beric A: Altered sensation and pain in spinal cord injury. Recent Achievements in Restorative Neurology, Vol. 3, Altered Sensation

and Pain. Edited by Dimitrijevic MR, Wall PD, Lindblom U. Basel, Karger, 1990, pp. 27-36

37. Davis R, Lentini R: Transcutaneous nerve stimulation for treatment of pain in patients with spinal cord injury. Surg Neurol 4:100-101, 1975
38. Friedman AH, Nashold BS: Pain of spinal origin, Neurological Surgery. Edited by Youmans J. Philadelphia, W.B. Saunders, 1989, pp. 3950-3959
39. White JC, Sweet WH: Pain and the Neurosurgeon. Springfield, IL, Charles C. Thomas, 1969

PREVENTION OF POST-HERPETIC NEURALGIA

A. P. Winnie

While the pain of herpes zoster usually disappears with or shortly after the healing of the skin lesions, the most common (and dreaded) complication of the disease is persistent pain, termed post-herpetic neuralgia. Post-herpetic neuralgia can vary in degree from a mild, bothersome discomfort to severely debilitating and agonizing pain. Severe post-herpetic neuralgia, most frequently described as a burning pain, is unique in that it may occur spontaneously and continuously without stimulation, though it is exacerbated by light tough and/or temperature changes. Post-herpetic neuralgia produces significant physical, mental, and emotional incapacitation, and is associated with a high rate of drug addiction and suicide (1).

The therapeutic benefit of sympathetic blocks in herpes zoster was discovered by coincidence by Rosenak (2), who was utilizing lumbar paravertebral sympathetic blocks to treat a patient with severe peripheral vascular disease. The patient also had developed painful, acute herpes zoster in the gluteal area two days earlier, and following the blocks, the patient had dramatic relief of the zoster pain with drying and crusting of the vesicles within 48 hours. Startled by the seemingly illogical but dramatic effect of sympathetic blocks on acute herpes zoster, Rosenak undertook further trials of this therapeutic modality, and in 21 subsequent patients he obtained relief of pain in 19, with prompt drying and crusting of the vesicles. In one case the sympathetic block was incomplete on the first attempt; and when it was repeated, the patient obtained complete relief. Rosenak's only failure was a patient who had a six-year history of recurrent neuralgia which was frequently accompanied by a rash, and it may be that this patient had zosteriform herpes simplex (3) rather than repetitive episodes of acute herpes zoster. Nonetheless, Rosenak still

T. H. Stanley and M. A. Ashburn (eds.), Anesthesiology and Pain Management, 253–264.

achieved a 95% success rate in his series, an impressive finding in a disease for which there had previously been no treatment whatsoever.

Since Rosenak's original publication a multitude of reports concerning the use of sympathetic nerve blocks for the treatment of acute herpes zoster have appeared sporadically in the literature (2,4-27). Because most of these studies were uncontrolled, Tenicela (28) reconfirmed the efficacy of sympathetic blocks in terminating acute herpes zoster in a double-blind, randomized study. It is important to realize that the data presented in most of the studies cited were obtained in patients treated within one month of the onset of their pain. Colding, who has the largest series of cases in the literature (12,14), has stated that it would appear from his data that the earlier this treatment is started, the more successful it will be. In fact, in his second paper (14) Colding reported that 90% of those patients treated before the eruption was 2 weeks old exhibited a dramatic response to sympathetic block, whereas only 40% of those treated more than 2 weeks after onset, responded to this treatment. Anyone with significant experience treating acute herpes zoster with sympathetic blocks is certainly aware that there is, indeed, a time after which the blocks cease to be effective in terminating acute herpes zoster and preventing post-herpetic neuralgia.

A recent study was undertaken at our institution to determine more precisely the relationship between the time of treatment of acute herpes zoster and the prevention of post-herpetic neuralgia and to utilize this clinical data to support our theory as to the mechanism by which sympathetic blocks provide their therapeutic benefit (20).

The charts of 122 patients treated in the University of Illinois Pain Control Center for pain related to herpes zoster were reviewed retrospectively. Only the records of patients with complete follow-up, whether by personal or telephone interview, were utilized for the study. All patients with complete follow-up were included, regardless of their response to treatment. The technique by which sympathetic blockade was provided, of course, depended on the location of the patient's pain. Patients who had trigeminal, cervical, brachial, or high thoracic nerve involvement received stellate ganglion blocks by the anterior approach; while patients with a thoracic, lumbar, or sacral distribution received epidural blocks. In a few cases where the herpetic lesions did not extend all the way to the midline, intercostal blocks were utilized for thoracic involvement. The local anesthetic agents utilized in the epidural (and intercostal) blocks were administered in a sufficient concentration to produce sensory as well as sympathetic blockade in order to confirm that the level of the blockade was appropriate for the level of the patient's pain. The agents utilized for the blocks included bupivacaine, mepivacaine, lidocaine, and 2-chloroprocaine, all without epinephrine.

In order to assess the importance of time of treatment on the efficacy of sympathetic blockade in terminating acute herpetic pain and in preventing post-herpetic neuralgia, great care was taken to accurately determine the duration of the patient's symptoms prior to the initial treatment and to note carefully the timing of subsequent treatments. Thus, patients were grouped according to the duration of their symptoms prior to the initiation of treatment as follows: Group A consisted of those patients whose treatment occurred less than two weeks following the onset of symptoms; Group B represents those patients treated at least 2 weeks but less than 1 month after the onset of symptoms; Group C patients were treated at least 1 month but less than 2 months after the initial onset of symptoms; the patients in Group D were treated at least 2 months but less than 6 months following their first symptoms; Group E patients were treated at least 6 months but less than 1 year after the initial symptoms; and the patients in Group F were all treated at least 1 year after the onset of their symptoms. In all cases the first sympathetic block was administered on the first visit to the Pain Control Center. The patient was told to return immediately if and when their pain returned for a second block. If a second block was carried out, again the patient was told to return if and when their pain recurred for a third block. If their pain returned after a third block, with rare exceptions, further sympathetic blocks were not administered.

Similarly, the various responses to treatment were grouped as follows: a Type I response indicates complete and permanent relief was achieved after a single block. A Type II response indicates that the first treatment provided pain relief, but though the relief outlasted the effect of the anesthetic (by as long as several days), the pain subsequently returned. However, when it returned, it was significantly less severe, and with this type of response repeated blocks (usually two or three) did provide

permanent pain relief. A Type III response indicates that temporary pain relief was provided by each treatment; but the relief only lasted as long as the local anesthetic, and when the pain returned, the intensity was the same as before the block. However, in this type of response **subsequent** to the series of blocks these patients had a slow, gradual improvement in their pain until they were ultimately (and permanently) pain free. It is significant to note that all of those who exhibited a Type I, II, or III response ultimately became and remained pain free, unlike those exhibiting a Type IV or Type V response: A Type IV response, like the Type III response, indicates that temporary pain relief was provided by each treatment, relief which only lasted as long as the local anesthetic. But **unlike** the Type III response, patients exhibiting a Type IV response, though improved, still had residual pain at the time of follow-up. A Type V response indicates no apparent improvement whatsoever with treatment and residual pain at the time of follow-up. So all patients exhibiting a Type IV or V response continued to have pain in spite of the treatment.

All patients included in this study were followed up by telephone. In addition to the data concerning age, sex, distribution of lesions, duration of symptoms prior to treatment, number of treatments and response to treatment, information was obtained concerning any complications of the treatment, any co-existent diseases and any medications being taken concomitantly.

The results of this study were analyzed using a contingency table (Table 1), which gives the number of patients in each group (A-F), and within each group, the number exhibiting each type of response (I-V). This table was then analyzed by a chi-square approximation (29). The results are tabulated in Table 1 and presented graphically in Figure 1, which indicates dramatically the relationship between the type of response to treatment and the time interval between the initial symptoms and the initiation of treatment. Of the 21 patients in Group A, all 21 (100%) had complete relief of their pain at the time of follow-up: 7 in this Group demonstrated a Type I response, 11 demonstrated at Type II response, and 3 a Type III response. Of the 13 patients in Group B, 12 (92.3%) were pain free at the time of follow-up, and one was improved, though he did still have some residual pain: 3 of the patients in this Group exhibited a

Table 1. Number of patients of each group demonstrating each type of response.

	Type of Response					
	I	II	III	IV	V	I, II, III Combined
Group A n=21	7(33.3%)	11(52.4%)	3(14.3%)	—	—	100%
Group B n=13	3(23%)	7(54%)	2(15%)	1(8%)	—	92.3%
Group C n=15	—	10(67%)	2(13.3%)	1(6.7%)	2(13.3%)	80%
Group D n=28	2(7%)	2(7%)	1(4%)	9(32%)	14(50%)	18%
Group E n=19	2(10.5%)	2(10.5%)	—	4(21%)	11(58%)	21%
Group F n=26	—	1(3.5%)	—	4(15.5%)	21(81%)	4%
Combined Groups	Prevented Post-herpetic Neuralgia			Developed Post-herpetic Neuralgia		Prevented Post-herpetic Neuralgia

Except for the combined groups (far right column) and the relationship between the type of response and the development of post-herpetic neuralgia (bottom line), this table represents a contingency table giving the number of patients classified into response Classes I-V and into Groups A-F (defined by time elapsed between onset of symptoms and institution of treatment). When analyzed by a chi-square approximation of a 5 x 6 contingency table (21), chi-square = 91.24 with 20° of freedom (P<0.0001), demonstrating that the effect of time elapsed between onset of symptoms and institution of therapy has a highly significant effect in the type of response.

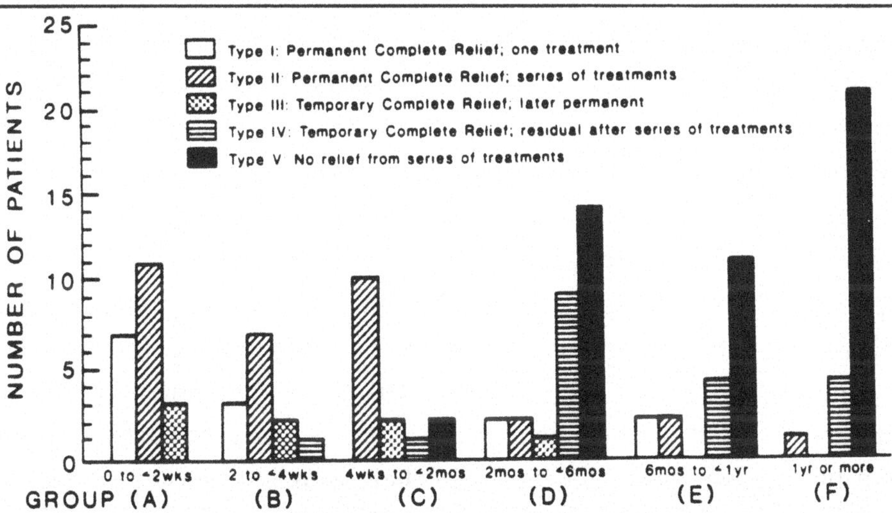

Figure 1. Graphic representation of the relationship between time of treatment and type of response (see text).

Type I response, 7 a Type II response, and 2 a Type III response, and 1 a Type IV response.

Of the 15 patients in Group C, 12 (80%) were pain free at the time of follow-up, while 3 had residual pain; of the patients who were pain free at the time of follow-up, none exhibited a Type I response, 10 exhibited a Type II response, and 2 a Type III response. Of those who still had pain at the time of follow-up, 1 represented a Type IV response, while 2 exhibited a Type V response.

Of the 28 patients in Group D, 5 (18%) were pain free at the time of follow-up, while 23 still had pain: of the 5 who were pain free at the time of follow-up 2 had exhibited a Type I response, 2 a Type II response, and 1 a Type III response. Of those who had persistent pain at the time of follow-up, 9 represented a Type IV response and 14 a Type V response.

Of the 19 patients in Group E, 4 (21%) were pain free, and 15 had persistent pain: of the patients who were pain free at the time of follow-up, 2 had exhibited a Type I response and 2 a Type II response. Of those patients with persistent pain at the time of follow-up, 4 represented a Type IV response and 11 a Type V response.

Of the 26 patients in Group F, only 1 (4%) was pain free, with all of the other 25 complaining of persistent pain: the patient who was pain free at the time of follow-up had exhibited a Type II response, while 4 of the patients with persistent pain represented a Type IV response and 21 a Type V response.

With respect to complications specifically related to the treatment, only 3 of the 134 patients who received epidural blocks developed hypotension, and in each case the hypotension responded promptly to intravenous fluid therapy and/or small doses of ephedrine without further sequelae. In two of the patients treated with epidural injections, the dura was inadvertently punctured. Of these two, one had no sequelae and went home after remaining supine several hours, while the other experienced a severe spinal headache with nausea and vomiting and ultimately required an epidural blood patch to obtain relief. Interestingly, in spite of having had such a severe headache, this patient remained enthusiastic about the treatment, because it had provided complete relief from her herpetic pain. Of the 135 stellate ganglion blocks carried out, only one resulted in undesirable side effects, which in this case consisted of hoarseness, blurred vision, and nausea, all of which resolved spontaneously without treatment.

Certainly the above study corroborates Colding's impression that the earlier sympathetic blocks are initiated, the more successful they will be in terminating the acute phase of the disease and preventing post-herpetic neuralgia.

As may be seen in Table 1 (I, II, III Combined column, far right), 100% of the patients in Group A were pain free at the time of follow-up. However, only 85% were pain free upon completion of their last sympathetic block. In Group B 92.3% of the patients were pain free at the time of follow-up, though again, only 77% were pain free at the time of their last block. In Group C, while the overall success rate decreased somewhat, nonetheless, 80% of the patients were pain-free at the time of follow-up, 67% of whom were free of pain following their last block. It is important to note that when the initial treatment was delayed beyond two months, as was the case in Groups D, E, and F, the overall success rate fell drastically to 18%, 21%, and 4%, respectively. Interestingly enough, at six months and beyond, it is only those patients who obtained relief at the time of the last treatment that are pain free at the time of follow-up, i.e., there are no Type III responses.

From these data it would appear that while success in terminating acute herpes zoster is greatest when the patient is treated within the first few weeks, if treatment is begun within two months, the chance of preventing post-herpetic neuralgia is still almost 80%. To test statistically the difference between treatment before and after two months in terms of preventing post-herpetic neuralgia (i.e., whether 2 months is the latest that this therapy will provide a reasonable expectation of preventing post-herpetic neuralgia), the data were analyzed using a contingency table (Table 2) and applying the Fisher Exact test (30). Such analysis indicates the highest statistical significance ($P<0.000001$). Nonetheless, in spite of the low incidence of Type I and Type II responses to sympathetic blocks when they were administered, more than 2 months after the initial onset of symptoms, this form of therapy should be tried no matter how late after the initial symptoms the patient is seen, since the occasional success achieved represents 100% success to that patient. And even if the treatment fails, it is innocuous in competent hands, as attested to by the fact

Table 2. Relationship between time of treatment and prevention of post - herpetic neuralgia (residual pain).

Time Elapsed Between Initial Symptoms and Treatment	No Residual Pain	Residual Pain	Totals
4 weeks to < 2 months	45	4	49
> 2 months	10	63	73
Totals	55	67	122

In order to test the effect of considering 60 days as the longest elapsed time (between the on set of symptoms and the institution of therapy) which will give reasonable expectation of not having residual pain after cessation of therapy, the data were analyzed using a contin gency table giving the numbers of patients classified on the basis of response (no residual pain or residual pain) and time of treatment (60 days or less or more than 60 days). This table was analyzed by the Fisher Exact Test (22), giving a P value of <0.000001. Thus, the proportion of patients treated within 60 days of onset of disease who do not have residual pain after cessation of treatment is highly significantly greater than those who are treated more than 60 days after the onset of the disease.

that we experienced no serious complications in our entire study, in spite of the fact that most of the blocks were performed by residents and fellows.

Any theory as to how sympathetic blockade terminates the acute phase of herpes zoster must also explain how sympathetic blockade prevents the development of post-herpetic neuralgia if a patient is treated early enough and why it fails to do so when treatment is delayed. We feel that such a theory is as follows: It is well established that shortly after reactivation, the Varicella-Zoster virus moves rapidly out along the course of the involved nerve(s), producing an inflammatory reaction that is responsible for the initial hyperesthesia, dysesthesia, pain, and ultimately, the characteristic vesicular eruption (31). Such an inflammatory response typically produces intense sympathetic stimulation, and Selander has recently demonstrated experimentally that sympathetic stimulation can reduce blood flow in the intraneural capillary bed by as much as 93% (32). Furthermore, Lundborg has shown that when such ischemia is prolonged, there is anoxic damage to the endoneurial capillary endothelium with leakage of albumen, and the formation of endoneurial edema. This edema, in and of itself, can cause increased intrafascicular pressure and result in even greater impairment of endoneurial blood flow and ultimately irreversible nerve damage (33). In addition to the production of hypoxic damage, such a reduction in blood flow results in glucose deprivation, which like hypoxia produces preferential destruction of large nerve fibers with survival and/or recovery of the less metabolically active small fibers (34).

It would appear, then, from the available laboratory data that in the acute phase of herpes zoster the virus (or its toxin) is capable of producing severe sympathetic stimulation which results in ischemia of the involved nerves; and it would appear from our clinical data that, after the first few weeks, the reversal of the results of the ischemia (the hypoxic, hypoglucic, and toxic damage to large fibers) takes progressively longer and requires a greater number of sympathetic blocks. And finally, also from our clinical data, it would appear that after two months the ischemic damage becomes irreversible.

Both Fink and Lundborg have demonstrated experimentally in animals that, unlike large fibers, small fibers are able to survive prolonged periods of ischemia and still recover full function (33,35). That this is also true in man is supported histologically by the work of Noordenbos (36), who many years ago compared cross-sections of post-herpetic and normal nerves under the light microscope and found that in the post-herpetic nerve, the vast majority of the large nerve fibers have been destroyed and replaced by fibrous tissue. As a result, unlike the situation in a normal nerve, where the population of nerve fibers is predominately composed of large fibers, Noordenbos found that in the post-herpetic nerve there was a predominance of small fibers, a phenomenon he referred to as "fiber dissociation." Correlating these histological findings with the clinical picture of spontaneous pain in the post-herpetic patient, Noordenbos postulated that large fibers tend to inhibit the entry of noxious impulses into the central nervous system, while small fibers tend to enhance such entry. Therefore, in the post-herpetic nerve, "fiber dissociation" abolishes the normal inhibitory effect of large fiber predominance with the result that not only is the entry of noxious impulses into the spinal cord enhanced, many impulses that are not ordinarily noxious are interpreted as noxious by the altered large/small fiber balance.

The similarity of Noordenbos' theory to the Gate Control Theory conceptualized by Melzack and Wall 6 years later (37) is remarkable in itself; but more importantly, it is critical to our hypothesis as to the mechanism by which sympathetic blocks produce their therapeutic benefit.

Since the characteristic lesion in post-herpetic neuralgia is the death and replacement of large nerve fibers within the nerve, clearly, if the sympathetic response responsible for the ischemic state of the nerve is interrupted before the changes in the large fibers become irreversible, the symptoms of acute herpes zoster disappear, and the development of post-herpetic neuralgia is avoided. It would appear from the data obtained in the present study that this is precisely what has happened in those patients who had a favorable response to sympathetic blocks. It would also appear from this study that if this therapy is instituted within the first few weeks of the onset of the disease, in most cases, reversal of the ischemic changes is almost immediate, whereas if treatment is delayed, the changes secondary to the ischemia become progressively more severe; and after about two months, large fiber death and fiber dissociation make the process virtually irreversible.

Interestingly, the advent of acyclovir for the "specific" treatment of herpes zoster at first appeared to represent a replacement for the nerve block therapy of this disease. However, it now has been shown that while acyclovir is effective in terminating the acute phase of herpes zoster in a high percentage of cases, it does not prevent against the development of post-herpetic neuralgia (38). As a matter of fact, it may even enhance this possibility, since in those patients in whom acyclovir fails to terminate the acute phase of the disease, the time required for a course of acyclovir only serves to delay the institution of sympathetic blocks by several weeks. Thus, because the effectiveness of sympathetic blocks in terminating the disease process is related to the time of therapy, the delay to administer acyclovir could reduce the efficacy of the sympathetic blocks, once they are administered.

REFERENCES

1. Bonica JJ: Thoracic segmental and intercostal neuralgia, The Management of Pain, Chapter 26. Philadelphia, Lea & Febiger, 1953, p. 865
2. Rosenak S: Procaine injection treatment of herpes zoster. Lancet 2:1056-1058, 1938
3. Juel-Jensen BE, MacCalum FO: Herpes simplex varicella and zoster, Clinical Manifestations and Treatment. Philadelphia, JB Lippincott, 79-116, 1972

4. Leger L, Audoly P: Traitement du zona par l'infiltration stellaire. La Presse Med 50:588, 1942
5. Street A: The use of sympathetic nerve block in: (1) herpes zoster (2) Bell's palsy. Mississippi Doctor 20:480-481, 1943
6. Verhaeghe A, Merlen J, Lagache G. Sur un cas d'algies brachiales post-zonateuses gueries par infiltration stellaire. La Presse Med 194351:249,
7. Findley T, Patzer R: The treatment of herpes zoster by paravertebral procaine block. JAMA 128:1217-1219, 1945
8. Rougues L: Traitement du zona par l'infiltration des ganglions sympathiques. La Presse Med 53:716, 1945
9. Lovell WW: The treatment of herpes zoster. South Med J 39:777-779, 1946
10. Ferris LM, Martin GH: The use of sympathetic nerve block in the ambulatory patient with special reference to its use in herpes zoster. Ann Intern Med 32:257-260, 1950
11. Marmer MJ: Acute herpes zoster: Successful treatment by continuous epidural analgesia. Calif Med 103:277-279, 1965
12. Colding A: The effect of regional sympathetic blocks in the treatment of herpes zoster. Acta Anaesth Scand 13:133-141, 1969
13. Tamesa T, Wakasugi B, Yuda Y, et al: Nerve block therapy in the treatment of herpes zoster. Masui 20:903-905, 1971
14. Colding A: Treatment of pain: Organization of a pain clinic: Treatment of acute herpes zoster. Proc R Soc Med 66:541-543, 1973
15. Gale DA: The management of neuralgias complicating herpes zoster. Practitioner 219:794-798, 1973
16. Motegi K, Bamba S, Shimizu M, et al: A case of topical application of rifampicin with blocks of the infraorbital nerve and stellate ganglion in the treatment of herpes zoster. J Jpn Stomatol Soc 40:80-84, 1973
17. Miyazaki T, Masaharu O: The nerve block treatment of herpes zoster. Am Soc Anesthesiol Annual Meeting Abstracts, pp. 173-174, 1974
18. Tamesa T, Wakasugi B, Yuda Y: Nerve block therapy in the treatment of herpes zoster in the pain clinic. Masui 22:333-339, 1974
19. Masud KZ, Forster KJ: Sympathetic block in herpes zoster. Am Family Physician 12:142-144, 1975
20. Mani M, Keh L, Lee KN, et al: Sympathetic blockade for herpes zoster and postherpetic neuralgia. Am Soc Anesthesiol Annual Meeting Abstracts, p. 469, 1976
21. Rickles JA: Ambulatory use of sympathetic nerve blocks: Present day clinical indications. Angiology 28:394-400, 1977
22. Perkins HM, Hanlon PR: Epidural injection of local anesthetic and steroids for relief of pain secondary to herpes zoster. Arch Surg 113:253-254, 1978
23. Bauman J: Treatment of acute herpes zoster neuralgia by epidural injection or stellate ganglion block. Anesthesiology 51:S223, 1979

24. LaFlamme MY, Labrecque B, Mignault G: Zona ophthalmique: Traitement de la nevralgie zonateuse par infiltrations stellaires repetees. Can J Ophthalmol 14:99-101, 1979
25. Schreuder M, Fothergill WT: Shingles: a belt of roses from hell. Brit Med J 1:5, 1979
26. Bettinger R, Patrick L, Thompson R: Outpatient therapy prevents or relieves herpes zoster pain. Anesth News 7:1, 1981
27. Riopelle JM, Naraghi M, Grush KP: Chronic neuralgia incidence following local anesthetic therapy for herpes zoster. Arch Dermatol 120:747-750, 1984
28. Tenicela R, Lovasik D, Eaglstein W: Treatment of herpes zoster with sympathetic blocks. Clin J Pain 1:63-67, 1985
29. Brownlee KA: Statistical Theory and Methodology in Science and Engineering. New York, John Wiley & Sons, 1960, p. 155
30. Conover WJ: Practical Nonparametric Statistics. New York, John Wiley & Sons, 1971, pp. 140-149
31. Burgoon CF, Jr, Burgoon JS: The natural history of herpes zoster. JAMA 164:265-269, 1957
32. Selander D, Mansson LG, Karlsson L, Svanvic J: Adrenergic vasoconstriction in peripheral nerves of the rabbit. Anesthesiology 62:6-10, 1985
33. Lundborg G: Structure and function of the intraneural microvessels as related to trauma, edema formation, and nerve function. J Bone & Joint Surg 57-A:938-948, 1975
34. Fink BR, Cairns AM: A bioenergetic basis for peripheral nerve fiber dissociation. Pain 12:307-317, 1982
35. Fink BR, Cairns AM: Differential tolerance of mammalian myelinated and unmyelinated nerve fibers to oxygen lack. Reg Anes 7:2-6, 1982
36. Noordenbos W: Pain. Elsevier, Amsterdam, 1959
37. Melzack R, Wall PD: Pain mechanisms: New theory. Science 150:971-979, 1965
38. McKendrick MD, McGill JI, Wood MJ: Lack of effect of acyclovir on postherpetic neuralgia. Br Med J 298:431, 1989

OPIOIDS AND THE MANAGEMENT OF NON-MALIGNANT CHRONIC PAIN

Bradford D. Hare, M.D., Ph.D.

Systemic opioid analgesics are of critical importance in the treatment of acute pain and the pain resulting from malignancy. On the other hand, the role for opioids in the management of non-cancer chronic pain (NCCP) is controversial (1); some authorities contend that for most NCCP the opioids are not helpful (2,3) and yet others feel that opioids can be safe and effective for long term use, at least in certain subgroups of this population (4,5). This chapter will explore arguments on both sides and attempt to give some practical guidelines for opioid management in this patient population.

Most physicians treating NCCP find certain patients for whom long term opioid treatment is effective and appropriate (6). Little published information suggests how these patients might be selected. Portenoy reports a series of patients with mostly neurogenic pain who experienced good pain relief with opioids with long-term treatment and yet show little tendency toward tolerance or escalation of dose (4). He concludes that NCCP can be successfully treated with opioids and that opioids are not more widely used in this setting because of physician fears and misconceptions about prescribing sufficient opioid doses. He implies that more aggressive treatment of NCCP with opioids would result in greater benefits. But many patients seeking help for NCCP are already using substantial doses of opioids, alone or in combination with other mood-altering drugs. Yet relief judged by patient self-report is no better than similar patients not taking opioids (7) and is insufficient to allow a desired level of comfort and function. Thus further help and other interventions are sought. In view of limited efficacy for pain, why do patients continue to receive and take these medications? Several possible reasons are listed in Table 1 and explained more fully in the following text.

T. H. Stanley and M. A. Ashburn (eds.), Anesthesiology and Pain Management, 265–272.

Table 1. Reasons other than pain relief to explain opioid use in NCCP.

1.	Relief of "distress" (a combination of nociception, stress, anxiety, depression, etc.)
2.	Only treatment option made available to patient
3.	Patient fears return of pain if medication is stopped
4.	To sustain opioid habituation and dependency

1. While reported pain relief may be limited, these medications may result in an overall improvement in the patient's level of distress (a combination of nociception, stress, anxiety, and depression). "Pain" rating may better reflect the patient's distress rather than nociception *per se* (2, 3). As opioids have multiple pharmacologic effects, the patient can conceivably get relief from either the analgesic effects or many of the other non-analgesic effects of these compounds. As variable combinations of pain, depression and anxiety usually coexist in the chronic pain patient, it is often hard to determine which pharmacological effect might be most important in relieving distress in these patients. If analgesia is not the primary effect, opioids should be avoided as depression and anxiety can be more appropriately treated by other means without the risks of long term opioid use.

2. The prescribing physician may give the patient no alternative to opioids to control pain thus the patient feels that having a small degree of control with opioids is better than nothing. Physicians may be prone to act rather than state they have no treatment to offer and when treatment options seemingly have been exhausted, medications are resorted to as an attempt to give the patient some relief, even when the results are marginal.

3. The patient reports fear of when opioids are discontinued pain may worsen. Under these circumstances the cessation of medications may lead to increasing pain due to heightening of anxiety and anticipatory fear and the patient finds his/her beliefs reinforced. Certainly as the short-acting analgesics wear off the patient may find a heightened sensitivity to nociception, another reinforcing factor.

4. Opioid habituation and dependency can occur in the chronic pain patient. Frequent and escalating opioid dosage may be necessary to prevent signs of withdrawal and worsening of symptoms. The patient

may report taking larger doses of opioids and a need to awaken during the night to take additional analgesics; the patient is likely awakened by early signs of withdrawal. Some NCCP patients, although in our experience their numbers are relatively small, do have a primary medication abuse problem and use pain as an excuse to obtain opioids or other desired medications. This problem will be addressed later.

The primary indication for opioid therapy is in the treatment of pain which is opioid sensitive. Opioid sensitivity may be defined as a source of pain which can be predictably and effectively treated with opioids while still preserving a selective analgesic effect. In the treatment of acute and cancer pain, opioid sensitivity for many types of pain has been demonstrated and yet even in these categories there are certain painful conditions not well treated with opioids. The opioid sensitivity of the various types of NCCP is recognized largely by clinical experience. The textbook review by Bonica and others (8) would suggest that most NCCP is not predictably sensitive to treatment with opioids and many other more successful treatments are available. Yet for some patients opioids may be helpful. Neither the etiology of pain nor the patient's characteristics are a good predictor of a positive response. Patients with NCCP are often quite complex and nociception may be only one component of their overall problem. Even if opioids are successful in treating the nociceptive component, other symptoms leading to distress may persist and if not addressed can overshadow a partial success with opioids.

In summary, there are many reasons why NCCP patients may use opioids in the long term. Specific analgesic effect can be important but may only partially explain this use. For many patients the pharmacologic side-effects which suppress co-existing symptoms may be a better explanation for this long term use (9). Yet in some NCCP patients opioid use may be beneficial and safe but few guidelines exist for their successful selection. The following section will attempt to deal with this problem.

CHOOSING THE PATIENT APPROPRIATE FOR OPIOID TREATMENT

The NCCP patient must first be evaluated from a multi-disciplinary view point as not only nociception but many other factors may contribute to the chronic pain problem. These must be recognized and a comprehensive treatment plan formulated which addresses the various contributors to the overall problem. Records should be obtained and reviewed regarding past and present treatments. A complete history and physical examination is performed with an emphasis on the pain problem and issues which may be contributing to the pain problem. Psycho-social information should be obtained not only to evaluate the impact of the pain but also to identify the important factors which may contribute to or perpetuate the pain complaints. The medication history will reveal that most patients have tried opioid analgesics and their response may be a crude indication of opioid sensitivity. In other words, the patient who obtained only a small degree of relief while on hefty doses of opioids will probably respond better to non-opioid therapy. On the other hand, the patient who clearly gets considerable relief that corresponds well to the pharmacologic effects of opioids, i.e., appropriate onset and duration of relief, etc., may show potential long term benefit from opioid use. The history may indicate that the patient was better relieved with muscle relaxants, barbiturates or benzodiazepines than with opioids. As these substances are not analgesics but can act as anti-anxiety drugs, this report would suggest the patient's primary problem may be anxiety rather than pain (nociception) and opioids would not have any specific analgesic effect in these patients. Based on the evaluation of the patient, therapy should be aimed at improving the patient's function and hopefully, comfort level, by effecting "curative" changes. From a behavioral, rehabitational and medical standpoint, opioid therapy must always be considered as <u>symptomatic</u> relief and is unlikely, particularly alone, to alter the debilitating problems of NCCP.

If opioid use is found to be significant at the time of the initial evaluation, the role of these medications in the patient's overall condition must be better identified. While the patient may indicate these medications offer some degree of relief, the negative side of the medications must likewise always be considered. Is the relief obtained more than offset by the detrimental effects of these medications? A straight forward way to answer this question is to reassess the patient when medication-free on an in-patient or out-patient basis depending on the degree of medication use. The patient can be tapered off opioids and other medications which may not be appropriate. Generally the patient is monitored as to medication intake for 48 hours and then is withdrawn from these medications using a "pill taper." Likewise, the medications may be converted to an equivalent amount of methadone which is withdrawn at approximately 20% a day. Pain diaries should be kept by the patient during this period to indicate the patient's subjective response to drug withdrawal. This process is reviewed elsewhere (10,11). After this process the patient may fall into one of three categories:

Category 1: The patient refuses to be withdrawn from medications despite assurances that discomfort will be minimized, pain is not likely to be worse, and new therapies are likely to be more beneficial. If the patient has demonstrated a long history of opioid use for this problem or others, they insist that the medication is not a problem for them and particularly if they have demonstrated illegal activities to obtain drugs, a primary drug problem must be considered. Table 2 gives some indicators as to history and patient behavior that increase the likelihood that primary substance abuse is the problem rather than a NCCP with dependency on medications. A primary drug problem is best initially treated in a substance abuse program. Once a patient has demonstrated compliance in a drug rehabilitation program, the pain problem can be reassessed if needed (pain may no longer be a problem). Few NCCP patients fit into this category, but those who do must be recognized.

Table 2. Characteristics of a primary substance abuse problem. [From Hare and Lipman (10)]

1. Obtained by deception or illegal activity
2. Compulsive drug use—securing medication is primary goal
3. History of or ongoing alcoholism or illicit drug use
4. Unwilling to consider or comply with non-medication therapy
5. Patient's unreasonable insistence that he has no drug problem
6. Medications taken not as directed and to excess
7. Failed drug treatment program

Category 2: The detoxification process results in no change or a decrease in subjective pain report and function is maintained or improved. One can conclude that the pain problem is not opioid sensitive and opioids should not be a part of therapy in the future. The same would hold true for other psychoactive medications withdrawn. This category represents the largest group of patients.

Category 3: The patient experiences increased pain as opioids are withdrawn. This group can be challenging and difficult to assess. If the patient reports increased pain but observational data would suggest no reduction in function or level of comfort, opioids should not be reinstituted for only the complaint of pain. If, on the other hand, there is a clear reduction of function as apparently related to increased nociception, then opioid therapy might be considered, particularly if no other means of reducing nociception is available or if other options have been exhausted.

The reintroduction of opioids into the patient's therapy should only be done when treatment has otherwise been optimized. In other words, the multidisciplinary approach has been effective in addressing other aspects of the patient's care, including coexisting depression, anxiety, physical deconditioning and environmental factors which may be contributing to the pain problem. Once these are no longer felt to be important factors and yet the patient is still complaining of pain which is opioid sensitive, even though improvement has been realized in other areas, then opioids may be reintroduced. Assuming a rather constant source of pain, the patient should be placed on time contingent opioids at a dose which has been titrated to efficacy but not over medication. At this point it is important, not only to consider the patient's subjective report of pain relief, but also their level of function and the side effects produced by the medication. When pain relief and function improve and side effects do not lead to a significant compromise then the opioids may prove to be an important part of long term therapy. If only subjective pain relief is obtained and yet there is no improvement in function then it is difficult to justify long term use of these medications (2,3,12). Another similar approach is described by Chabal, et al (13).

If opioids are to be used, the following guidelines in Table 3 should be followed: 1) Minimal, effective opioid doses should be used. 2) Long-acting drugs (i.e., methadone) or time-release dose forms (i.e., MS-

Table 3. Guidelines for long-term opioid administration for continuous pain.

1. Use minimal, effective dose
2. Use long-acting dose forms
3. Use time-contingent administration, not PRN
4. Avoid parenteral routes of administration unless patient is NPO
5. Spinal routes of administration is inadvisable

Contin®) should be used for the patient with continuous pain. Short-acting drugs would be appropriate only in the patients with pain predictably related to activity or other factors where these medications could be taken in anticipation of these events. Short-acting opioids for continuous pain give uneven therapeutic effect and need to be taken frequently. This is disruptive to the patient in terms of consistency in pain relief and disruption of sleep at night when medications must be taken. 3) For continuous pain these medications should be used on a time contingent schedule, not PRN. 4) Parenteral routes of administration should be avoided unless the patient is unable to take oral medications. Intramuscular and intermittent intravenous administration is to be avoided as the drug effects are transient and inconsistent. The transdermal fentanyl patch, an expensive dose form, achieves consistent serum levels with long-term use, but is not necessary or advantageous when the patient can take oral medications. 5) The use of spinal opioids is inadvisable in the NCCP. The efficacy of spinal opioids in treating this difficult patient population has not been well demonstrated, and the long-term use of spinal opioids results in problems with tolerance, escalating dose, and loss of efficacy. In addition, equipment failure and the potential for infection makes management of these patients very complicated.

The role of opioids in the management of acute and cancer pain is well established, but is not yet defined for the NCCP patient. The majority of these patients will respond to a multi-disciplinary treatment program aimed at improved function and pain. For most patients, opioids will not improve their overall condition. A small identifiable group of patients may get relief from opioids when pain is otherwise not addressed by the above approach. This group can be stabilized on small opioid doses, receive relief and yet experience minimal side effects with little problem of tolerance or escalation of dose.

REFERENCES:

1. Turk DC, Brody MC. Chronic opioid therapy for persistent noncancer pain: Panacea or oxymoron? APS Bulletin 1:1-6, 1991
2. Fordyce WE. On opioids and treatment targets. APS Bulletin 1:1-4, 1991
3. Fordyce WE. Opioids, pain and behavioral outcomes. APS Journal 1:282-284, 1992
4. Portenoy PK. Chronic opioid therapy in non-malignant pain. J Pain Symptom Manage 5:S46-S62, 1990
5. Zenz M, Strumpf M, Tryba M. Long-term oral opioid therapy in patients with chronic nonmalignant pain. J Pain Symptom Manage 7:69-77, 1992
6. Turk DC, Brody MC. What positions do APS's physician members take on chronic opioid therapy? APS Bulletin 2:1, 1992
7. Chabal C, Mariano AJ, Chaney EF. Patterns of narcotic, sedative, hypnotic and adjunctive medication use on intake and after six months of pain clinic treatment (abstract). American Pain Society Meeting, San Diego, CA, October 1992, p. 52
8. Bonica JJ, Loeser JD, Chapman CR, Fordyce WE. The management of pain. Philadelphia, Lea & Febiger, 1990
9. Turner JA, Calsyn DA, Fordyce WE, Ready LB. Drug utilization patterns in chronic pain patients. Pain 12:357, 1982
10. Hare BD, Lipman AG. Uses and misuses of medication in the management of chronic, noncancer pain. Problems in Anesthesia. 4:577-589, 1990
11. Buckley FP, Sizemore WA, Charlton JE. Medication management in patients with chronic non-malignant pain. A review of the use of a drug withdrawal protocol. Pain 26:153, 1986
12. Brena SF, Sanders SH. Opioids in nonmalignant pain: Question in search of answers. Clin J Pain 7:342, 1991
13. Chabal C, Jacobson L, Chaney EF, Mariano AI. Narcotics for chronic pain: Yes or no? A useless dichotomy. APS Journal 1(4):276, 1992

EPIDURAL STEROIDS

A. P. Winnie

INTRODUCTION

Injection into various parts of the peridural space has been advocated for the management of sciatica since 1930 (1), but with the findings of Mixter and Barr (2) in 1934, linking the signs and symptoms of sciatica with a herniated nucleus pulposus, surgery has continued to be the definitive therapy for this problem. However, over the years, except in patients with a rapidly progressive neural deficit, surgery has provided disappointing therapeutic results, so efforts to find a non-surgical therapeutic approach have continued. From a theoretical point of view, two approaches to the problem of non-surgical therapy have been developed, one aiming to remove the etiologic mechanism and the other aiming to modify the response to that mechanism.

CHEMONUCLEOLYSIS

The approach which attempts to remove the disc without surgery was first described by Lyman Smith (3), who in 1963 reported a procedure which he termed "chemonucleolysis," in which chymopapain was injected percutaneously into the involved disc. By depolymerizing the cementing protein of the chondromucoid complex, chymopapain was said to reduce the molecular size and viscosity of the nucleus pulposus, resulting in chemical decompression. While Smith was able to provide complete relief in slightly over 80% of his patients (4), not all reports indicated similar success rates (5). Though chemonucleolysis appeared to be a simple procedure in expert hands, it painful and required the administration of a general anesthetic. In addition, for the first 12 to 36 hours following the injection, there was a significant incidence of severe lumbar

T. H. Stanley and M. A. Ashburn (eds.), Anesthesiology and Pain Management, 273–280.

muscle spasm. Most importantly, there was a 1-2% incidence of anaphylaxis associated with this procedure (6).

EPIDURAL AND INTRATHECAL STEROIDS

The other approach to non-surgical therapy seeks not to treat the etiologic mechanism itself but rather the radiculopathy which results. This was the approach of Lievre and his associates (7), who in 1953, reported on the beneficial effect of hydrocortisone injected into the epidural space in 20 patients. Subsequently, others began to try this technique in selected cases. Cappio (8) reviewed the early literature abroad and reported that good results were obtained in 67% of the first 80 of these cases. Later, in the United States, Goebert and his co-workers at the Cleveland Clinic treated 113 patients with painful radiculopathies with hydrocortisone and procaine injected caudally and obtained good results in 72% of the patients (9).

After first determining its safety in laboratory animals (10), the Cleveland Clinic group then went on to record an improved success rate following the injection of 40 mg of methylprednisolone and 40 mg of procaine intrathecally (11). They reported no complications following the injection of steroids with procaine into either the extradural or intradural compartments.

In spite of the simplicity of this therapeutic approach to the management of discogenic pain and its freedom from side effects and complications, the present author, like many others, was initially skeptical of its efficacy. Therefore, in 1968 we initiated a preliminary study to evaluate the efficacy of methylprednisolone as a therapeutic modality for discogenic pain and to compare the result obtained when the drug was injected epidurally with the result obtained when the drug was injected intrathecally, with both injections consisting of methylprednisolone alone (without local anesthetic) and both injections being made as close to the level of the lesion as possible. The data obtained in that study indicated that methylprednisolone is an effective therapeutic modality in the management of discogenic pain in about 80% of the patients so treated, and that the success rate is almost identical regardless of whether the drug is injected intrathecally or epidurally, as long as the injection is made as close to the level of the disc as possible (12).

Following publication of this study in 1972, we have continued to obtain a high degree of success using this therapeutic regimen. Unfortunately, most of the patients with sciatica are referred first to surgeons, so there has been little data available indicating the success rate of epidural and/or intrathecal steroids as a primary course of therapy, since most surgeons consider it a "last resort" in the management of discogenic pain in patients in whom laminectomy, with or without fusion, has failed to provide relief. As a result, much of the published data has been obtained in a mixture of patients consisting of a few who refused surgery and many who had failed to obtain relief following surgery.

Therefore, in the mid 1970's we undertook a study of 30 patients with discogenic pain in whom only intrathecal and/or epidural Depo-Medrol was utilized as the primary form of therapy (13). This study indicated three important findings: First, of the 30 patients receiving only epidural and/or intrathecal Depo-Medrol, 29 obtained complete and apparently permanent relief. The one patient who did not obtain relief underwent surgery and no disc was found. Second, in the majority of the cases (14 out of 30), one injection of Depo-Medrol was insufficient. Thirteen required two injections and 3 required three. Finally, contrary to the report of Abram, if one route of injection fails to provide relief, the other route of injection may provide success. Such was the case in 8 of the 30 patients in this study.

MECHANISM OF ACTION OF EPIDURAL/INTRATHECAL STEROIDS

When Mixter and Barr first demonstrated the relationship between disc protrusion and radicular pain (2), they believed that the signs and symptoms of sciatica were due to the mechanical compression of the nerve root by the protruded disc. This mechanical explanation of sciatica is what prompted surgeons to consider laminectomy to be curative. However, the results of surgery failed to support this hypothesis.

Recently, Olsson (14) experimentally produced cervical disc protrusion in dogs and found that the size of the disc and the amount of compression were less important in the production of symptomatology than the accompanying inflammation. The etiologic role of inflammation in sciatica is supported by the observation during lumbar laminectomy under local anesthesia that inflamed spinal nerves adjacent to a prolapsed disc are very sensitive to minor manipulations, whereas uninflamed nerves can be manipulated with very little discomfort (15). Inflammation of nerve roots in patients with low back pain has been demonstrated myelographically (16) and visually at the time of surgery (17) and has been confirmed on histological examinations of biopsy specimens taken from nerve roots during surgery (18-20). Indeed, improvement in clinical symptoms has been shown to coincide with the resolution or diminution of nerve root edema in the presence of persistent herniated intervertebral disc (16).

Once it was established that "sciatica" is the result of an inflammatory process of the involved nerve root(s), it was a logical step to utilize corticosteroids in the vicinity of the inflamed nerve root(s) to counteract the inflammation. As already pointed out, our own studies, which simply applied this information clinically by treating discogenic pain with intrathecal and epidural steroids supports the "inflammatory hypothesis" (12,13).

The success rate is similar with the intrathecal and epidural approaches. In addition, no complications have been reported in the literature following intrathecal steroid injections, **provided:** (1) reasonable dosages were administered; (2) the number of injections was reasonable; and (3) the patient was free of central nervous system disease, i.e., multiple sclerosis. However, because of the increasing concerns of anesthesiologists about the litigious state of medicine, intrathecal steroid injections gave way to epidural injections.

CONTROVERSIAL ASPECTS OF EPIDURAL STEROIDS

Other investigators have been unable to reduplicate our high success rates. Carron has challenged the credibility of our reports; but we are convinced that the success rate will depend, to a large degree, upon the accuracy of the diagnosis. If the patient has truly and only discogenic pain, then the chances of success are great. Our studies have also been criticized for not providing concurrent controls and/or randomization, and this is true. However, Dilke and his co-workers (21) had already reported on a randomized study of 100 consecutive patients with low back pain and radicular pain in the lower extremity, in which 10 ml of normal saline and 80 mg of methylprednisolone were injected epidurally in the study group, while the control group received an injection of 1 ml of sterile saline in the intraspinous ligament in the lumbar area. Of the patients who received Depo-Medrol, 46% reported complete pain relief one week after the injection, compared with 11% of the control group. More recently Cuckler (22) and his co-workers have carried out a prospective, randomized, and double-blind study comparing methylprednisolone and saline in patients with radicular pain due to a herniated nucleus pulposus or due to spinal stenosis. They detected no statistically significant difference between the control and experimental groups, whether the pain was due to acute disc herniation or spinal stenosis.

The problem with both of these studies is the fact that only a single dose of steroid was utilized and the success or failure of the technique was based on this one therapeutic intervention. Our studies have shown rather conclusively that two and in many cases three injections are necessary, and that for some reason, in certain patients one route of injection (intrathecal or epidural) succeeds where the other has failed. In view of the simplicity and safety of this technique, with the virtual absence of significant side effects, it would appear that in patients with an acute herniated nucleus pulposus, this form of therapy should be carried out **before** any other. The early use of epidural/intrathecal steroids could markedly reduce the loss of income resulting from prolonged bed rest and traction, and may even save the expense of a CAT scan if the therapy is successful.

As a matter of fact, there is good evidence that the earlier this treatment is initiated the greater will be the chance of success. Brown (23) was the first to report that the success rate was related to the duration of symptoms at the time of treatment; noting 100% efficacy in those patients treated within the first three months, and only 20% when treated later. Ryan & Taylor (24) tried to make an even more precise correlation between the time of treatment and success rate, finding in their study of 108 patients the following results: Patients who were treated within the first two weeks of symptoms achieved a 77% success rate, from 2 to 4 weeks a 72% success rate, from 4 to 6 weeks a 60% success rate, and over 6 weeks a 43% success rate. However, unlike their predecessors, the latter investigators actually injected 40 mg of methylprednisolone intrathecally, followed by 40 mg epidurally. Nonetheless, these two investigators felt that their data and the obvious relationship between time of treatment and incidence of success provided clinical support for the theory that epidural steroids are effective in disc protrusion with "irritative" [inflammatory] neuropathy, but not "compressive neuropathy." In other words, they felt that the reason for the progressive decrease in success with time was due to the fact that as time progresses, the continued inflammatory response produced progressively increasing intraneural fibrosis and ischemic changes that become irreversible, and that will not be affected by steroids.

CONCLUSIONS

In short, for optimal results with epidural steroids, it is critically important that the diagnosis be correct, (i.e., that one is dealing with an inflammatory neuropathy), that the treatment is instituted early (while the process is predominantly inflammatory), and that the sequence and timing of the injections are appropriate. The use of the proper steroid is equally important, if not for success, for preventing complications: We have only utilized Depo-Medrol, since Gardner showed this to be the safest agent when used intrathecally, though others have achieved results similar to ours using dexamethasone. Hydrocortisone should never be utilized, as it is irritating to the meninges and can cause grand-mal seizures (25,26). The beauty of this form of therapy is that if it does not provide the expected relief, other therapeutic modalities can still be carried out. However, if this therapeutic approach were followed routinely in patients having their first acute herniated disc, very few would ever need to undergo a laminectomy and discectomy.

REFERENCES

1. Evans W: Intrasacral epidural injection in the treatment of sciatica. Lancet 2:1225-1229, 1930
2. Mixter WJ and Barr JS: Rupture of the intervertebral disc with involvement of the spinal canal. J Neurosurg 21:74-81, 1934

3. Smith L: Enzyme dissolution of the nucleus pulposus in humans. JAMA 187:137-140, 1964
4. Smith L: Chemonucleolysis. Clin Orthop 67:72-80, 1969
5. Ford LT: Clinical use of chymopapain in lumbar and dorsal disc lesions. Clin Orthop 67:81-87, 1969
6. Massie WK: Editorial comment. Clin Orthop 67:2-5, 1969
7. Lievre JA, Block-Michel H and Attali, P: L'injection trans-sacree. Etude clinique et radiologigue. Bull et Mem Soc Med Hop Paris 73:1110-1118, 1957
8. Cappio M: Il trattamento idrocortisonico per via epidurole sacrole delle lombroscaitalgie. Reumatismo 9:60-70, 1957
9. Goebert HW Jr, Jallo SJ, Gardner WJ et al: Painful radiculopathy treated with epidural injections of procaine and hydrocortisone acetate: Results in 113 patients. Anesth Analg 40:130-134, 1961
10. Sehgal AD, Tweed DC, Gardner WJ et al: Laboratory studies after intrathecal corticosteroids. Arch Neurol 9:64-68, 1963
11. Gardner WJ, Goebert HW Jr, Sehgal AD: Intraspinal corticosteroid in the treatment of sciatica. Trans Am Neurol Assoc 86:214-215, 1961
12. Winnie AP, Hartman JT, Meyer HL Jr, et al: Pain Clinic II: Intradural and extradural corticosteroids for sciatica. Anesth Analg 51:990-999, 1972
13. Winnie AP and Ramamurthy S: Steroids for discogenic pain. Paper presented at the VI World Congress of Anesthesiology, Mexico City, Mexico, April 1976
14. Olsson SE: The dynamic factor in spinal cord compression. A study of dogs with special reference to cervical disc protrusion. J Neurosurg 15:308-321, 1958
15. Murphy RW: Nerve roots and spinal nerves in degenerative disc disease. Clin Orthop 129:46-40,1977
16. Berg A: Clinical and myelographic studies of conservatively treated cases of lumbar intervertebral disc. Acta Chir Scand 104:124-129, 1958
17. Roaf J: Some observations regarding 905 patients operated upon for protruded lumbar intervertebral disc. Am J Surg 97:388-399, 1959
18. Lindahl O, Rexed B: Histologic changes in spinal nerve roots of operated cases of sciatica. Acta Orthop Scand 20:215-225, 1950
19. Irsigler FJ: Nikroskopische Befunde in den Ruckenmarkswurzeln beim lumbalen und lumbosakrolen (dorsolateralen) Diskusprolaps. Acta Neurrochir (Wien) 1:478-516, 1951
20. Marshall LL, Trethwie ER: Chemical irritation of nerve root in disc prolapse. Lancet 2:230, 1973
21. Dilke TFW, Burry HC and Grahame R: Extradural corticosteroid injection in the management of lumbar nerve root compression. Br Med J 2:635-637, 1973
22. Cuckler JM, Bernini PA, Wiesel SW, et al: The use of epidural steroids in the treatment of lumbar radicular pain. J Bone Joint Surg 67-A:6366, 1985

23. Brown FW: Management of diskogenic pain using epidural and intrathecal steroids. Clin Orthop 129:72-78, 1977
24. Ryan MD and Taylor KF: Management of lumbar nerve-root pain by intrathecal and epidural injections of Depo Methylprednisolone Acetate. Med J Aust 2:532-534, 1981
25. Oppelt WW and Rall DP: Production of convulsions in the dog with intrathecal corticosteroids. Neurol 11:925-927, 1961
26. Ildirim I, Furcolow ML et al: A possible explanation of posttreatment convulsions associated with intrathecal corticosteroids. Neurol 20:622-625, 1970

MULTIDISCIPLINARY EVALUATION AND MANAGEMENT OF CHRONIC PAIN

T. M. Murphy

INTRODUCTION

Pain has afflicted patients and frustrated therapists since time began.

Nociception is the transmission of tissue damaging energy along the A delta and C fibers of the sensory nervous system with specific cortical projections.

This "straight through" system almost certainly operates in the majority of acute pain situations, but as pain becomes more chronic, this "direct" pathway becomes modified by interaction of this incoming signal both with other non-nociceptive incoming signals, and with descending inhibitory or facilitatory effects.

Patients presenting to pain clinics usually have a chronic pain complaint that can span the whole spectrum from say, an extensive malignant tumor, to a predominant behavioral problem.

CLASSIFICATION OF CHRONIC PAIN

Although incompletely understood, chronic pain has been divided into four broad categories.

Nociception

Pain originating usually from tissue damage, includes the pain of injury, cancer, chronic degenerative arthritic diseases, etc., is perhaps the best understood.

T. H. Stanley and M. A. Ashburn (eds.), Anesthesiology and Pain Management, 281–285.

Central Pain States

Imperfectly understood, believed to arise as a result of abnormalities in the central nervous system, probably some "short circuit." A variety of centrally acting medications and stimulus produced analgesia have been tried with various reports of success.

Psychological Pain

A mislabeling of aversive or unpleasant sensations whereby the patient uses the language and behavior as though nociception was occurring in response to what are primarily believed to be psychological forms of suffering such as anxiety, depression, neurosis, hysteria, etc.

Behavioral Pain

"Learned pain behavior" can outlast the healing process and persist purely as a behavioral phenomenon.

DIAGNOSIS OF CHRONIC PAIN

Pain clinics will at a very early stage have to evaluate and assess the relative contributions of the above factors to an individual's pain complaint and offer treatment accordingly.

This evaluation is usually done by a concurrent medical evaluation and ideally a coincident psychological and behavioral analysis. With all of the above information to hand, treatment can be planned accordingly.

TREATMENT OF CHRONIC PAIN

Accept the patient's pain complaint as real.

Protect the entrenched chronic pain patient from unnecessary invasive testing and surgeries where there is no clear indication for same.

Medication Treatment for Chronic Pain

Most non-malignant chronic pain is best treated with the non-opioid analgesics in an appropriate dose, at time contingent intervals. If more significant nociceptive impulse (e.g., an invading carcinoma), then progression to the more powerful opioid medication is not only justified but indicated. It is referable to use an orally acting opioid, probably methadone is the optimal drug, (in terminal cancer, oral morphine might pose some advantages).

Tricyclic antidepressants have been much used in recent years.

Stimulation Produced Analgesia

Effectively done using transcutaneous electrical nerve stimulators with an adequate trial over a two to three week period.

These are virtually risk free, have no side effects and apart from the expense appear to be a useful form of therapy.

Biofeedback

Biofeedback is a relaxation form of therapy, often worth a trial in muscle tension pain and vascular headaches.

Nerve Blocks

These can run the whole gamut from simple infiltration by either "dry" needling and/or injection of local anesthetic, through to destructive neurolytic blocks, but these latter are reserved for terminally ill patients.

Sympathetic Blocks

In the condition of reflex sympathetic dystrophy (RSD), injection of the sympathetic ganglia can often be spectacularly effective and, if good relief obtained, such treatment should be coupled with active physical therapy during the period the block is effective.

Somatic Nerve Blocks

Can be useful diagnostically in attempting to decide if nociception is a significant aspect of the patient's problem. Permanent neurodestruction may be needed in cases of terminal cancer. Since the advent of epidural opioids there has now been less need to invoke these irreversible neurodestructive procedures although they still have a place in selected patients.

Neuraxial Narcotics

This is an exciting new field which has much potential for providing pain control in the terminal cancer patient and, maybe as the technique is refined, in chronic non-cancer pain.

Psychological and Behavioral Therapies

The spectrum of therapies here can vary from the prescribing of some appropriate psychoactive agent, e.g., anti-depressants, etc. through to expensive intensive inpatient behavioral modification programs. These programs can be spectacularly effective initially and do seem to be effective at reducing health care utilization in the future.

CONCLUSIONS

Chronic pain and the resulting disability have been a frustrating and major problem for both patients and society for a long time. A variety of pharmacological and technological analgesic options have been tried over time, but, alas, have not resolved the problem, often leaving a legacy of angry and frustrated patients (1).

Since the advent of the gate theory, the complex interactions of nociceptive input and its modification by ascending and descending influences within the central nervous system has led to a new concept in the therapeutic approach based on improving cognitive understanding, coping strategies and maximizing physical rehabilitation. Pioneered by Fordyce (2), this approach continues to undergo modification and runs the whole gamut from exclusively inpatient residential treatment through to more innovative (and less costly) outpatient programs.

They are modestly effective in reducing pain and appear to be the best method available for re-establishing function (3-6). Peters and Large (7) in New Zealand noted more marked gains in inpatient therapy groups compared with outpatients but both were better than an untreated control group.

Until we can successfully prevent chronic pain, its treatment will continue to be a major frustration and expense. The entrenched chronic pain patient is a complex mixture of depression, anger, and frustration (1) and requires both sympathy and firmness in management and both control of and comprehensive understanding of the environment in which the patient suffers (8). Without both patient and environmental cooperation, chronic pain continues to be frustratingly difficult to treat.

REFERENCES

1. Wade JB, Price DD, Hamer RM, et al: An emotional component analysis of chronic pain. Pain 40:303-310, 1990
2. Maruta T, Swanson DW, McHardy MJ: Three year follow-up of patients with chronic pain who were treated in a multidisciplinary pain management center. Pain 41:47-53, 1990
3. Fordyce WE, Fowler RS Jr, Lehmann JF, et al: Operant conditioning in the treatment of chronic pain. Arch Phys Med Rehabil 54:399-408, 1973
4. Sturgis ET, Schaefer CA, Sikora TL: Pain control follow-up study of treated and untreated patients. Arch Phys Med Rehabil 54:301-303, 1984
5. Kames LD, Rapkin AJ, Naliboff BD, et al: Effectiveness of an interdisciplinary pain management program for the treatment of chronic pelvic pain. Pain 41:41-46, 1990
6. Cott A, Anchel H, Golberg WM, et al: Non-institutional treatment for chronic pain by field management: An outcome study with comparison group. Pain 40:183-194, 1990
7. Peters JL, Large RG: A randomised control trial evaluating in- and outpatient management programs. Pain 41:283-293, 1990
8. Murphy TM: Treatment of Chronic Pain, Anesthesia. Edited by Miller RD. New York, Churchill Livingstone, 1990, pp. 1927-1950

CANCER PAIN SYNDROMES

K. M. Foley

Recognizing and treating the cause of pain in the patient with cancer should be the initial approach to the management of this common symptom. Careful analysis of patients with cancer and pain has led to the elucidation of common pain syndromes unique to this disease process (Table 1). They are often misdiagnosed because health care professionals are unfamiliar with their clinical presentation. In each of these syndromes, pain is the overriding symptom which prompts medical attention. The three major categories of pain syndromes include: pain associated with direct tumor involvement, pain associated with cancer therapy, and pain not associated with the cancer or the cancer therapy (1-5).

PAIN ASSOCIATED WITH DIRECT TUMOR INVOLVEMENT

In those patients with pain associated with direct tumor involvement, studies at Memorial Sloan-Kettering Cancer Center (MSKCC) demonstrate that 78% of the pain problems in an inpatient cancer population and 62% of pain problems in an outpatient cancer pain clinic fall into this category. Metastatic bone disease, nerve compression or infiltration or involvement of the viscera by either obstruction of the hollow viscus or diffuse peritoneal seeding are the most common causes of pain from direct tumor involvement.

Tumor Infiltration of Bone

Primary or metastatic tumor involvement of bone produces pain in one of two ways, by direct involvement of the bone and activation of the nociceptors locally; or by compression of the adjacent nerves, soft tissues or vascular structures. Pain is the most common syndrome associated with tumor infiltration of bone and bone pain represents the most common cause of pain in patients with cancer.

T. H. Stanley and M. A. Ashburn (eds.), Anesthesiology and Pain Management, 287–303.

Table 1. Common cancer pain syndromes.

PAIN SYNDROMES ASSOCIATED WITH DIRECT TUMOR INVOLVEMENT

I. Tumor Infiltration of Bone
- A. Metastases to the Base of Skull
  1. Orbital Syndrome
  2. Parasellar Syndrome
  3. Middle Fossa Syndrome
  4. Jugular Foramen Syndrome
  5. Occipital Condyle Syndrome
  6. Clivus Metastases
  7. Sphenoid Sinus Metastases
  8. Odontoid Fracture
- B. Vertebral Body Syndromes
  1. C7-T1 Syndrome
  2. T12-L1 Syndrome
  3. Sacral Syndrome
- C. Metastases to Long Bone and Joints

II. Tumor Infiltration of Nerves
- A. Peripheral Nerve Syndromes
  1. Intercostal Neuropathy
  2. Thoracic Radiculopathy
- B. Plexopathy Syndromes
  1. Brachial Plexopathy
  2. Lumbosacral Plexopathy
- C. Spinal Cord Syndromes
  1. Epidural Spinal Cord Compression
  2. Leptomeningeal Metastases
  3. Intramedullary Metastases

III. Tumor Infiltration of Viscera
- A. Pleural Effusion Syndrome
- B. Peritoneal Carcinomatosis
- C. Bowel and Bladder Obstruction
- D. Ureteral Obstruction

PAIN SYNDROMES ASSOCIATED WITH CANCER THERAPY

I. Acute Syndromes Common in Patients Following Chemotherapy, Surgery, or Radiation Therapy
- A. Corticosteroid Withdrawal Pain
- B. Post-Procedure Pain
  1. Bone marrow aspiration
  2. IM, IV, epidural injections
  3. Lumbar puncture headache
- C. Post-Operative Pain
- D. Acute Herpes Zoster
- E. Chemotherapy-Induced Pains
  1. Vincristine myalgia and neuralgia
  2. IT methotrexate headache & meningismus
  3. Trans-retinoic acid bone pain
  4. Hormonally-induced pain flares
  5. Oral mucositis
- F. Radiation-Induced Pain
  1. Oral mucositis
  2. Skin Irritation
  3. Gastrointestinal and bladder spasms

II. Chronic Pain Syndromes Following Cancer Therapy
- A. Post-surgical Pain Syndromes
  1. Post-radical neck dissection
  2. Post-mastectomy
  3. Post-thoracotomy
  4. Post-nephrectomy
  5. Post-limb amputation
- B. Post-Chemotherapy Pain Syndromes
  1. Peripheral neuropathy
  2. Steroid pseudorheumatism
  3. Aseptic necrosis of bone
  4. Post-herpetic neuralgia
- C. Post-Radiation Therapy Pain Syndromes
  1. Radiation fibrosis of the brachial plexus
  2. Radiation fibrosis of the lumbosacral plexus
  3. Radiation myelopathy
  4. Radiation-induced peripheral nerve tumors

Table 1. Common cancer pain syndromes (Cont.).

PAIN UNRELATED TO THE CANCER OR THE CANCER THERAPY	
I. Lumbar Disc Disease	III. Diabetic Neuropathy
II. Osteoporosis	IV. Trigeminal Neuralgia

Metastases to Base of Skull

The syndromes associated with metastases to the base of skull are commonly seen in patients with nasopharyngeal tumors but may occur with any type of tumor that metastases to the bone (6), most commonly breast and prostate cancer. The syndromes in this group all share three common features: 1) pain is the earliest complaint, often preceding neurologic signs and symptoms by several weeks to months; 2) documentation by plain x-ray film is usually not possible, requiring the use of computerized tomography (CT) or magnetic resonance imaging (MRI); 3) early treatment is associated with the greatest improvement of neurologic function suggesting that early diagnosis will have a significant impact on outcome.

Orbital Syndrome. The first symptom of this syndrome is progressive continuous pain in the supraorbital area of the affected eye. Blurred vision is followed by diplopia. Examination reveals proptosis of the involved eye and external ophthalmoplegia. There may be decreased sensation in the ophthalmic division of the trigeminal nerve or a palpable orbital tumor.

Parasellar Syndrome. This syndrome presents as unilateral supraorbital and frontal headache in up to 83% of patients and adds diplopia without proptosis. There may be an associated ocular paresis or papilledema.

Middle Fossa Syndrome. Most patients with middle fossa syndrome present with numbness, paresthesias, or pain referred to the second and third division of the trigeminal nerve. Over one-half of the patients experience a dull ache in the cheek or the jaw. Pain similar to trigeminal neuralgia but without trigger points, has also been reported as a presentation of this disorder. Sensory symptoms in the trigeminal distribution proceed other symptoms by weeks to months. Diplopia, headache, dysarthria, and dysphagia can then develop. Headache occurs in 28% of patients with middle fossa syndrome. Examination of this group of patients reveals sensory loss in the trigeminal nerve distribution as well as signs of weakness in the pterygoids and masseters, signs of abducens palsy, and other ocular palsies.

Jugular Foramen Syndrome. The presenting symptom in patients with the jugular foramen syndrome is hoarseness or dysphagia. Patients may have an associated glossopharyngeal neuralgia and syncope. Unilateral pain behind the ear with neurologic signs that include unilateral weakness of the palate, vocal cord, sternocleidomastoid, trapezius, and tongue are commonly seen in this syndrome.

Occipital Condyle Syndrome. This syndrome is characterized by severe unilateral occipital pain worsened with neck flexion and associated with stiffness of the neck. Examination reveals tenderness to palpation over the occipital area and XII cranial nerve paralysis. Both weakness of the sternocleidomastoid and dysarthria may be associated with this syndrome.

Clivus Metastasis. Presentation of this lesion is typically with a vertex headache exacerbated by neck flexion with dysfunction in the lower cranial nerves, specifically, cranial nerves VI through XII. These signs initially begin unilaterally but may progress to bilateral involvement.

Sphenoid Sinus Metastases. These metastases often present with bifrontal headache radiating to the temples and intermittent retroorbital pain that may be associated with nasal congestion and diplopia. Examination commonly reveals the presence of unilateral or bilateral sixth nerve palsies.

Odontoid Fractures. Lesions in the odontoid may simulate a base of skull metastasis (7). The pain typically radiates over the posterior aspect of the skull to the vertex and is exacerbated by neck movement, particularly flexion. Fractures of the odontoid process are usually secondary to the destruction of the atlas. Pathological fracture may result in secondary subluxation and spinal cord or brain stem compression. Pain is the earliest symptom and neurologic signs of progressive sensory, motor and autonomic dysfunction involving the upper extremities may be present.

The combination of CT scanning with bone windows as well as axial and sagittal MRI studies are the diagnostic procedures of choice to define both alignment as well as bony disease.

Vertebral Body Syndromes

Vertebrae are the most common sites of bone metastases. Neck and back pain are the most common symptoms in patients with tumor infiltration of bone in these areas. Diagnostic studies including plain x-rays, bone scans, CT scanning and MRI are most useful to define the degree of bony involvement with evidence to suggest that both CT and MRI are more sensitive than bone scanning and MRI in certain tumor types may be more sensitive than CT in defining early tumor infiltration of bone. There are several specific vertebral body syndromes that are often missed on plain x-ray because of overlapping bony structures or lack of understanding of referred pain patterns.

C7-T1 Vertebral Syndrome. This syndrome commonly occurs in patients with lung and breast cancer and results from tumor either arising predominantly in bone or spreading to bone from contiguous paraspinal lymph nodes or spreading from contiguous paraspinal tumors. The pain is most commonly referred to either the shoulder or interscapular region and is associated with radicular symptoms in the arm with pain referred to the elbow. The referred pattern of interscapular or elbow pain is often not recognized as emanating from the C7-T1 area. Similarly, plain x-rays are not useful in defining the anatomy of this area because of overlapping bony structures on lateral views, specifically, the shoulder joint. Both Pancoast tumors and tumor-induced brachial plexopathies are commonly associated with bony disease at this site (8,9).

T12-L1 Vertebral Body Syndromes. These syndromes often present with a referred pain characterized by deep aching pain over either the right or left sacroiliac joint. This is a commonly referred site for T12 or L1 root and patients may have little pain at the site of bony involvement. Recognition of the referred pattern of pain from this vertebral body site can help to direct the appropriate diagnostic study.

Sacral Pain Syndrome. Tumor infiltration of the sacrum is often not readily diagnosed on plain x-rays, and again requires more sophisticated studies with either CT or MRI scanning. Pain is characterized by an aching sensation in typically either both buttocks, perineum, or posterior thighs. It is often exacerbated by sitting or lying and relieved by standing and walking. The pain may also be referred to the hips or anterior thighs and careful assessment of the sacrum and the pelvis is necessary to define the full extent of tumor infiltration in this site.

Epidural Spinal Cord Compression. This is a commonly associated complication of tumor infiltration of bone, although it may occur in the absence of bony infiltration from extension, from a paraspinal mass, or by tracking along the nerve root into the epidural space (10,11). This neurologic complication of cancer occurs in 10-15% of patients. Early diagnosis is critical because the efficacy of treatment is determined most commonly by the degree of neurologic impairment the patient reports at the time therapy is initiated. Seventy-five percent of patients who begin treatment while ambulatory remain so, but only 30-50% for those who begin treatment while markedly paretic and less than 10% for those patients who are paraplegic at the time of presentation. Again, back pain is the overriding symptom in 96% of patients. In 10% of patients, it is the only symptom at the time of diagnosis. Detailed algorithms for the assessment and treatment of patients with back pain and epidural spinal cord compression have been published and are beyond the scope of this discussion.

Metastases to Long Bones and Joints

The most common long bones involved with tumor include the humerus and the femur, most typically at their proximal ends. Again, early diagnosis is critical to prevent and to reduce the development of fractures. The treatment for patients with proximal humerus involvement is often radiation therapy and/or rod placement and, as in patients who have infiltration in the acetabulum, hip replacement is often considered as a mode of therapy to effectively treat pain. Plain x-rays are typically not useful in this population of patients requiring the use of sophisticated MRI or CT scanning techniques to define the extent of tumor infiltration.

Pain Syndromes Associated with Tumor Infiltration of Nerve

The pain syndromes in this group are caused by either direct tumor infiltration of nerve or by progressive compression of nerve structures, by sudden compression, or by metastatic fracture of bone adjacent to a nerve or nerve root. The neuropathology of these lesions has not be correlated with the nature of the pain. The neurophysiologic evidence suggests that persistent mechanical and noxious stimulation of peripheral nociceptors combined with damage of axons and myelin sheaths may be associated with the development of typical neuropathic pain.

Peripheral Neuropathy. The peripheral nerve is most commonly infiltrated by tumors which invade the intercostal, paravertebral, or retroperitoneal space. Constant burning pain with dysesthesias in an area of sensory loss is the usual clinical presentation. The pain is radicular and often unilateral. Careful sensory examination can delineate the site of nerve compression. The most common examples include metastatic tumor involvement of rib, producing intercostal nerve entrapment. At the present time, the use of CT and MRI scanning and can help to define the appropriate diagnosis.

Brachial Plexopathy. Pain is the most common presentation in this group of patients commonly associated with progressive neurologic dysfunction (8,9,12). A series of very specific pain signs and symptoms have been developed to distinguish tumor infiltration of the brachial plexus from other causes of neurologic dysfunction involving the upper extremity. These are listed in Table 2. Again, early diagnosis is critical to prevent the development of irreversible neurologic injury. Of importance, tumor can infiltrate all levels of the brachial plexus. Breast cancer, lymphoma and lung cancer are the most common types of tumor infiltration. In patients with carcinoma of the breast, tumor can infiltrate the brachial plexus initially presenting with pain in the shoulder, biceps region, elbow or hand. Burning dysesthetic sensations in the index finger or thumb are common in patients who develop tumor in a supraclavicular region. Patients who develop pain in the shoulder, elbow, and 4th and 5th fingers have tumor infiltration of the lower cord of the plexus. In those patients who have undergone previous radiation therapy to the brachial plexus,

Table 2. Clinical features of brachial plexus syndrome in patients with breast cancer.

Feature	*Tumor Infiltration*	*Radiation Fibrosis*	*Reversible Radiation*	*Acute Ischemic Brachial Plexopathy*
Incidence of Pain	89%	18%	40%	Painless
Location of pain	Shoulder, upper arm, elbow, radiating to 4th and 5th fingers	Shoulder, wrist, hand	Hand, forearm	Hand, forearm
Nature of pain	Dull aching in shoulder; lancinating pain in elbow and ulnar aspect of hand; occasional dysesthesias, burning, or freezing sensations	Aching pain in shoulder; paraesthesias in C5-6 distribution in hand	Aching pain in shoulder Paresthesias in hand and forearm	Paresthesias in hand and forearm
Severity of pain	Moderate to severe (severe in 98% of patients)	Milder to moderate; severe in 35% of patients	Mild	
Course	Progressive neurologic dysfunction; atrophy and weakness with C7-T1 distribution; persistent pain; Horner syndrome	Progressive weakness with C5-6 distribution; stabilizing pain with appearance of weakness	Transient weakness and atrophy affecting C6-7, T-1; complete resolution of motor findings	Acute nonprogressive weakness and sensory changes
CT scan findings	Circumscribed mass diffuse infiltration of tissue planes	Diffuse infiltration of tissue planes	Normal	Normal angiography shows subclavian artery segmental obstruction
MRI	High signal intensity in circumscribed mass on T2-weighted images may enhance with gadolinium	Diffuse low signal intensity on T2-weighted images; no change with gadolinium	No data	Normal
EMG findings	Segmental slowing; no myokymia	Myokymia	Segmental slowing; no myokymia	Segmental slowing; no myokymia

the onset of pain with neurologic symptoms in the arm strongly suggests tumor infiltration rather than radiation injury.

Pancoast Syndrome in which tumor occurs in the superior pulmonary sulcus produces a brachial plexopathy. Pain is the initial symptom in 95% of patients and is characterized by an aching sensation in the shoulder and paraspinal region. Of interest, only 50% of patients present with a Horner's syndrome but by the time of final diagnosis more than 80% of patients will have involvement of the sympathetic nervous system. From the available literature, misdiagnosis of this syndrome occurs commonly with patients not obtaining an appropriate diagnosis for up to 7 or 8 months following the initial pain symptomatology. Both CT scanning and MRI scanning can be of benefit in defining the anatomic changes in this area. From our experience however, CT scanning appears to be more widely used effectively in determining the degree of tumor infiltration.

Lumbosacral Plexopathy. This pain syndrome is one of the most disabling complications of pelvic tumors because of incapacitating pain and leg weakness which immobilizes the patient (13). At times it can be difficult to distinguish a lumbosacral plexopathy from lesions of the spinal cord, the cauda equina or the nerve roots. From studies of this syndrome, the evidence suggests that any primary tumor can metastasize to the lumbosacral plexus, although this syndrome appears to occur more commonly in patients with colorectal tumors and genitourinary tumors. The diagnostic studies most useful in delineating the nature of pain in this group of patients is both the CT and MRI scan. Evidence suggests that about 35% of patients who develop significant leg weakness will have epidural extension of tumor, further suggesting that both MRI of the lumbar spine and MRI or CT of the pelvis are necessary to define the extent of tumor producing these symptoms. A series of specific pain syndromes including an upper and lower panplexopathy have been described and these are detailed in Table 3.

Table 3. Symptoms and signs by level of lumbosacral plexopathy.

Clinical Level	*Upper Plexopathy*	*Lower Plexopathy*	*Pan Plexopathy*
Pain distribution:			
Local	Lower abdomen	Buttock, perineum	Lumbosacral
Radicular	Anterolateral thigh	Posterolateral thigh & leg	Diffuse buttock and legs
Referred	Flank, iliac crest	Hip and ankle	Lower abdomen, buttocks & legs
Numbness/ paresthesias	Anterior thigh	Perineum, thigh, sole of foot	Anterior thigh, leg and foot
Motor and reflex changes	L2-L4	L5-S1	L2-S2
Sensory loss	Anterolateral thigh	Posterior thigh, sole of foot	Esp. anterior thigh, leg
Tenderness	Lumbar	Sciatic notch, sacrum	Lumbosacral area
Positive SLRT			
Direct	Common	Common	Always
Reverse	Rare	Common	Common
Leg Edema	Common	Common	Common
Rectal Mass	Uncommon	Uncommon	Uncommon
Sphincter weakness	Uncommon	Common	Uncommon

Spinal Cord Pain Syndromes

Epidural spinal cord compression, leptomeningeal metastases and intramedullary metastases are the most common tumor-related pain syndromes which involve the spinal cord.

Epidural spinal cord compression has been previously discussed. Leptomeningeal metastases results from tumor infiltration of the leptomeninges. Pain occurs in 40% of patients and is generally of two types, either headache or back pain. The back pain is most commonly localized to the low back and buttock regions. The use of MRI scanning with gadolinium can define the extent of this tumor and lumbar puncture is the procedure of choice to detect neoplastic cells in the cerebrospinal fluid of these patients.

Intramedullary metastases occur rarely but commonly present with unilateral or bilateral pain of a central origin associated with symmetric motor and sensory findings. Patients often complain of hyperesthesia, dysesthesia and allodynia and areas of sensory loss. MRI scanning with gadolinium is the diagnostic procedure of choice. Patients with intramedullary metastases commonly have associated leptomeningeal metastases.

Pain Syndromes Associated with Tumor Infiltration of Viscera

There are a series of common pain syndromes in this category in which pain arises from either compression, destruction, inflammation, or obstruction of pulmonary, gastrointestinal, genitourinary, and endocrine structures. Tumor infiltration of the pleura produces significant pain on inspiration or expiration and is often associated with a cutaneously referred pain. Diffuse abdominal carcinomatosis produces both compression and obstruction giving rise to abdominal pain that is often intermittent, colicky, cramping, and severe in nature. Tumor infiltration of the pancreas produces a classical mid-epigastric pain often referred posteriorly to the back and of a dull, aching and persistent quality. Tumor infiltration of the bladder produces referred pain to the right or left lower quadrant but may commonly refer pain to both upper quadrants and may be associated with a prominent sympathetic syndrome characterized by headache, diaphoresis, and hypotension. Ureteral obstruction produces a unilateral pain commonly referred to the groin region or to the umbilicus and is often acute, severe, and cramping in nature and may or may not be intermittent.

In summary, recognition of these various visceral pain syndromes requires an understanding of the referred patterns of abdominal pain and a careful assessment of the other associated signs and symptoms.

PAIN ASSOCIATED WITH CANCER THERAPY

In those patients with pain associated with cancer therapy, 19% of pain problems in an inpatient adult cancer pain population and 25% of pain problems referred to an outpatient cancer pain clinic comprise this category. Pain occurring during the course of or as a result of chemotherapy, surgery, or radiation therapy are included in this population of patients. Each of these primary therapeutic modalities is associated with a series of both acute and chronic pain syndromes including oral mucositis of chemotherapy, postsurgical pain syndromes following thoracotomy, as well as acute postoperative pain. Each of these syndromes has a characteristic clinical presentation and needs to be carefully differentiated from tumor-induced pain.

PAIN NOT-ASSOCIATED WITH CANCER OR CANCER THERAPY

Pain not associated with the cancer or the cancer therapy represents the third major category. Experience from MSKCC suggests that 3% of patients had pain unrelated to their cancer or its treatment. This figure increases to 10% when assessing an outpatient cancer pain population. Accurate diagnosis in this group of patients clearly alters both therapy and prognosis.

STRATEGY FOR ASSESSMENT AND TREATMENT

In developing a strategy to manage the patient with pain and cancer, identification of the nature of the pain (somatic, visceral, or neuropathic) and the specific pain syndrome can facilitate the development of an approach for pain relief. Therefore, it is not only critical that the identification of the cancer pain syndrome be made, but that an attempt to define the potential pathophysiology is pursued. It is now recognized that these various clinical pain syndromes have a complex neurophysiologic and neuropharmacologic inter-relationship. Two broad categories of pain have been described and are referred to as nociceptive pain which includes both somatic and visceral pain and non-nociceptive pain or neuropathic pain.

Somatic pain is the most common type of pain in patients with cancer with bone metastases as the most prevalent cause. Somatic pain is characterized as well-localized, intermittent or constant, and described as aching, gnawing, throbbing or cramping. Such metastases are characterized by bone destruction with concurrent new bone formation. Both myelinated and unmyelinated afferent fibers are present in bone and their density is greatest in the periosteum. Prostaglandins play a major role in the mechanisms of bone metastases as osteolysis and osteoblast formation occurs. They are postulated as the agents that sensitize nociceptors and produce hyperalgesia and pain. It is well recognized that the drugs that interfere with prostaglandin synthesis inhibit bone pain by inhibiting the sensitization and may also inhibit tumor growth. Other factors such as the osteoclasts activating factor also sensitize nociceptors that produce increased sensitization to pain. Infiltration of soft tissue, muscle and of skin can activate a variety of substances that lead to sensitization of peripheral nociceptors and secondary pain. These substances include potassium ions, adenosine triphosphate, bradykinin, the prostaglandins and leukotrienes. Tumor infiltration and compression causes both mechanical and chemical activation of nociceptors.

Visceral pain is pain mediated by discrete nociceptors in the cardiovascular, respiratory, gastrointestinal, and genitourinary system. It is usually described as deep, squeezing or colicky, and commonly referred to cutaneous sites which may be tender. This referral pattern is thought to be related to the fact, that somatic and visceral structures have dual innervation by common afferent fibers. These fibers converge together in the dorsal horn of the spinal cord. The pain of a visceral site may be misrepresented as a cutaneous one. Shoulder pain resulting from diaphragmatic irritation from a pleural effusion is an example of a cutaneous referral of a visceral pain. Visceral pain results from mechanical or chemical activation of nociceptors by tumor compression or visceral distension or obstruction.

Both somatic and visceral pain result from stimulation of nociceptors without actual injury to the receptors or to the afferent fiber. Somatic and visceral pain respond to a wide variety of pain management approaches including pharmacologic, anesthetic, and neurosurgical procedures.

Neuropathic pain is the second type of pain that is common in cancer patients. It results from injury to the peripheral receptor, afferent fiber or central nervous system. Such injury is associated with spontaneous and ectopic firing in the peripheral nerve as well as at the level of the dorsal horn. Reorganization of the nervous system occurs and spontaneous neural activity can be measured at the level of the thalamus. Neuropathic pain is clinically described as a burning, dysesthetic, squeezing sensation with paroxysms of shock-like pain. Tumor infiltration of the brachial and lumbar plexus are the most common causes of neuropathic pain. Such pain can also result from injury to the peripheral nerve as occurs in postmastectomy and postthoracotomy pain. In contrast to somatic and visceral pain, neuropathic pain is only partially responsive to available approaches. Some authors have described this pain as opioid unresponsive pain, but there is good evidence to suggest that opioids may, in fact, be partially active in treating these pain syndromes.

Once both the specific pain syndrome as well as the potential pathophysiologic mechanisms have been determined, the strategy for the patient's assessment and treatment can move forward to include: an individualization of the therapeutic approach; assuring available expertise to provide therapeutic strategies to patients; continual reassessment of the degree of pain relief and impact on mood, functional status, patient and family acceptance and patient's overall quality of life; the need to chose the simplest approach prior to the use of complicated and expensive techniques; and the critical need for ongoing communication between the physician and the patient in defining the options for therapy and the potential risk/benefit ratios of any of the therapeutic approaches.

IMPACT OF A COMPREHENSIVE EVALUATION ON THE MANAGEMENT OF CANCER PAIN

Although the need for a comprehensive medical and neurological evaluation in the treatment of cancer pain is well described, the full impact of such an approach has been formally studied by the MSKCC Pain Service, in a retrospective review of 226 consultations in a total of 190 patients, and in 50 consultations evaluated prospectively in 46 patients (14). Based on the history, examination, and results of imaging procedures, a pain diagnosis was derived which included the delineation of a somatic, visceral, or neuropathic lesion. Sixty-percent of the consultations were requested in patients with known metastatic disease. A new lesion was identified through the pain evaluation performed by the consultant in 64% of retrospectively studied consultations and 64% of consultations evaluated prospectively. More than 50% of diagnoses were neurological with the most common diagnosis being epidural spinal cord compression. The Pain Service evaluation resulted in changes of treatment and provided an opportunity for primary antineoplastic therapies to be considered. Radiation therapy was offered to 19% of the retrospective group and to 12% of prospective study patients. Two-percent of patients from both studies received chemotherapy; and 1% of retrospective study patients and 4% of prospective study patients were referred to surgery on the basis of the pain evaluation. The prospective survey also tabulated specific neurological diagnoses both related and unrelated to the pain complaint. Thirty-four percent (17 patients) had a neurological diagnosis prior to evaluation by the pain consultant. Nine of the 17 diagnoses were confirmed and the consultation led to a new neurological diagnosis in an additional 18 patients. Thus, neurological evaluation by the pain consultant confirmed neurological diagnoses in 54% of patients, and the most prevalent of these were epidural spinal cord compression in nine patients and lumbosacral plexopathy in another nine patients. Eight new cases of malignant lumbosacral plexopathy were identified by the pain consultant, far more than any other neurological condition in this group of patients.

This study supports the construct that new pathology is commonly identified through a comprehensive assessment of pain in cancer patients. Equally important, many of these lesions are amenable to primary therapy which may have direct analgesic consequences. Approximately one-fifth of the patients received primary antineoplastic therapy based upon the pain evaluation, and another 6% received antibiotics. Although the high prevalence of neurological diagnosis may represent a bias in the MSKCC study, it is essential to recognize that neurological lesions comprise a substantial proportion of painful lesions in the cancer population (15).

In a prospective study of the neurological symptoms, neurological diagnoses, and primary tumors in all patients with a history of systemic cancer (referred to the MSKCC Department of Neurology's consultation service), the three most common symptoms in 851 patients were:

(1) back pain (18%)

(2) altered mental status (17.1%)

(3) headache (15.4%)

The most common neurological diagnosis was brain metastasis (15.9%) followed by metabolic encephalopathy (10.2%), pain associated with bone metastasis only (9.9%), and epidural extension or metastasis of tumor (8.4%), as has been emphasized previously. Physicians evaluating patients with cancer pain need to have sufficient knowledge of the neurological complications of cancer to evaluate and treat this group of patients appropriately.

REFERENCES

1. Foley KM. Pain syndromes in patients with cancer. In: Bonica JJ, Ventafridda V (eds.) Advances in Pain Research and Therapy, Vol. 2, Raven Press, New York, 59-75, 1979
2. Foley KM. Pain syndromes in patients with cancer. In: Foley KM, Payne R (eds.) Medical Clinics in North America, Vol. 71, No. 2, W.B. Saunders, Philadelphia, 169-184, 1987
3. Elliott K, Foley KM. Neurologic pain syndromes in patients with cancer. In: Portenoy RK (ed) Neurologic Clinics, Pain: Mechanisms and Syndromes, W.B. Saunders, Philadelphia, Vol. 7:333-360, 1989
4. Cherny N, Portenoy RK. Practical management of cancer pain. In: Wall PD, Melzack R (eds.) Textbook of Pain, 3rd Ed. Churchill Livingstone, Edinburgh, In Press
5. Portenoy RK. Cancer pain: pathophysiology and syndromes. Lancet 339:1026-1031, 1992
6. Greenberg JS, Deck MDF, Vikram B, et al. Metastasis to the base of the skull: Clinical findings in 43 patients. Neurology 31:530-537, 1981
7. Sundaresan N, Galicich JH, Lane JM, et al. Treatment of odontoid fractures in cancer patients. J Neurosurg 54:187-192, 1981
8. Kori SH, Foley KM. Computed tomography evaluation of bone and soft tissue metastases. In: Weiss L, Gilbert HA (eds.) Bone Metastases. Metastases Monograph Series, Vol. 4, Chap. 12, G.K. Hall, Boston, 245-257, 1981
9. Cascino TL, Kori S, Krol G, Foley KM. CT scanning of the brachial plexus in patients with cancer. Neurology 33:1553-1557, 1983
10. Greenberg JS, Kim JH, Posner JB. Epidural spinal cord compression from metastatic tumor: results with a new treatment protocol. Ann Neurol 8:361-366, 1980
11. Portenoy RK, Lipton RB, Foley KM. Back pain in the cancer patient: an algorithm for evaluation and management. Neurology 37:134-138, 1986
12. Foley KM. Brachial plexopathy in patients with breast cancer. In: Harris Jr, Hellman S, Henderson IC, Kinne D (eds.) Breast Diseases. JP Lippincott, Philadelphia, 722-729, 1991

13. Jaeckle KA, Young DF, Foley KM. The natural history of lumbosacral plexopathy in cancer. Neurology 35:8-14, 1984
14. Gonzales GR, Elliott KJ, Portenoy RK, Foley KM. Impact of a comprehensive evaluation in the management of cancer pain. Pain, 47:141-144, 1991
15. Clouston PD, DeAngelis LM, Posner JB. The spectrum of neurological disease in patients with systemic cancer. Ann Neurol 31:268-73, 1992

MANAGING THE UNMANAGEABLE

T. M. Murphy

Chronic pain complaints are ubiquitous in society. Approximately 80% of the population suffer from low back pain at some time or another. Headaches are probably even more common! The majority of such suffering is coped with by the majority of patients, often with simple self-administered measures, and rarely involves professional therapeutic efforts. However, a significant subset of individuals with such problems seeks formal professional help and, for the most part, is catered to, and appropriately cared for by a variety of analgesic therapies.

The individuals that do not achieve relief with such appropriate therapy are those who are usually referred to pain clinics. Most of these will then often benefit from a variety of novel treatments that have been developed by pain clinics for pain patients over the last few decades. Alas there is, however, a subgroup of such chronic sufferers for whom neither the conventional, nor the novel therapies seem to bring resolution to the problem and although these patients only constitute a relatively small percentage of the population, they often consume a great deal of medical involvement and effort, some of which can make the problem worse, rather than better. Any pain clinic will have a subset of such individuals and it is helpful to both identify them as early as possible and to formulate an appropriate treatment strategy.

Even before the first clinic visit occurs, it has often been preceded by a variety of anxious referral contact, which, although initially may be in the printed form, is more often by telephonic communication, maybe by a patient but more often by patient advocates (relatives, medical attendants, etc.), all anxious to refer the patient on! As with most pain patients, it is critical to obtain as much information as possible about the patient's previous background, and in such patients it will often reveal a platter of

T. H. Stanley and M. A. Ashburn (eds.), Anesthesiology and Pain Management, 305–309.

frustrating unsuccessful interactions with a variety of practitioners inside and outside conventional, medical and surgical practice.

History is critical, usually much more important than the physical examination.

These difficult patients often come in different types (1). The medically-dependent individual is often encountered although less frequently than in the past, since modern physicians and modern prescribing patterns have tended to identify and reduce this problem in recent years (2). If the pain problem is generated by out-of-control medication, then this is usually easily resolved with conventional pain clinic activities. However, if this individual is a medication-dependent individual, it can lead to significant and ongoing prescription arrangements, described below.

Another type of individual is the confounder. These are usually a fairly small percentage of patients who can be easy to identify if an appropriate history and initial evaluation are undertaken. Usually no medical help is ever able to solve an ongoing problem and these include hysterics (more likely to be female patients), sociopathic patients (they are more likely to be male) and Münchausen's patients. This latter group, however, although they may establish an initial consultation contact with pain clinics, rarely become a management problem because pain clinics with their de-emphasis for surgical resolution of pain problems have little appeal to this type of patient. True malingerers are actually encountered relatively infrequently in tertial referral clinics, probably because of the effective screening processes that occur; however, they will be encountered more frequently further down the referral chain.

Every patient presenting with a pain problem warrants an appropriate evaluation (i.e., a conventional medical history and physical and, in addition, a "behavioral" analysis whereby assessment of the patient's functioning as opposed to his complaints is obtained) and this is usually done through the collection of pain clinic diaries and interviewing witnesses from the patient's environment (3). In addition, a psychological profile can be obtained relatively simply from an MMPI and, more comprehensively, from a formal psychological interview. As a result of this, most pain patients will be channeled into appropriate pain treatment therapies, but for the group under discussion today, the vast majority either are not suitable for some, or have previously been involved in such therapies and have usually failed.

Initially these patients should be reassured that you believe in their pain problem—challenging the existence of pain in such patients leads to loss of credibility as the therapist. These patients should be seen regularly on a formal schedule arranged in advance at the previous visit and "p.r.n." returns should be actively discouraged. For the most difficult patients, I always schedule return visits on a Friday (to hopefully prevent "decompensation" over the weekend)! A determined effort is made to avoid dependency producing drugs. Ideally, such patients may often be better attended to with no medication, but in the society in which we live, the transfer of a prescription at the end of a patient/physician interaction appears to be an established fact and, therefore, we should prescribe medications that will minimize ongoing disability (i.e., avoid sedating and dependency producing medications). Despite these good intentions, however, many chronic nonmalignant patients are maintained using such drugs, but very strict control is necessary, that is why this author prefers the administration in a masked vehicle (pain cocktails, pain tablets, etc.) rather than conventional opioid or sedative-hypnotic tablets. The use of conventional tablets tends to escalate in these patients as they attempt to bring some resolution to their ongoing distress and can easily become part of the problem rather than part of the solution.

The managing physician should actively support and maximize any nonpain behavior. I actively encourage socialization, outdoor activities, and consider and freely use formal physical therapy appointments for active (not passive) therapy. The managing physician should minimize spending time and attention on the pain complaint at follow-up visits. Such patients will usually discuss this ad nauseam, if given the opportunity. Freely utilize social and environmental reinforcement by involving family members in such an effort and do not hesitate to employ vocational rehabilitation specialists, if there is a glimmer of hope at returning dysfunctional individuals to the work place. Pilowsky (4) has described the classic triad of patients with chronic pain (i.e., that of illness conviction, somatic focus and denial). These people hold a conviction, despite frequent medical evidence to the contrary, that some significant disease process is at work in their bodies. Although they need to be constantly reassured with regard to the absence of serious disease, it is usually futile to adversely challenge this belief. Freely discuss the process of the disease in terms of muscle and connective tissue rehabilitation rather than "nerves" and "bones" and "discs" and, if need be, use somatically focused therapies in this regard such as needling procedures, stimulation-produced analgesia, hands-on manipulative help, etc., to cater to this illness conviction and somatic focus. Although the other aspect of Pilowsky's triad is that of denial of other problems in life, these are quite often rampant in this group of unmanageable patients. Enlisting the assistance of social workers and other agencies can be very helpful in addressing what may well be the core problem of unhappy marriages, job dissatisfactions, interpersonal rivalries and other social circumstances which often can be attended to if they are identified by asking the right questions. In this latter context, vocational issues are frequently critical, especially in the majority of disabled low back pain sufferers in their middle years. Every effort could and should be made to resolve this, although, alas, medical school training and the talents of many physicians, unfortunately, is often lacking in bringing resolution to this very important issue, although we are frequently called upon to license and validate such disability (5).

Because of this illness conviction and somatic focus, and the current pharmacological focus of society, prescribing inevitably occurs for such patients. It is important that this be appropriate, and although it may not resolve the pain complaint, it should not make it worse! Currently there is significant use of the tricyclic compounds and other antidepressants, which do seem to have an analgesic effect. They may potentiate other analgesics or by blocking reuptake of neurotransmitters lead to an increase in the patients own endogenous analgesics. If ongoing formal analgesic prescription is needed, it is optimal to utilize the non-opioid analgesics, and acetaminophen seems to be well tolerated over time more so than the whole variety of nonsteroidal anti-inflammatory drugs (NSAIDs) which are equally effective analgesics but come with a spectrum of side effects that can create many problems in this somatically focused group of individuals. Alas, the prescribing of "simple" drugs fail to satisfy the perceived needs of many such patients and their "advocates" and for this reason when such drugs are presented in a "pain cocktail" format, they are often better accepted, although pharmacologically identical to tablet form.

The ongoing prescribing of opioids has been appropriately and traditionally de-emphasized in this group of individuals, although every pain clinic is aware of patients who can utilize these drugs all of the time in a responsible fashion. Certainly consideration of such drugs as methadone, which are potent analgesics and lend themselves to better controlled use over time, can and should be considered in those patients who cannot be managed by simpler pharmacology. These drugs can be easily incorporated into masking vehicles (pain cocktails) if need be (and they usually are): The managing physician should have a list of appropriate medications which can be utilized for such patients without compromising function or adding to dependency as crises occur from time to time (and they will).

The physician must not only be prepared to do what is right, but also to make the patient, the attendants and the externals cooperate. With "unmanageable" patients adherence to such principles is the appropriate management strategy. Alas, spectacular therapeutic success will often not be forthcoming, however, at this moment in time such strategies appear to be the optimal way of managing these unmanageable patients for whom, despite the claims of many zealous therapists, there does not appear to be alternative solutions.

REFERENCES

1. Sternbach RA: Pain Patients, Traits and Treatment. New York, Academic Press, 1974
2. Murphy TM: Treatment of chronic pain, Anesthesia. Edited by Miller RD. New York, Churchill Livingstone, 1990, pp. 1927-1950
3. Wade JB, Price DD, Hamer RM, et al: An emotional component analysis of chronic pain. Pain 40:303-310, 1990
4. Pilowsky I: Pain and chronic illness behavior, The Management of Pain. Edited by Bonica JJ. Philadelphia, Lea & Febiger, 1990, pp. 300-309
5. Sullivan MD, Loeser JD: The diagnosis of disability. Treating and rating disability in a pain clinic. Arch Intern Med 152:1829-1835, 1992
6. Murphy TM: Psychoactive drugs for pain control. Pain Reviews 1(1) 1993

ISSUES IN OPIOID THERAPY FOR THE TREATMENT OF CANCER PAIN

K. M. Foley

Evaluation and treatment of pain in the patient with cancer has now evolved to encompass a series of clinical guidelines which define a comprehensive approach to the management of this difficult medical problem. Current knowledge in cancer pain includes the description of the common cancer pain syndromes in this population, as well as their postulated neurophysiologic mechanisms; a classification of the types of patients with pain, the different types of pain (acute, chronic, breakthrough) and the psychological factors that contribute to and alter the pain complaint; the development and implementation of well-validated pain measurement methodologies to assess pain intensity, degree of relief, and mood (psychological distress); the modeling of pharmacokinetic pharmacodynamic relationships to correlate opioid drug distribution with pain relief and side-effects; and refined use of anesthetic and neurosurgical approaches and the broader integration of cognitive-behavioral approaches (1-16).

These advances have focused attention on the cancer patient as the clinical model of pain, and have led to improved pain management in patients with medical illness. Moreover, this patient population has offered the unique opportunity as a natural experiment to study the chronic administration of analgesic drugs, specifically the opioids, to non-addict populations, providing insight, as well as controversy, in their appropriate use for different types of pain and the phenomenon of clinical tolerance, and physical and psychological dependence.

Based on several national and international surveys, one-third of patients in active therapy and two-thirds of patients with advanced disease report pain. Tumor infiltration of bone, nerve, soft tissue or viscera are the most common causes of pain accounting for 65-75% of patients. Pain

T. H. Stanley and M. A. Ashburn (eds.), Anesthesiology and Pain Management, 311–331.

as a result of cancer therapy from surgery, chemotherapy, or radiation accounts for 15-25% of pain, with 5-10% of patients reporting pain independent of their cancer or cancer therapy. Various factors influence the prevalence of pain including the primary tumor type; stage and site of disease; and patient variables, especially psychological variables (17-22).

A GLOBAL CANCER PAIN RELIEF PROGRAM

Data from the World Health Organization Cancer and Palliative Care Unit reports that 4.3 million cancer patients die each year with inadequate control of cancer pain (1-2). To remedy this situation, the WHO has created a Cancer Pain Relief Programme and through a series of expert panels has developed guidelines for the treatment of cancer pain. The Program has achieved a broad international consensus based on the concept that analgesic drug therapy is the mainstay of treatment for the majority of patients with cancer pain. Field testing of the WHO Guidelines in conjunction with clinical experience has shown that 80-90% of cancer patients' pain can be controlled using a simple, inexpensive method described as a Three Step Analgesic Ladder (23). This approach is based on the use of a combination of non-opioid, opioid, and adjuvant drugs, titrated to the individual needs of the patient, according to the severity of pain and its pathophysiology. Implementation of the analgesic guidelines; assurance of drug availability—specifically, opioids; the education of health care professionals; and designating cancer pain a priority for all national cancer control programs are the major goals of the WHO effort. Dr. Jan Stjernsward, Head of the WHO Cancer and Palliative Care Unit has repeatedly emphasized that nothing would have a greater impact on the treatment of cancer pain for patients in developing and developed countries than implementation of existing knowledge (24).

BARRIERS TO EFFECTIVE CANCER PAIN TREATMENT

These health care policy programs and scientific advances notwithstanding, the undertreatment of cancer pain remains a serious medical problem. Numerous barriers have been documented that prevent patients from receiving effective treatment and health care professionals from providing such care. The knowledge and attitude of health care professionals toward pain and its impact on the patient is particularly important since both these factors definitely influence the priority both they and their patients place on pain treatment. Recent studies of medical students, physicians, nurses, and state medical boards demonstrate a significant lack of knowledge on both the theoretical and practical understanding of the use of analgesic drugs, particularly the opioids, in cancer pain management (25-31).

Patient-physician communication about pain symptoms has been shown to be problematic, particularly when patients report pain as moderate or severe. Physicians consistently underestimate patients' physical pain and overemphasize its psychological components. In one study of cancer patients' reports of pain and the concurrent physicians' and nurses observations, the correlates of the nurse, house officer and oncology fellow differed significantly from that of the patient with an overall correlation of 13% for patients reporting moderate to severe pain (31). These observations have been confirmed by the Van Roenn et al. study which obtained responses from 1177 physicians (65% response rate) through a survey of the Eastern Cooperative Oncology Group (ECOG). Eighty-five percent of the respondents who care for over 70,000 cancer patients agreed that the majority of cancer patients with pain were undermedicated with poor pain assessment (76%) and lack of knowledge about analgesic drug therapy as common barriers to inadequate treatment (27).

Limited availability of opioids, excessive regulation of opioids, and the lack of use of alternatives to systemic analgesics--such as nerve blocks, palliative neurosurgery, and behavioral treatments--also prevent adequate treatment. Recent cancer pain initiatives in the Philippines, China, Japan and Argentina have facilitated opioid drug availability (32,33). For example in Japan, there has been a 17-fold increase in morphine consumption since the introduction of the WHO Cancer Pain Relief Programme. The increase in opioid availability worldwide for medical use has not been associated with an increase in diversion of morphine to the illicit market.

In a special report of the International Narcotics Control Board (INCB) which addressed the demand and supply of opioid drugs for medical and scientific needs, the INCB strongly endorsed the WHO Cancer Pain Relief Programme and recommended that governments develop guidelines for the rational use of opioids for treatment of painful medical conditions (34).

This cumulative survey data provide a powerful incentive for the implementation of educational efforts to improve both health care professionals' and patients' knowledge about cancer pain and its treatment. Attempts to remedy this situation include major educational efforts of various professional societies including the American Pain Society, the American Society of Clinical Oncology, the Oncology Nursing Society, etc. An interdisciplinary group of national organizations—the National Coalition for Cancer Pain Relief—has been formed to make prevention and relief of cancer pain an integral part of cancer care. As well, 25 states have started cancer pain initiatives to increase awareness and disseminate information for patients and health care professionals. In contrast, undergraduate and graduate medical programs have not yet implemented formal curricula to meet these educational needs (35).

Recent reviews of therapeutic strategies for cancer pain patients demonstrate that multimodality therapy with anesthetic and neurosurgical approaches as well as home based supportive care programs significantly impact the quality of life and degree of analgesia of advanced cancer pain patients (36-38). Implementation of national palliative care programs and quality assurance programs to monitor cancer pain management as a standard of care are current approaches to implement therapeutic strategies in pain (39).

CONTROVERSIES IN THE CLINICAL USE OF OPIOIDS IN CANCER PAIN

Analgesic drug therapy is the mainstay of treatment, yet opioid use remains a controversial issue. A brief review of some of the major controversial issues influencing this pharmacotherapy are discussed.

Types of Pain

Recent attention has focused on the observation that the pathophysiologic mechanisms of pain influence analgesic responsiveness

(40-48). Based on neuroanatomical and neurophysiologic correlates, three types of pain, somatic, visceral, and neuropathic, occur in cancer patients. Each type results from activation and sensitization of nociceptors and mechanoreceptors by compression, infiltration, or disruption from injury induced by surgery, chemotherapy, or radiation therapy. Cancer patients commonly have multiple sites and types of pain. It has been suggested that neuropathic pain which accounts for 10-20% of difficult to manage pain problems is "opioid resistant" and that opioid drugs are ineffective and should not be used (40). From studies in cancer patients with both nociceptive and neuropathic pain, as well as from controlled studies in nonmalignant neuropathic pain syndromes, neuropathic pain demonstrates a variable response (43). The concept of a continuum of opioid responsiveness rather than an all or none quantal phenomenon has been clearly observed. Opioid responsiveness is defined as the degree of analgesia achieved during dose escalation to either intolerable side effects or adequate analgesia. Patient characteristics, pain-related factors, as well as drug selective effects influence this variability in responsiveness. A wide range of adjuvant analgesics including the tricyclic antidepressants, anticonvulsants, corticosteroids, benzodiazepines, oral and parenteral local anesthetics, etc. have been suggested to provide analgesia. Controlled studies assessing the efficacy of opioids and the adjuvant analgesics in various cancer pain syndromes are critical to resolving the controversy and to providing scientifically-based guidelines for analgesic drug therapy.

Choice of Opioid Drug

The WHO Cancer Unit designated morphine as the drug of choice in its Cancer Pain Relief Programme (1). This choice was based on practical not scientific considerations. At the time of this decision in 1982, morphine was on the Essential Drug List of the WHO, was familiar to physicians for acute pain management, had been demonstrated to be effective in hospices for treatment of chronic cancer pain, and its clinical pharmacology was thought to be fully defined. These considerations were incorrect.

The introduction of the WHO program rapidly demonstrated morphine's limited availability worldwide for oral dosing for chronic cancer pain. Moreover, morphine's expanded use combined with new formulations and new information about the analgesic activities of morphine metabolites focused renewed attention on the clinical pharmacology of morphine with recognition of morphine-6-glucuronide as an active metabolite (49-52). Morphine's major metabolites include morphine-6-glucuronide (M-6-G) and morphine-3-glucuronide (M-3-G). From animal studies, M-6-G but not M-3-G binds to the opiate receptor, and compared to morphine it is twice as potent subcutaneously, 90 times as potent intracerebroventricularly and 650 times as potent intrathecally (53-55). From human studies, M-6-G is analgesic in man and appears in the plasma and cerebrospinal fluid of patients receiving morphine systemically (56). The T-1/2 half-lives of morphine and M-6-G are 108 and 120 minutes, respectively, with clearances of 132 and 1093 ml/per minute, respectively (unpublished data). The small clearance for M-6-G reflects its limited volume of distribution compared to morphine. Current studies demonstrate that the M-6-G to morphine ratio (mean molar ratio: = 1.2) is independent of morphine dose in patients with normal renal function (57,58). In renal dysfunction, M-6-G undergoes both an increase in elimination half-life and a decrease in clearance confirming a true delay in elimination of the compound and leading to an increase in M-6-G:morphine ratio during chronic therapy (59-64). Adverse effects (nausea and respiratory depression) have been attributed to plasma concentrations of the metabolite, particularly in patients with renal failure (62,63). Plasma levels of M-6-G predict cerebrospinal fluid distribution (59). Although the steady-state levels of M-6-G are always greater than morphine (approximately twice as much), the distribution of M-6-G in cerebrospinal fluid averages only one-third to one-fifth as much as morphine. These data are consistent with the physio-chemical property differences between the parent and metabolite and the observation that, in animals, M-6-G is much more potent when introduced directly into the cerebrospinal fluid. To date, there is no evidence of CNS production of M-6-G after intrathecal morphine or peripheral conversion of M-6-G back to morphine.

Various factors may influence the levels of both M-6-G and M-3-G including: route, (increased M-6-G following oral administration), age, greater than 70 years (increased M-3-G and M-6-G), male sex (decreased morphine and M-6-G plasma concentrations), concurrent use of tricyclic antidepressants (increased M-3-G), ranitidine (increased morphine) (63).

Controlled release oral morphine preparations are currently available in a wide dose range, from 15 to 200 mg for every 12 hours administration. These preparations provide comparable analgesia to preparations administered every 4 hours, but offer increased convenience, improved compliance, and reduction in patient time spent in pain. Cost benefit issues focusing on quality of life appear to support the use of these preparations. Although the oral, intramuscular, subcutaneous, and intravenous routes are the common routes of morphine administration, preparations are currently available for rectal, epidural, intrathecal, and intraventricular administration.

Methadone. Methadone has also been proposed as the drug of choice for cancer pain management (65). By using an intravenous infusion technique to evaluate the clearance of methadone and a minimal effective analgesic concentration (MEAC) for pain relief, some pharmacologists titrate patients to effective pain control (66). Such methodologic expertise is not widely available and the effectiveness of methadone is highly variable with significant adverse effects having been reported in cancer patients receiving methadone by various routes. Methadone's bioavailability is 85% and from single dose studies, its oral to parenteral ratio is 1:2. Its plasma half-life is 17 to 24 hours (reported up to 50 hours in some patients), but its duration of analgesia is only 4 to 8 hours (67). Repetitive doses of methadone lead to drug accumulation resulting in adverse effects. This discrepancy between its analgesic duration and its plasma half-life make it a drug that requires careful titration. It has been proposed that methadone be considered as a second line drug in patients after they have had prior exposure to opioids. Methadone is one of the cheapest of the oral analgesic preparations but its name has negative connotations for cancer patients who view methadone as a drug used to treat addicts. More recently, there have been a number of case reports that have highlighted the possibly greater analgesic potency of methadone than the often quoted 1:1 equivalency of methadone to morphine. Rogers reported a 50-year-old female, a patient with chronic cancer pain, who was poorly controlled on an equivalent daily dose of parenteral morphine of 300 mg (69). Good pain control was achieved with methadone at a dose of 90 mg. Galer et al., in five case reports on the subject of individual variability in response to different opioids, reported three patients switching from levorphanol and morphine to methadone due to inadequate pain control. In all cases, the amount of methadone required was far below the equianalgesic dose (46). Methadone can be administered by a variety of routes including subcutaneously, intravenously, rectally, epidurally, and intrathecally. A variety of studies have demonstrated its efficacy by these routes of administration. At the current time, the remaining controversy is the equianalgesic dose and the appropriate interval for administration (70). The major controversy is the fact that adverse effects appear to be reported with this drug and that there is a need to use the drug cautiously with doses tailored according to the individual patient's response, with a need for future studies to address both the issue of equianalgesic dose and appropriate interval of administration.

Oxycodone. Oxycodone is another important drug that is commonly used to manage cancer pain. Its most common use is in the patient with moderate to severe pain, often prior to the use of morphine or hydromorphone. In this population of patients, oxycodone is the active component of a series of combination drugs and is typically used in these combinations. A series of recent studies has shed further light on the pharmacokinetics of oxycodone and has suggested that it may produce less sedation and less hallucinatory effects as compared to morphine in treatment of postoperative pain (70-72). Although these are preliminary studies, they suggest that oxycodone may have a more acceptable spectrum of side effects as compared to morphine or methadone and therefore may play a role in chronic dosing in certain populations of patients such as the elderly. There is a strong impetus for further studies to help determine the role of oxycodone in populations of patients, e.g., those with renal disease and, e.g., those who have shown an intolerance to morphine or methadone (73).

Hydromorphone. Hydromorphone, like oxycodone, is a morphine congener, is five times more potent than morphine and is a highly water soluble salt. Its bioavailability varies from 30 to 40% with an oral to parenteral ratio of 5:1. Studies to date report its ability to produce excellent analgesia with a shorter latency to effect and reduced incidence of side-effects when compared with morphine (74). There is some evidence to suggest that it may play an important role in the management of patients, specifically the elderly, because of its short half-life. More recent observations indicate that hydromorphone has many metabolites that may play a role in producing CNS toxicity (75). This at the present time is only a hypothesis and has not been clearly demonstrated in the clinical situation.

Levorphanol. Levorphanol is a synthetic opioid analgesic and a congener of morphine. It is used commonly as a second line agent in patients with chrónic pain who cannot tolerate morphine because of inadequate analgesia with excessive side-effects. Dose titration needs to be done carefully, particularly in the opioid naive patient, because it produces analgesia for only 4 to 6 hours. Recently animal studies of levorphanol, have suggested that it is one of the morphine congeners that has a greater affinity for the delta receptor (76).

Making choices among these congeners of morphine or between morphine and its congeners and methadone remains problematic because of the lack of comparative studies in patient populations. Although the WHO suggested that morphine should be the drug of choice, in fact, there is no best choice of drug.

Meperidine. There is good evidence to suggest that meperidine, which is a synthetic opioid with anticholinergic properties, probably should not be used on a chronic basis in the management of patients with pain and cancer. Repetitive dosing of meperidine with doses greater than 250 mg per day can lead to normeperidine accumulation which is an active toxic metabolite resulting in central nervous system (CNS) hyperexcitability (77). This is characterized initially by subtle mood effects followed by tremors, multi-focal myoclonus and occasionally seizures. The CNS hyperexcitability occurs commonly in patients with renal disease yet it can occur following repeated administration in patients with normal renal function. The factors associated with CNS excitation due to meperidine include the plasma normeperidine level, the plasma normeperidine:meperidine ratio, compromised renal function, duration of meperidine administration, and meperidine dose. Naloxone does not reverse meperidine-induced seizures and its use in meperidine toxicity is controversial. There have been some case reports during meperidine intoxication that the use of naloxone has precipitated generalized seizures in individual patients. Lastly, in rare instances, CNS toxicity characterized by hyperpyrexia, muscle rigidity, and seizures has been reported following the administration of a single dose of meperidine to patients being treated with monoamine oxidase inhibitors.

Fentanyl. A drug that recently has been used effectively in the cancer patient because of its novel route of administration, is fentanyl. This is a synthetic opioid that interacts predominantly with the mu receptor. It has been widely used to manage acute intra- and postoperative pain. It is used by the intravenous, epidural, transmucosal, and transdermal routes. The recent development of a transdermal patch has broadened its clinical usefulness to the management of patients with chronic cancer pain by this novel route. The half-life of fentanyl shows signs of variability, ranging from 3 to 12 hours (78). It is metabolized in the liver and n-dealkylated to nor-fentanil and other inactive metabolites. Seventy-five percent of the dose is excreted in urine. Its relative potency compared to parenteral morphine varies from 1:20 to 1:30 in the non-tolerant acute pain patients.

In countries where many of these drugs are not available, the WHO has worked hard to make oral morphine available, but in many countries limited availability forces practitioners to use any analgesic opioid as the first-line agent. In trying to further clarify these issues in opioid pharmacology, further studies on both the clinical pharmacology of the drugs, as well as on the epidemiology of their use, will be helpful.

In practice, there is no "best" opioid drug. Individualized therapy is the critical factor to ensure effective analgesia and numerous other opioid drugs have been used to manage cancer pain. Current pharmacologic guidelines have been described in the literature. The general approach is to use oral analgesics titrated to the needs of the individual patient, based on the age of the patient, the nature of the pain, the prior opioid exposure, the degree of hepatic and renal compromise, and the accessible route.

Route of Administration

A third controversy includes the route of administration. Although the oral route represents the simplest and most commonly used approach, the impetus for the development of these novel routes of administration has come from the goal to maximize analgesia, minimize side effects, and provide convenient dosing schedules for patients who require parenteral drug administration. Survey data demonstrate that the majority of patients with progressive disease and pain will require at least two and, in at least 25% of cases, three routes of drug administration (79). What remains controversial is the logic of both patient selection and timing and implementation of these alternative routes (79-81).

Risk/benefit and cost/benefit analyses are beginning to address these issues. Various factors including the availability of oral opioids, the expertise of the treating physician (internists, oncologists versus anesthesiologists), the nature of the pain, and the financial resources of the patient have confounded the true assessment of the "best approach."

The key concept in considering alternative routes is the effectiveness of an intervention and its appropriateness. The crucial part of appropriateness for novel routes is the incidence of adverse effects. The golden rule for comparison of adverse effects of two analgesic interventions is that the comparison should be made at the same level of analgesic effect. This comparison of equianalgesic medications adminstered systemically versus via the spinal or other novel routes has not been completed (80).

The Development of Tolerance

The chronic use of opioids in cancer pain patients has provided for the first time the unique natural experiment to study tolerance development to opioid analgesia and side effects in a medical setting. Previous studies of tolerance in humans have focused on the neuroadaptation of mood and autonomic effects in addict populations and have not addressed tolerance to analgesia in acute and chronic pain patients. From a series of studies assessing the patterns of opioid drug use in cancer pain patients, it is evident that the role of tolerance development varies enormously among patients and is influenced by numerous environmental, behavioral, pharmacologic, pain and patient related factors (82-87). Several patterns of opioid use have been described:

1. rapidly escalating doses of opioids associated with escalating pain and/or psychological distress.
2. stable doses of opioids for long periods of time (weeks to months) with effective analgesia without dose escalation or reduction.
3. reduction in or discontinuation of opioid drugs with effective analgesia from anti-cancer therapies or anesthetic or neurosurgical approaches.

These patterns have been described in various patient populations including hospice programs, home care and supportive care programs, hospitalized settings and outpatient cancer pain clinics.

These clinical observations are in marked contrast to the suggestions in the pharmacologic textbooks and information culled from the medical literature suggesting that such patients would continue to escalate their requirements for opioid analgesia on the basis of tolerance alone. These observations are in concert with an extensive animal literature demonstrating the wide variability of tolerance development on the basis of behavioral, environmental and pharmacologic factors. In the cancer patient with pain in contrast to the animal paradigm, the pain stimulus is changing. Discerning the relative contributions of a change in pain state from that due directly to tolerance is confounding. From the clinical data, the overriding factor in dose escalation is progression of disease. Other factors that play a role include the patient's prior opioid exposure, the endpoint measured for opioid effect, and the type of pain. In a series of studies, Houde et al. demonstrated that pharmacologic tolerance occurs in cancer patients and is characterized by a shift in the dose response curve to the right (88). These studies also demonstrated that cross-tolerance is incomplete and that dose escalation often requires a doubling of the dose because of the log dose effect relationship. There is no limit to tolerance. These aspects of tolerance have clinical implications. It is now well recognized that a wide range of opioid analgesics are used in cancer pain management. Although numerous studies have demonstrated that the majority of patients may be managed in a dose range of 30 to 700 mEq of morphine per 24 hours (79). There are however, a series of patients who may require very large doses for adequate control and who require rapid dose escalation and doubling or tripling of their initial dose regimen. These high doses are often misinterpreted as inappropriate by inexperienced physicians who undermedicate patients because of their reliance on only standard doses rather than using the concept of opioid responsiveness as their endpoint.

Tolerance develops at different rates to the respiratory depressant, analgesic, emetic, pupillary constrictor, and slowly, if at all, to the constipatory effects of the opioids. This differential rate of development explains the safe use of large doses of opioids in cancer patients without compromising their respiratory status.

The fact that cross-tolerance is incomplete is reflected in part by the individual variability in response to opioid analgesics. This concept is the basis for switching to alternative opioids to provide analgesia. The mechanism of this phenomenon is that tolerance develops independently at each receptor subtype. For example, D-Ala2-D-Leu5-enkephalin, a delta selective opioid peptide, produced significant analgesia following intrathecal administration in cancer patients tolerant to morphine (85).

The mechanisms underlying tolerance are complex and include actions at the level of the receptor and effector systems as well as activation of antagonist systems and/or downregulation of facilitatory ones. At the current time at the molecular level, it is postulated that a functional decoupling of opioid receptors from G proteins may be the underlying explanation. Recent studies have demonstrated the role of NMDA receptors in the development of morphine tolerance (85-87). MK801, an NMDA antagonist, not only reverses morphine tolerance but prevents its development without reducing morphine analgesia. This dissociation of tolerance from pain inhibition (analgesia) suggests that different mechanisms account for these phenomena and, in part, help to explain why patients may continue to obtain analgesia even when tolerant to opioids. These studies also suggest that both non-opioid and opioid mechanisms are involved in tolerance development. Of particular clinical relevance is the fact that combinations of excitatory amino acid antagonists with opioid analgesics might facilitate the clinical usefulness of opioid drugs by limiting the development of tolerance to the analgesic effects of the drug.

At the current time there are multiple ways to provide analgesia to patients who are tolerant to opioid analgesics, such as the use of adjuvant analgesics; the use of oral, intravenous and epidural local anesthetics; and the use of specific anesthetic and neurosurgical approaches to interrupt pain pathways. The potential for drug combinations with an excitatory amino acid antagonist to manage this clinical situation offer important future approaches.

CONFUSION BETWEEN THE RELATIONSHIP OF PAIN MANAGEMENT TO PATIENT REQUESTS FOR PHYSICIAN-ASSISTED SUICIDE AND EUTHANASIA

In one survey 69% of cancer patients reported that they would consider committing suicide if their pain was not adequately treated (25). Uncontrolled pain is an important contributing factor in cancer patients assessed to be at risk for suicide (92). Persistent pain interferes with a patient's quality of life and this, in turn, influences a patient's choice about suicide or physician-assisted suicide (93). Pain relief in oncology cannot be isolated from the overwhelming need to manage the multitude of physical as well as psychological symptoms that occur in this population of patients. It is the responsibility of the treating physician to manage pain in this patient population. The intent, goal, and conditions in which physicians and patients interact are directed toward the management of symptoms and should not be construed as euthanasia. Aggressive treatment of pain with increasing doses of opioids to provide analgesia should not be referred to as "hastening death." Its intent and rationale are to manage uncontrollable or unendurable symptoms. The prevalence of and treatment for physical symptoms of pain, dyspnea, delirium and psychological distress in the dying patient have become controversial issues. Their expert management using opioids and sedative drugs is misconstrued as active euthanasia. Lack of understanding of the concept of tolerance, the dearth of pharmacologic data on drugs to provide terminal sedation and the ambivalence on the part of patients, families and physicians because of ethical concerns have thwarted the provision of appropriate medical care for this population of patients. At the present time, there are few highly trained physicians in cancer pain management, psycho-oncology or palliative care whose main interest is to place a high priority on pain management, symptom control and psychological support for patients with advanced disease. Any debate that focuses on the needs of the dying patient and their options for care at the end of life must recognize that the education and training of physicians, as well as patients and families, is the first step in providing patients with access to care that will facilitate their choice of options (94-96).

REFERENCES

1. Cancer Pain Relief. World Health Organization, Geneva, 1986
2. Cancer Pain Relief and Palliative Care, World Health Organization, Geneva, 1990
3. Bonica JJ: Cancer pain, The Management of Pain, JJ Bonica (ed). Philadelphia, Lea & Febiger, 400-34, 1990
4. Foley KM: The treatment of cancer pain. N Engl J Med 313:84-95, 1985
5. Elliott K, Foley KM: Neurologic pain syndromes in patients with cancer. Neurologic Clinics, Pain: Mechanisms and Syndromes, Vol. 7, Portenoy RK (ed). WB Saunders, Philadelphia, 1989, pp. 333-360
6. Portenoy RK: Cancer pain: pathophysiology and syndromes. Lancet 339:1026-1031, 1992
7. Portenoy RK, Hagen NA: Breakthrough pain: definition and management. Oncology 3(Suppl):25-29, 1989
8. Ahles TA, Blanchard EB, Ruckdeschel JC: The multidimensional nature of cancer related pain. Pain 17:277-289, 1983
9. Breitbart WS, Holland J: Psychiatric aspects of cancer pain, Advances in Pain Research and Therapy, Vol. 16. Foley KM, Bonica JJ, Ventafridda V (eds). Proceedings of the Second International Congress on Cancer Pain. Raven Press, New York, 1990, pp. 73-88
10. Fishman B, Pasternak S, Wallenstein SL, et al: The Memorial Pain Assessment Card: a valid instrument for the evaluation of cancer pain. Cancer 60:1151-1158, 1987
11. Daut RL, Cleeland CS, Flanery RC: The development of the Wisconsin Brief Pain Questionnaire to assess pain in cancer and other diseases. Pain 17:197-210, 1983
12. Graham C, Bond SS, Gertrovitch MM, Cook MR: Use of the McGill Pain Questionnaire in the management of cancer pain--replicability and consistency. Pain 8:377-387, 1980
13. Inturrisi CE, Colburn WA, Kaiko RF, Houde RW, Foley KM: Pharmacokinetic and pharmacodynamics of methadone in patients

with chronic pain. Clin Pharmacology & Therapeutics 41:392-401, 1987

14. Hill HF, Chapman CR, Saeger LS, Bjurstrom R, Walter MH, Schoene RB, Kippes M: Steady-state infusions of opioids in humans: II. Concentration-effect relationships and therapeutic margins. Pain 43:69-80, 1991
15. Cousins MJ: Anesthetic approaches in cancer pain, Advances in Pain Research and Therapy, Vol 16. Foley KM, Ventafridda V, Bonica JJ (eds). Second International Congress on Cancer Pain. New York, Raven Press, 1990, pp. 249-274
16. Arbit E: Neurosurgical management of cancer pain, Advances in Pain Research and Therapy, Vol 16. Foley KM, Ventafridda V, Bonica JJ (eds). Second International Congress on Cancer Pain. New York, Raven Press, 1990, pp. 289-300
17. Foley KM: Controversies in cancer pain--medical perspective. Cancer 63:2257-2266, 1989
18. Portenoy RK, Foley KM, Inturrisi CE: The nature of opioid responsiveness and its implications for neuropathic pain: new hypotheses derived from studies of opioid infusions. Pain 43:273-286, 1990
19. Foley KM: Clinical tolerance to opioids, Towards a New Pharmacotherapy of Pain. Dahlem Konferenzen. Basbaum, AI, Besson JM (eds). Chichester: John Wiley & Son, 1991, pp. 181-204
20. Foley KM: Pain syndromes in patients with cancer, Advances in Pain Research and Therapy, Vol. 2. Bonica JJ, Ventafridda V (eds), New York, Raven Press, 1979, pp. 59-75
21. Daut RL, Cleeland CS: The prevalence and severity of pain in cancer. Cancer 50:1913-1918, 1982
22. Spiegel D, Bloom JR: Pain in metastatic breast cancer. Cancer 52:341-345, 1983
23. Ventafridda V, Tamburini M, Caraceni A, DeConno F, Naldi F: A validation study of the WHO method for cancer pain relief. Cancer 59:850-856, 1987
24. Stjernsward J: WHO cancer pain relief programme. Cancer Surv 7:195-208, 1988
25. Cleeland CS: Pain control: public and physician attitudes, Advances in Pain Research and Therapy, Vol- 11. Hill CS Fields WS (eds). Raven Press, New York 1989, pp. 81-89
26. Weissman DE, Dahl JL: Attitudes about cancer pain: A survey of Wisconsin's first year medical students. J Pain Symptom Manage 5:345-349, 1990
27. Van Roenn JH, Cleeland CS, Gonin R, Hatfield A, Pandya KJ: Physicians' attitudes toward cancer pain management survey: results of the Eastern Cooperative Oncology Group Survey. Ann Int Med In press, 1993
28. Ferell B, McGuire DB, Donovan MI: Knowledge and beliefs regarding pain in a sample of nursing faculty. J Prof Nurs In press, 1993

29. Joranson DE, Cleeland CS, Weissman DE, Gilson AM: Cancer pain, opioids and the law: a survey of state medical board members. Fed Bulletin: The Medical Journal of Licensure and Discipline In press, 1993
30. Peteet J, Tay V, Cohen G, Macintyre J: Pain characteristics and treatment in an outpatient cancer population. Cancer 57:1259-1265, 1986
31. Grossman SA, Sheidler VR, Swedeen K, Mucenski J, Pianladosi S: Correlation of patient and care giver ratings of cancer pain. J Pain Symptom Manage 6:53-57, 1991
32. McDonald N: Initiatives in China, WHO News. Palliative Medicine 6:6-8, 1992
33. Takeda F: Changing attitudes toward narcotic use in cancer pain management in Japan. Postgrad Med J S31-34, 1992
34. Report of the International Narcotics Control Board for 1989. Demands for and Supply of Opiates for Medical and Scientific Needs. United Nations, New York, 1989
35. Dahl JL, Joranson DE: The Wisconsin Cancer Pain Initiative, Advances in Pain Research and Therapy, Vol. 16. Foley KM, Ventafridda V, Bonica JJ (eds). Second International Congress on Cancer Pain. New York, Raven Press, 1990, pp. 499-503
36. Ventafridda V, Tamburini M, DeConno F: Comprehensive treatment of cancer pain, Advances in Pain Research and Therapy, Vol. 9. Fields HL, Dubner R, Cervero F (eds). Raven Press, Ltd., New York 617-628, 1985
37. Ventafridda V, DeConno F, Ripamonti C, Gamba A, Tamburini M: Quality-of-life assessment during a palliative care programme. Annals of Oncology 1:415-420, 1990
38. Scott JF: Palliative Care 2000: What's Stopping Us? J Pall Care 8:5-8, 1992
39. Committee on Quality Assurance Standards: American Pain Society quality assurance standards for relief of acute pain and cancer pain. Proceedings of VIth World Congress on Pain. Bond MR, Charlton JE, Woolf CJ (eds). Amsterdam, Elsevier 1991, 185-189
40. Arner S, Meyerson BA: Lack of analgesic effect of opioids on neuropathic and idiopathic forms of pain. Pain 33:11-23, 1988
41. Hanks GW, Justins DM: Cancer pain management. Lancet 339:1031-1035, 1992
42. Cherny NI, Thaler HT, Friedlander-Klar H, Lapin J, Portenoy RK: Opioid responsiveness of neuropathic cancer pain: combined analysis of single dose analgesic trials. Proc ASCO 11:383, 1992
43. Portenoy RK, Foley KM, Inturrisi CE: The nature of opioid responsiveness and its implications for neuropathic pain: new hypotheses derived from studies of opioid infusions. Pain 43:273-286, 1990
44. Foley KM: The role of opioid analgesics in neuropathic pain, Lesions of the primary afferent fibers as a tool for the study of clinical pain.

Besson JM, Guilbaud G (eds). Amsterdam, Elsevier Science Publ 1991, pp. 277-292

45. Rowbotham MC, Fields HL: Post-herpetic neuralgia: the relation of pain complaint, sensory disturbance, and skin temperature. Pain 39:129-144, 1989
46. Galer BS, Coyle N, Pasternak GW, Portenoy RK: Individual variability in the response to different opioids: report of five cases. Pain 49:87-91, 1992
47. Portenoy RK: Issues in the management of neuropathic pain, Towards a New Pharmacotherapy of Pain. Basbaum A, Besson J-M (eds). New York, John Wiley & Sons, 1991, pp. 393-416
48. Macaluso C, Foley KM: Adjuvant analgesic drugs in cancer pain management, Relief of Chronic Pain. Aronoff GM (ed). Addison Wesley Pubs., Boston, Mass., In Press, 1992
49. Sawe J: Morphine and its 3- and 6-glucuronides in plasma and urine during chronic oral administration in cancer patients, Advances in Pain Research and Therapy, Vol. 8. Foley KM, Inturrisi CE (eds). Raven Press, New York 1986, pp. 45-55
50. Osborne RJ, Joel SP, Slevin ML: Morphine intoxication in renal failure: the role of morphine-6-glucuronide. Br Med J 292:1548-1549, 1986
51. Osborne RJ, Joel SP, Trew D, Slevin ML: The analgesic activity of morphine-6-glucuronide. Lancet i:828, 1988
52. Osborne RJ, Joel SP, Trew D, Slevin ML: Morphine and metabolite behavior after different routes of morphine administration: demonstration of the importance of the active metabolite morphine-6-glucuronide. Clin Pharmacol Ther 47:12-19, 1990
53. Shimomura K, Kamata O, Ueki S, et al: Analgesic effect of morphine glucuronides, Tohoku J Exp Med 105:45-52, 1971
54. Pasternak GW, Bodnar RJ, Clark JA, Inturrisi CE: Morphine-6-glucuronide, a potent mu agonist. Life Sci 41:2845-2849, 1987
55. Paul D, Standifer KM, Inturrisi CE, Pasternak GW: Pharmacological characterization of morphine-6-glucuronide, a very potent morphine metabolite. J Pharmacol Exp Ther 251:477-483, 1989
56. Poulain P, Moran-Ribon A, Hanks GW, Hoskin PJ, Aherne GW, Chapman DP. CSF concentrations of morphine-6-glucuronide after oral administration of morphine. Pain 5 (Suppl):S194, 1990
57. Hand CW, Blunnie WP, Claffey LP, et al: Potential analgesic contribution from morphine-6-glucuronide in CSF Lancet ii:1207-1208, 1987
58. Portenoy RK, Thaler HT, Inturrisi CE, Friedlander-Klar H, Foley KM: The metabolite, morphine-6-glucuronide, contributes to the analgesia produced by morphine infusion in pain patients with normal renal function. Clin Pharm Ther 51:422-431, 1992
59. Portenoy RK, Khan E, Layman M, Lapin J, Malkin MG, Foley KM, Cerbone DJ, Inturrisi CE: Chronic morphine therapy for cancer pain:

Plasma and cerebrospinal fluid morphine and morphine-6-glucuronide concentrations. Neurology 41:1457-1461, 1991
60. Portenoy RK, Foley KM, Stulman J, Khan E, Adelhardt J, Layman, Cerbone DF, Inturrisi CE: Plasma morphine and morphine-6-glucuronide during chronic morphine therapy for cancer pain: plasma profiles, steady-state concentrations and the consequences of renal failure: Pain 47:13-19, 1991
61. Petreson GM, Randall CTC, Paterson J: Plasma levels of morphine and morphine glucuronides in the treatment of cancer pain: relationship to renal function and route of administration. Eur J Clin Pharmacol 38:121-4, 1990
62. Hagen N, Foley KM, Cebrone DJ, Portenoy RK, Inturrisi CE: Chronic nausea and morphine-6-glucuronide. J Pain Symptom Manage 6:125-128, 1991
63. McQuay HJ, Caroll D, Faura CC, Gavaghan DJ, Hand CW, Moore RA: Oral morphine in cancer pain: influences on morphine and metabolite concentration. Clin Pharmacol Ther 48:236-244, 1990
64. Breda M, Bianchi M, Ripamonti C, Zecca E, Ventafridda V, Panerai AE: Plasma morphine and morphine-6-glucuronide patterns in cancer patients after oral, subcutaneous, sublingual, and rectal short-term administration. Int J Clin Pharmacol Res 11:93-97, 1991
65. Fainsinger R, Schoellrs T, and Bruera E: Methadone in the management of cancer pain: a review. Pain 52:137-147, 1993
66. Grochow L, Sheidler V, Grossman S, et al: Does intravenous methadone provide longer lasting analgesia than intravenous morphine? A randomized double-blind study. Pain 38:151-157, 1989
67. Inturrisi CE, Colburn WA, Kaiko RF, Houde RW, Foley KM. Pharmacokinetic and pharmacodynamics of methadone in chronic pain patients. Clin Pharmacology & Therapeutics, 41:392-401, 1987
68. Ettinger DS, Vitale PJ, Trump DL: Important clinical pharmacologic considerations in the use of methadone in cancer patients. Cancer Treat Rep 63:457-459, 1979
69. Rogers AG: The use of methadone in opioid tolerant patients. J Pain Symptom Manage 3:45, 1988
70. Kalso E, Poyhia R, Onnela P, Lanko K, Tigersledt I, Tammusto T: Intravenous morphine and oxycodone for pain after abdominal surgery. ACTA Anaesthesiol Scand 35:642-646, 1991
71. Poyhia R, Olkkola KT, Seppala T, Kalso E: The pharmacokinetics of oxycodone after intravenous injection in adults. Br J Clin Pharmac 32:516-518, 1991
72. Poyhia R, Seppala T, Olkkola KT, Kalso E: The pharmacokinetics and metabolism of oxycodone after intramuscular and oral administration to healthy subjects. Br J Clin Pharma 33:617-621, 1992
73. Rogers A: The under utilization of oxycodone. J Pain Symptom Manage 6:452, 1991
74. Moulin DE, Kreeft JH, Murray-Parsons N, Bouquillon AL: Comparison of continuous subcutaneous and intravenous

hydromorphone infusions for management of cancer pain. Lancet 337:465-468, 1991

75. Babul N, Darke AC: Palliative role of hydromorphone metabolites in myoclonus. Pain 51:260-261, 1992
76. Moulin DE, Ling GSF, Pasternak GW: Unidirectional analgesic cross-tolerance between morphine and levorphanol in the rat. Pain 33:233-239, 1988
77. Kaiko RF, Foley KM, Grabinski PY, et al: Central nervous system excitatory effects of meperidine in cancer patients. Ann Neurol 131:180-185, 1985
78. Portenoy RK, Southam MA, Gupta SK, Lapin J, Layman M, Inturrisi CE, Foley KM: Transdermal fentanyl for cancer pain: repeated dose pharmacokinetics. Anesthesiology 78:36-43, 1993
79. Coyle N, Adelhardt J, Foley KM, Portenoy RK: Character of terminal illness in the advanced cancer patient: pain and other symptoms in the last 4 weeks of life. J Pain Symptom Manage 5:83-93, 1990
80. Mather LE. Novel methods of analgesic drug delivery, Proceedings of the Vlth World Congress on Pain. Bond MR, Charlton JEO, Woolf CJ (eds). Amsterdam, Elsevier 159-174, 1990
81. McQuay HJ: The logic of alternative routes. J Pain Symptom Manage 5:73-136, 1991
82. Twycross RG: Clinical experience with diamorphine in advanced malignant disease. Int J Clin Pharm 9:184-198, 1974
83. Portenoy RK, Moulin DE, Rogers AG, Inturrisi CE, Foley KM. Continuous intravenous infusion of opioids in cancer pain: Review of 46 cases and guidelines for use. Cancer Treat Rep 7:575-581, 1986
84. Kanner RM, Foley KM. Patterns of narcotic drug use in a cancer pain clinic. Research developments in drug and alcohol use. Ann NY Acad Sci 362: 161-172, 1981
85. Moulin DE, Max MB, Kaiko RF, Inturrisi CE, Maggard J, Yaksh T, Foley KM: The analgesic efficacy of intrathecal D-Ala2-D-Leu5-enkephalin in cancer patients with chronic pain. Pain 23:213-221, 1985
86. Foley KM: Clinical tolerance to opioids, Toward a New Pharmacotherapy of Pain. Dahlem Konferenzen. Basbaum AI, Besson JM (eds). Chichester, John Wiley & Sons, 181-204, 1991
87. Foley KM: Changing concepts of tolerance to opioids. What the cancer patient has taught us, Current & Emerging Issues in Cancer Pain: Research & Practice. Chapman CR, Foley KM (eds). New York, Raven Press, pp. 331-349, 1993
88. Houde RW, Wallenstein SL, Beaver WT: Evaluation of analgesics in patients with cancer pain, Clinical Pharmacology. Section 6, Vol. 1. International Encyclopedia of Pharmacology and Therapeutics. Lasagna L (ed). Oxford, Pergamon 1966, pp. 9-98
89. Trujillo KA, Akil H: Opiate tolerance and dependence: recent findings and synthesis. The New Biologist 3:915-923, 1991

90. Trujillo KA, Akil H: MK801 prevents the development of opioid tolerance. Science 251: 85-88, 1991
91. Marek P, Ben-Eliyahu S, Gold M, Liebeskind JC: Excitatory amino acid antagonists (kynurenic acid and MK-801) attenuate the development of morphine tolerance in the rat. Brain Research 547:77-81, 1991
92. Breitbart W: Cancer pain and suicide. Advances in Pain Research and Therapy, Vol 16. Second International Congress on Cancer Pain, Foley KM, Ventafridda V, Bonica J (eds). New York, Raven Press, 399-412, 1990
93. Foley KM: The relationship of pain & symptom management to patient requests for physician-assisted suicide. J Pain Symptom Manage 6:289-297, 1991
94. Ventafridda V, Ripamonti C, DeConno F, Tamburini, M: Symptom prevalence and control during cancer patients' last days of life. J Palliative Care 6:7-11, 1990
95. Roy DJ: Need they die before they sleep? J Palliative Care 6:3-4, 1990
96. Mount B: A final crescendo of pain? J Palliative Care 6:5-6, 1990

NEUROLYTIC BLOCKS—CURRENT STATUS IN THE TREATMENT OF CANCER AND CHRONIC PAIN

M. J. Cousins

INTRODUCTION

In the management of cancer pain and chronic pain, the clinician now often relies on the systemic administration of centrally-acting drugs, the utility of which is determined by the balance between analgesic efficacy and side effects mediated by the central nervous system (CNS). Nonetheless, the potential for regionalized pain control as an alternative to this systemic approach has been recognized since the demonstration of nerve conduction block by Koller in 1884. The latter observation led to an explosion of reversible anesthetic techniques, which target with varying degrees of selectivity any region of the nervous system to provide pain relief with lesser risk of CNS side effects (1).

THE ROLE OF THE ANESTHETIST AND NEUROLYTIC TECHNIQUES IN PAIN MANAGEMENT

In the past, conduction blockade of peripheral nerves and sympathetic ganglia were the major tasks of the anesthetist in the management of cancer and chronic pain. Anesthetic approaches to pain control now compromise techniques that are designed to deliver drugs that (a) interacts with nociceptive receptors (local anesthetics and NSAID's) (b) block axonal transmission (local anesthetic or neurolytic blockade), (c) block sympathetic function (local anesthetic or neurolytic blockade), or (d) decrease CNS transmission of nociceptive information (e.g., spinal opioids and non-opioids). The approaches selected in any individual case may involve one or multiple sites of the nervous system. The anesthetist provides both technical skills and knowledge of the

T. H. Stanley and M. A. Ashburn (eds.), Anesthesiology and Pain Management, 333–342.

indications, contraindications and management strategies used in the application of these techniques. The appropriately trained anesthetist can, therefore, make considerable contributions to the management of the patient with chronic pain.

NEUROLYTIC BLOCKADE OF THE CENTRAL NERVOUS SYSTEM

In general, neurolytic blocks are best suited for patients with short life expectancy and well localized pain. These techniques are most effective in nociceptive pain (2), deafferentation pain (3) responds poorly despite initial temporary relief.

Ethyl alcohol and phenol are the most frequently used neurolytic agents. Glycerol also has been used, and may be advantageous in trigeminal ganglion block. Phenol has local anesthetic properties which can result in painless injection. Similar to local anesthetics, however, phenol may produce convulsions followed by CNS depression if injected intravascularly. Few data exist presently to determine an advantage of one agent over others.

SUBARACHNOID NEUROLYTIC BLOCK

Subarachnoid neurolytic block is an effective method of pain relief, which should be restricted to patients with advanced malignancy. The pain should be unilateral and limited to only a few segments. The aim is to produce a posterior rhizotomy to disrupt the pain pathways in the affected region.

The general progressive nature of the patients' underlying disease makes assessment of spinal neurolytic blockade difficult. In experienced hands, 60% of patients obtain good results (pain relief for more than one month). Complications have been reported in the range of 1 to 4%, with the lowest complication rate following injection into the thoracic region (4). Unilateral chest pain (e.g., due to mesothelioma) is an excellent application for thoracic subarachnoid neurolytic block. The key to efficacy and safety is needle placement close to the affected segments, usually placement of more than one needle and injection of small volumes (0.5 to

0.75 ml) via each needle. Correct position of the patient is vital, e.g. with alcohol (hypobaric) the patient is placed 45° semi-prone with affected side uppermost.

SUBDURAL OR EPIDURAL NEUROLYTIC BLOCK

Subdural or epidural neurolytic blockade may also be effective, although there have been no studies comparing the effects of subarachnoid blocks with subdural or epidural block. Epidural or subdural block may be preferable in the cervical segments, because subarachnoid injection is followed by rapid dilution of neurolytic agents in the CSF from the rapid circulation of adjacent intracranial CSF (4); it is also difficult to limit the spread of the neurolytic agent to the desired segments. Cervical subdural block has been used for pain in the region of the ear, nose and throat as well as tumors in the cervical region (4).

NEUROLYTIC TRIGEMINAL BLOCK

Neurolytic trigeminal nerve blockade has been effectively used in the management of chronic pain, and particularly for trigeminal neuralgia. Injection into the Gasserian ganglion with ethyl alcohol was widely used in the past, but newer therapies such as balloon compression, glycerol injection (5), open surgical procedures (e.g., Janetta), and thermogangliolysis (6) have superseded alcohol injection. Gasserian ganglion blockade is usually achieved via the foramen ovale approach using fluoroscopic control (7).

NEUROLYTIC BLOCKS OF THE PERIPHERAL NERVOUS SYSTEM

Neurolytic somatic neural blockade occasionally has a role in the management of cancer pain, despite a concern for neuralgia or motor blockade. Examples of such neurolytic blocks include intercostal, infraorbital, facial and obturator nerve blocks, brachial plexus block, and intralesional neurolytic injection for bony metastases (8). The incidence of inadequate analgesia can be lessened by careful technique, perhaps with the use of a nerve stimulator.

THE SYMPATHETIC NERVOUS SYSTEM, CHRONIC AND CANCER PAIN

Sympathetic nervous system blockade can produce significant analgesia depending on the etiology of the pain. The efferent sympathetic fibers and sympathetic ganglia are traversed by the visceral afferent nociceptive fibers (without synapse). In different clinical settings, therefore, sympathetic blockade may be used to block either the sympathetic efferent and/or the visceral nociceptive afferent fibers. Stellate ganglion block is the most common approach for pain in head, neck and upper extremity pain; celiac plexus block can be utilized for upper abdominal visceral pain; lumbar sympathetic block is used for lower abdominal visceral pain and lower extremity pain.

Recent work has drawn attention to the central, spinal component of sympathetically maintained pain, as well as the peripheral effect of sympathetic activity on nociceptors (9). It appears that nerve or soft tissue injury may cause expression of alpha-adrenergic receptors on nociceptors (10); subsequent sympathetic nervous system activity may activate those nociceptors. This nociceptor activity may sensitize the dorsal horn cells to respond to normally non-nociceptive stimuli, from a larger receptive field. This, in turn, may lead to a reflex increase in sympathetic discharge, creating a vicious cycle of sympathetically-maintained pain. In addition, there is some evidence of ephaptic connection between the sympathetic nervous system and nociceptive fibers (11). To abort or lessen these processes, sympathetic nerves may be blocked with local anesthetic or neurolytic techniques; however, the approach is only effective if used early in the course of chronic pain. Later the pathophysiology is predominantly spinal and supraspinal.

NEUROLYTIC SYMPATHETIC BLOCKADE

The demonstration of relief of neuropathic pain by local anesthetic sympathetic blockade is an important diagnostic test and indicates a potential benefit from neurolytic sympathetic blockade. In addition to the management of sympathetically-maintained pain, sympathetic blockade may be of benefit in the management of acute exacerbations of chronic problems, such as, ischemic crises in Raynaud's disease and other obliterative arteriopathies (12), and possibly in the management of established post herpetic neuralgia (12-14).

Neurolytic sympathetic block, including celiac plexus and lumbar sympathetic block, has great potential benefit in the management of patients with visceral pain. Mixed somatic and visceral pain syndromes are likely to have incomplete pain relief and appear to be best managed with spinal opioids. In such complicated cases, neurolytic sympathetic block may be useful in reducing pain and enhancing alternative therapy. The effects of one or more local anesthetic blocks should be very carefully assessed prior to deciding on neurolytic blocks.

NEUROLYTIC CELIAC PLEXUS BLOCKADE

Celiac plexus block provides a potent means of interrupting visceral nociceptive afferent fibers from the upper abdomen. The most significant role of neurolytic celiac plexus blockade (NCPB) is in the management of severe upper abdominal pain of malignant origin, especially carcinoma of the pancreas (15-20). NCPB has the potential to provide 70-80% of patients with good relief immediately (Table 1) and 60-75% until death. Chronic pancreatitis does not appear to be improved by NCPB due to the limited duration of analgesia and the role of other factors in such patients. However, it may rarely be used in selected cases to aid rehabilitation. NCPB is associated with temporary orthostatic hypotension and increased gastrointestinal motility. These side effects are usually mild and self-limiting. Fortunately, the incidence of more severe complications is low (Table 2). The true incidence and etiology of catastrophic complications are unknown, but in view of the several thousand patients who are reported to have safely undergone NCPB, the incidence appears to be extremely low. The most important factors in the application of NCPB are careful patient selection and meticulous technique with radiographic imaging to verify needle placement (20).

Table 1. Results of "classic" celiac plexus block with alcohol.

Author	Indication	Number of Cases	Results % Good	Fair	Poor
Brown (16)	Pancreatic Cancer	136	85*	-	15
Black (18)	Pancreatic Cancer	20	70	30	0
	Other abdominal Malignancy	37	70	17	13
Bridenbaugh (17)	Upper abdominal Cancer	41	73	24.5	2.5
Ischia (19)	Pancreatic Cancer	18	72	-	28[a]
		43	37	-	63[b]

* In 75% of patients, good relief lasted through remaining life. The success of repeated blocks was also 85%.

[a] Patients with duration of pain ≤ 2 months.

[b] Patients with duration of pain ≥ 2 months.

Table 2. Complications - celiac plexus blockade.

Complication	%
Weakness or numbness T_{10}-L_2	8%
Lower chest pain	3%
Failure of ejaculation	2%
Urinary retention	1%
Postural hypotension	1%*
Diarrhea, pneumothorax, paraplegia	?%

(Data from: Black A, Dwyer B. Coeliac plexus block. Anaesthesia and Intensive Care, 1973;1:315-318) (*temporary postural hypotension occurs in 30-60% of patients (18))

NEUROLYTIC LUMBAR SYMPATHETIC BLOCKADE

Ischemia due to peripheral vascular disease (PVD) is often associated with severe pain. This may lead to increased sympathetic discharge, resulting in sensitization of nociceptors (described above).

Neurolytic lumbar sympathetic block may cause vasodilation and interrupt the cycle of pain and reflex sympathetic discharge. Sympathetic blockade has been shown to reduce ischemic rest pain, increase blood flow, and enhance healing of chronic ulceration in inoperable PVD (21,22). Neurolytic sympathetic blockade is as efficacious as surgical sympathetic block but is less invasive and is associated with lower morbidity, mortality, lower cost and it is more easily repeated (21,22). Similar to surgical sympathetic blocks, neurolytic sympathectomy has a mean duration of effect of approximately six months (21).

Through blockade of pelvic visceral afferent fibers, lumbar sympathetic block may relieve the pain associated with pelvic cancer. Bilateral blocks may be useful in pain caused by tumors of the sigmoid colon, rectum, or urogenital organs, if the disease is confined to those viscera (12). Lumbar sympathetic blockade, in combination with NCPB, may provide pain relief for extensive intraabdominal spread (12,20).

NEUROLYTIC SUPERIOR HYPOGASTRIC PLEXUS BLOCK

Neurolytic superior hypogastric plexus block also has been reported to be effective in the management of pelvic cancer pain (23). This may provide a more selective block of afferent visceral fibers than lumbar sympathectomy. The role of superior hypogastric block in pelvic pain management requires further evaluation of its benefits and side effects.

PLACE OF NEUROLYTIC BLOCKS IN VIEW OF RECENT ADVANCES IN PAIN MANAGEMENT TECHNIQUES

During the last decade, the anesthetic management of chronic pain has undergone considerable change. Recent advances in the understanding of the neurophysiology and consequences of nociception and nerve damage (neuropathy), hold the potential for greater and more fundamental changes. Because of the 'plasticity' of the nervous system (i.e., alteration of function in response to previous neural activity), nociception and/or neuropathy may modify spinal cord function and may facilitate further pain transmission, leading to the development of severe, intractable pain (24-34). These changes appear to result in the temporal and spatial summation of nociceptive input, as well as changes in gene regulation in the dorsal horn, resulting in long term changes in response to noxious and non-noxious stimuli, anatomical re-organization and even cell death (24-34).

It is apparent that prompt, consistent, adequate pain relief is not simply a humane endeavor: there is now a growing body of evidence detailing the potential medical consequences of unrelieved pain (34), i.e., the development of severe cancer pain and chronic pain.

The availability of appropriate early management strategy, including neurolytic and non-neurolytic anesthetic techniques, has the potential for significantly reducing the incidence, severity, and consequences of chronic pain and cancer pain problems which become severe management problems (24-37).

REFERENCES

1. Cousins MJ, Cherry DA, Gourlay GK: Acute and chronic pain: Use of spinal opioids, Neural Blockade in Clinical Anesthesia and Management of Pain. 2nd ed. Edited by Cousins MJ, Bridenbaugh PO. Philadelphia, J. B. Lippincott, 1988, pp. 955-1029
2. Cousins MJ: Introduction to acute and chronic pain: Implications for neural blockade, Neural Blockade in Clinical Anesthesia and Management of Pain. 2nd ed. Edited by Cousins MJ, Bridenbaugh PO. Philadelphia, J. B. Lippincott, 1988, pp. 739-790
3. Brown AS: Current views on the use of nerve blocking in the relief of chronic pain, The Therapy of Pain. Edited by Swerdlow M. Philadelphia, J. B. Lippincott, 1981
4. Cousins MJ: Chronic pain and neurolytic neural blockade, Neural Blockade in Clinical Anesthesia and Management of Pain. 2nd ed. Edited by Cousins MJ, Bridenbaugh PO. Philadelphia, J. B. Lippincott, 1988, pp. 1053-1084
5. Hakanson S: Trigeminal neuralgia treated by injection of glycerol into the trigeminal cistern. Neurosurgery 9:638-646, 1981
6. Shapshay SM, Scott RM, McCann CF, Stoelting I: Pain control in advanced and recurrent head and neck cancer. Otolaryngol Clin North Am 13:551-560, 1980
7. Gomori JM, Rappaport ZH: Transovale trigeminal cistern puncture: Modified fluoroscopically guided technique. AJNR 6:93-94, 1985
8. Doyle D: Nerve blocks in advanced cancer. Practitioner 226:539-544, 1982
9. Wiesenfeld-Hallin Z, Hallin RG: The influence of the sympathetic system on mechanoreception and nociception: A review. Hum Neurobiol 3:41-46, 1984

10. Campbell JN, Raja SN, Meyer RA: Painful sequelae of nerve injury, Proceedings of the Vth World Congress on Pain. Edited by Dubner R, Gebhart GF, Bond MR. Amsterdam, Elsevier, 1988, pp. 135-143
11. Seltzer Z, Devor M: Ephaptic transmission in chronically damaged peripheral nerves. Neurology 29:1061-1064, 1979
12. Lofstrom JB, Cousins MJ: Sympathetic neural blockade of upper and lower extremity, Neural Blockade in Clinical Anesthesia and Management of Pain. 2nd ed. Edited by Cousins MJ, Bridenbaugh PO. Philadelphia, J. B. Lippincott, 1988, pp. 461-502
13. Tenicela R, Lovasik D, Eaglstein W: Treatment of herpes zoster with sympathetic blocks. Clin J Pain 1:63-67, 1985
14. Yanagida H, Suwa K, Corssen G: No prophylactic effect of early sympathetic blockade on postherpetic neuralgia. Anesthesiology 66:73-76, 1987
15. Saltzburg D, Foley KM: Management of pain in pancreatic cancer. Surg Clin North Am 69:629-649, 1989
16. Brown DL, Bulley CK, Quiel EL: Neurolytic celiac plexus block for pancreatic cancer pain. Anesth Analg 66:869-873, 1987
17. Bridenbaugh LD, Moore DC, Campbell DD: Management of upper abdominal cancer pain. Treatment with celiac plexus block with alcohol. JAMA 190:877-880, 1964
18. Black A, Dwyer B: Coeliac plexus block. Anaesth Intensive Care 1:315-318, 1973
19. Ischia S, Ischia A, Polati E, Finco G: Three posterior percutaneous celiac plexus block techniques. A prospective, randomized study in 61 patients with pancreatic cancer pain. Anesthesiology 76:534-540, 1992
20. Thompson GE, Moore DC: Celiac plexus, intercostal and minor peripheral blockade, Neural Blockade in Clinical Anesthesia and Management of Pain. 2nd ed. Edited by Cousins MJ, Bridenbaugh PO. Philadelphia, J. B. Lippincott, 1988, pp. 503-532
21. Cousins MJ, Reeve TS, Glynn CJ, et al: Neurolytic lumbar sympathetic blockade: Duration of denervation and relief of rest pain. Anaesth Intensive Care 7:121-135, 1979
22. Walsh JA, Glynn CJ, Cousins MJ, Basedow RW: Bloodflow, sympathetic activity and pain relief following lumbar sympathetic blockade or surgical sympathectomy. Anaesth Intensive Care 13:18-24, 1985
23. Plancarte R, Amescua C, Patt RB, Aldrete JA: Superior hypogastric plexus block for pelvic cancer pain. Anesthesiology 73:236-239, 1990
24. Jorum E, Holum E, Lundberg L, Torebjörk HE: Temporal summation in nociceptive systems (abstract). Pain 5:S314, 1990
25. Dickenson AH, Sullivan AF: Evidence for a role of the NMDA receptor in the frequency dependent potentiation of deep rat dorsal horn nociceptive neurones following C-fiber stimulation. Neuropharmacology 26:1235-1238, 1987

26. Davies SN, Lodge D: Evidence for involvement of N-methylaspartate receptors in 'wind-up' of class 2 neurones in the dorsal horn of the rat. Brain Research 424:402-406, 1987
27. Woolf CJ: Recent advances in the pharmacology of acute pain. Br J Anaesth 63:139-146, 1989
28. Woolf CJ, Shortland P, Coggeshall RE: Peripheral nerve injury triggers central sprouting of myelinated afferents. Nature 355:75-78, 1992
29. Katz J, Vaccarino AL, Coderre TJ, Melzack R: Injury prior to neurectomy alters the pattern of autonomy in rats. Behavioral evidence of central neural plasticity. Anesthesiology 75:876-883, 1991
30. Cousins MJ: NMDA antagonists, Proceedings of the VIth World Congress on Pain, Edited by Bond MR, Charlton JE, Woolf CJ. Amsterdam, Elsevier 249-305, 1991
31. Sonnenberg JL, Raunscher FJ III, Morgan JI, Curran T: Regulation of proenkephalin by Fos and Jun. Science 246:1622-1625, 1989
32. Almay BG, Johansson F, Von Knorring L, et al: Substance P in CSF of patients with chronic pain syndromes. Pain 33:3-9, 1988
33. Kehl LJ, Basbaum AI, Pollock CM, et al: The NMDA antagonist MK801 reduces noxious stimulus-evoked Fos expression in the mammalian spinal dorsal horn. Pain (Suppl) 5:S165, 1990
34. Cousins MJ: The treatment of postoperative pain, Proceedings of the VIth World Congress on Pain. Edited by Bond MR, Charlton JE, Woolf CJ. Amsterdam, Elsevier, 1991, pp. 41-52
35. Davar D, Maciewitz R: MK-801 blocks thermal hyperalgesia in a rat model of neuropathic pain. Neuroscience Abstracts 15:472, 1989
36. Woolf CJ, Wall PD: A dissociation between the analgesic and antinociceptive effects of morphine. Neuroscience Letters 64:238, 1986
37. Bach S, Noreng MF, Tjéllden NU: Phantom limb pain in amputees during the first 12 months following limb amputation, after preoperative lumbar epidural blockade. Pain 33:297-301, 1988

CHRONIC PAIN MANAGEMENT IN CHILDREN

D. C. Tyler

The purpose of this presentation is to review chronic pain and its management in children. In doing so, I shall define chronic pain, discuss the epidemiology of chronic pain in children, describe a method of evaluation of patients, and review treatment principles. Finally, I will discuss several common chronic pain problems seen in children.

ACUTE PAIN VS. CHRONIC PAIN

Just as in adults, it is important to distinguish between acute pain and chronic pain, as the two types of pain present different problems and should be treated differently. Anesthesiologists are familiar with acute pain, which is the type of pain typically associated with tissue injury and seen in the operating room and recovery room. Acute pain arises as a result of tissue damage and has the function of providing a warning about injury. Acute pain lasts for a short period of time, usually days, and it is amenable to treatment with physiologic or pharmacologic methods. Chronic pain, however, is defined as pain that lasts beyond the expected period of healing, has no function to the individual, has no expected end, and is not amenable to treatment with the usual methods. Typical examples of chronic pain in adults include headache and low back pain. It is well known that this sort of pain is difficult to treat and frequently recurs or continues in spite of treatment efforts. While having some similarities, chronic pain in children is quite different from that seen in adults. Different pain syndromes are involved, in that children usually have problems with headache, abdominal pain, limb pain, or chest pain, and unlike adults, are not troubled with low back pain. In adults, opioid dependence is frequently a problem in patients with chronic pain, but this

T. H. Stanley and M. A. Ashburn (eds.), Anesthesiology and Pain Management, 343–349.

is less often a problem with chronic pain in children. In children, the pain may be recurrent rather than continuous.

PSYCHOSOCIAL FACTORS INVOLVED WITH PAIN

While psychological and social factors are involved in the perception of acute pain, they are even more important in the patient's perception of chronic pain, and for the physician who is to help a patient with chronic pain, an understanding of the psychological and social factors that contribute to the child's perception of pain is necessary. It is important to recognize that pain is subjective; that is, different people will have different perceptions of the intensity of a standard noxious stimulus, and the same person will have different perceptions of the same stimulus delivered in different situations. Some of the influences that alter pain perception include family, culture, prior experiences of pain, expectations about the meaning of the pain, and expectations about the duration of the pain. In addition to these factors, in children there are additional influences of the child's age, his or her verbal and cognitive skills, the presence or absence of parents, the reaction of parents to the child's pain, the presence or absence of illness in the family, marital discord, school problems, and peer relationships. These factors need to be evaluated when a child with chronic pain is seen.

EVALUATION OF CHRONIC PAIN

Since chronic pain involves medical, psychological, social, and family issues, evaluation by one discipline or one doctor is usually not sufficient. With a complicated pain problem, no one individual has the skill or training to carry out a complete evaluation. Consequently, one common approach is a multidisciplinary evaluation, an approach that is felt to be the best method of trying to help patients with chronic pain. In our institution, this multidisciplinary evaluation includes a medical evaluation, a psychological evaluation, and an evaluation of the child's family and social situation. Our pain evaluation team consists of pediatrician-anesthesiologists, a child psychiatrist, an adolescent medicine pediatrician and a nurse. Each patient with chronic pain is seen by a pediatrician-anesthesiologist for a medical evaluation and a person trained in behavioral medicine for an evaluation of family-social issues. Each person evaluates the patient individually and then the team meets and discusses the patient. A team leader is chosen, and this person follows-up with the patient and carries out the treatment plan.

For the medical evaluation, the important issues are specific medical problems and chronic use of medications. Each medical problem is examined and treatment is evaluated. Untreated or inadequately treated problems are evaluated with respect to whether better treatment might improve pain management. Usually by the time children are seen in a chronic pain clinic, these sorts of medical issues have been dealt with, but they are worth evaluating again to ensure that there are not hidden problems or that obvious treatments have not been missed.

With respect to chronic medicine administration, it is important to note whether opioid or other medication use is a problem. For the most part, opioid administration does not help chronic pain and may be part of the problem. If chronic opioid use is a problem, then detoxification becomes a major issue. We use an oral route for detoxification. The general method is to determine over a one- to two-day period the patient's daily intake of opioid. Frequently, this will need to be done in an inpatient setting so that opioid use can be tracked accurately. After this evaluation has been undertaken, the total daily amount of opioid is calculated and converted to morphine equivalents. Methadone is substituted for morphine on a mg for mg basis. For instance, if a child was using 40 mg per day of morphine, he or she would be started on 40 mg per day of methadone. This dose can be divided into two to three doses and administered orally. The methadone dose is then decreased by 10% per day until the child has been weaned from medication.

From the psychological evaluation, we obtain information about psychological issues contributing to the pain and the way in which the child's pain affects his or her life. The psychological evaluation includes an examination of the behavioral setting in which the pain is occurring, looking particularly at whether pain is reinforced by events in the child's environment, looking to see if there are particular stressors in the environment or the family that are causing the child problems and whether there is psychopathology in either the child or the family that needs to be dealt with.

In terms of social and family issues, we look at friends, family and school and evaluate the ways in which these contribute to the pain and the way in which pain interferes with the child's activities. These family and social issues are very important in the evaluation of chronic pain in children. Usually the families are in turmoil and it is sometimes very difficult to tell whether this turmoil is the cause or the result of the child's pain. Other factors to evaluate are the social roles of the child in the family and the part that pain plays in the family relationships. It is also important to evaluate the child's relationships with peers and the child's performance and relationships in school.

Treatment will depend upon the findings on multidisciplinary evaluation. After the evaluation has been completed, the team members sit together and discuss the problems. Usually, it will become apparent whether the medical, psychological, or family issues are predominant in the individual child. Once the important issues have been determined, the member of the team who has expertise in that area becomes the overall team leader for that particular patient. With respect to medical treatment, it is necessary to ensure that the child is adequately detoxified and that appropriate diagnostic and therapeutic evaluations have been carried out to deal with any medical problems that are contributing to the pain.

For many children with chronic pain, behavioral treatment is an extremely important component of their therapy. This is especially true in headache where therapy such as hypnosis, imagery or biofeedback can be used with great benefit.

In some children with family disruption, family therapy to deal with the issues in the family is important and will yield great results in terms of pain management.

SPECIFIC COMMON PAIN PROBLEMS

Headache

Headache is a common problem in children (1). By the age of 15, 75% of adolescents have suffered with headache. Most headaches are not caused by serious medical problems, but one must remember that brain tumors in children often present as headache. Commonly, headaches are described as being either muscle tension headache or migraine, but since children may have a less well defined aura or may not be able to describe the aura, the diagnosis of migraine is more difficult in children.

Evaluation of a child with headache requires a thorough history and physical examination, looking for concomitant medical illness that may result in headache. Laboratory and imaging studies should be extensive enough to convince the physician, family, and patient that underlying pathology has not been missed. If medical or surgical problems are found, they should receive specific therapy. If no underlying pathology is found, a trial of behavioral treatment is appropriate, since a high percentage of patients responds to such therapy. This treatment may include hypnosis, self hypnosis, biofeedback, relaxation therapy, or a combination of these treatments (2).

Abdominal Pain

Abdominal pain is fairly common, occurring in approximately 10-15% of children (1,3). Many medical or surgical diseases have abdominal pain as part of their clinical presentation, and it is important for the physician to come to a clear diagnosis when possible. As with other forms of chronic pain in children, it is important to ensure that enough diagnostic evaluation has been carried out to ensure that treatable medical or surgical illnesses have not been missed and that the physician, patient and family are convinced that there is no undiagnosed medical problem. Abdominal pain without a clear medical or surgical diagnosis is notoriously difficult to treat. To make diagnosis and treatment somewhat easier, we feel that a psychological and family evaluation should also be carried out at the same time the medical evaluation is being carried out. It is generally helpful that the psychological factors be evaluated at the same time as the medical factors to avoid giving the family the idea that once the medical factors have been ruled out, the problem must be in the patient's head. In addition to these factors, one needs to assure that sexual abuse of either males or females is not occurring. This problem will not infrequently present with abdominal pain.

In those patients in whom medical or surgical illness is found, then treatment should be carried out in the most appropriate and expeditious manner. In those patients for whom no medical or surgical cause is found, then a trial of dietary fiber may be of help, since one study supports the beneficial effects of dietary fiber in this group of children (4). If dietary fiber has not been helpful, then a trial of behavioral treatment may be indicated.

Limb Pain

Another common pain problem in children is pain in the extremities. Pediatric textbooks have a long diagnostic list of problems that can result in pain in the extremities. One must also remember that referred pain, such as knee pain resulting from disease of the hip, is not an uncommon finding in children and one should look for these types of problems.

Some patients will have a type of reflex sympathetic dystrophy that bears some outward characteristics of reflex sympathetic dystrophy in adults (5,6,7). In addition to carrying out the physical or pharmacologic treatments for reflex sympathetic dystrophy, it is important to ensure that a family evaluation is also done. A significant number of children with reflex sympathetic dystrophy either have family problems or psychological problems as part of the cause of their illness or alternatively may develop family or psychological problems as a result of their illness. This type of complex mixture of psychological, social, and medical illness can best be evaluated and treated by a multidisciplinary team who can deal with both medical and psychological problems.

Chest Pain

Chest pain can be fairly common in adolescents (8,9,10,11). Again, a complete history and physical examination looking for treatable causes of chest pain should be undertaken. In addition, when appropriate, the patients should be reassured that although chest pain in adults can indicate cardiac disease, it is not so in children, and often reassurance will lead to some resolution of the problem. If these therapies have not been successful then a trail of behavioral treatment may be helpful.

REFERENCES

1. Øster J: Recurrent abdominal pain, headache and limb pains in children and adolescents. Pediatrics 50:429-436, 1972
2. Womack WM, Smith MS, Chen ACN: Behavioral management of childhood headache: A pilot study and case history report. Pain 32:279-283, 1988
3. McGrath PJ, Feldman W: Clinical approach to recurrent abdominal pain in children. J Dev Behav Pediatr 7:56-63, 1986
4. Feldman W, McGrath P, Hodgson C, et al: The use of dietary fiber in the management of simple, childhood, idiopathic, recurrent, abdominal pain. Results in a prospective, double-blind, randomized, controlled trial. Am J Dis Child 139:1216-1218, 1985
5. Fermaglich DR: Reflex sympathetic dystrophy in children. Pediatrics 60:881-883, 1977
6. Bernstein BH, Singsen BH, Kent JT, et al: Reflex neurovascular dystrophy in childhood. J Pediatrics 93:211-215, 1978
7. Sherry DD, Weisman R: Psychologic aspects of childhood reflex neurovascular dystrophy. Pediatrics 81:572-578, 1988
8. Selbst SM: Chest pain in children. Pediatrics 75:1068-1070, 1985
9. Selbst SM, Ruddy RM, Clark BJ, et al: Pediatric chest pain: A prospective study. Pediatrics 82:319-323, 1988
10. Pantell RH, Goodman BW Jr: Adolescent chest pain: A prospective study. Pediatrics 71:881-887, 1983
11. Driscoll DJ, Glicklich LB, Gallen WJ: Chest pain in children: A prospective study. Pediatrics 57:648-651, 1976

ALTERNATIVE DRUG DELIVERY SYSTEMS

J. B. Streisand

Anesthesiologists' major role in acute postoperative and chronic pain management has stimulated interest in developing novel analgesic delivery techniques. Recent advances in biopharmaceutical technology have produced sophisticated delivery systems that permit precise control of drug input into the body by unorthodox routes. In addition, new drug formulations that permit systemic drug delivery by these routes are undergoing development and clinical testing.

Optimal drug therapy includes the absorption and transport of drugs to specific receptor sites in the body, the maintenance of concentrations at these sites for as long as appropriate, and the rapid elimination of the drug when its effect is no longer desired. Time contingent oral or parenteral drug administration is often ineffective in achieving these goals. Oral administration of certain drugs is difficult and inefficient as they are broken down in the acid milieu of the stomach and by gastrointestinal enzymes. Bolus injections of drugs are painful, require trained medical personnel, and create peaks and valleys in plasma drug concentrations that are undesirable when prolonged, steady drug action is sought. This review will illustrate how some of the drawbacks of traditional drug administration are overcome by new analgesic drug delivery systems and how these systems fill certain niches in pain management.

TRANSDERMAL DRUG DELIVERY

Man has recognized the skin as a site for drug administration for centuries. In early transdermal drug delivery, creams and ointments were applied primarily for their local effect. The dose absorbed was quite variable and not easy to reproduce. In contrast, recently developed transdermal drug delivery systems are designed to deliver the active

T. H. Stanley and M. A. Ashburn (eds.), Anesthesiology and Pain Management, 351–372.

constituent through the skin at a sustained, predictable rate into the systemic circulation. Because transdermal delivery leads to sustained, uniform plasma drug concentrations, adverse effects associated with fluctuations in plasma concentration (typical of most time contingent, pulsed methods of drug administration) are minimized. Transdermal delivery circumvents gastrointestinal absorption and hepatic first pass metabolism and, therefore, provides greater bioavailability, a means of delivery for drugs that cannot be effectively administered by the oral route, and an effective alternative for patients not able to swallow. Finally, transdermal drug systems are convenient, noninvasive, painless, and easy to apply.

The stratum corneum, the thick, avascular, lipophilic, keratinized outermost layer of the skin, serves as a barrier to the intrusion of most toxins, chemicals, and microorganisms and retains the body's essential fluids (1). Thus most drugs have difficulty penetrating the skin and are not suitable for transdermal drug delivery. The skin changes in structure from the stratum corneum to a much more aqueous internal structure, the viable epidermis and dermis, which are the sites of uptake of drugs that get into the systemic circulation via the skin. Effective transdermal drug delivery requires that drug molecules have biphasic solubility; lipid solubility to pass through the stratum corneum and aqueous solubility to move through the dermis (2). Secondly, a drug must be potent enough to allow a therapeutic dose to pass through a small, convenient area of skin. Finally, the skin itself must be able to tolerate long-term contact with the drug.

Over 10 years of research, development and clinical testing has produced the first analgesic transdermal delivery system. The transdermal therapeutic system of fentanyl delivery (TTS-fentanyl) is a transparent, rectangular unit that is composed of 4 layers (Figure 1). The outermost layer, made of polyester film, provides an impermeable backing that prevents loss of drug from the system or the entry of foreign substances into the drug reservoir. The drug reservoir contains fentanyl, 2.5 mg/10 cm^2 patch, and alcohol, 0.1 ml/10 cm^2, jelled with hydroxyethyl cellulose. Alcohol is added to enhance the absorption of fentanyl. The microporous rate-controlling membrane is composed of an ethylene-vinyl acetate copolymer. The rate-controlling membrane limits the release rate of drug to a fraction of the uncontrolled rate of absorption

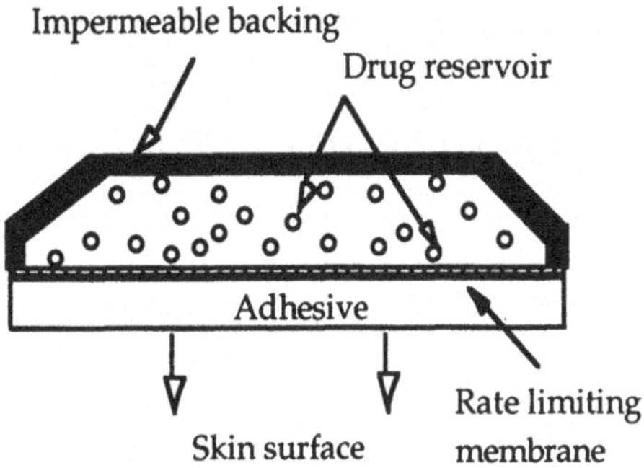

Figure 1. A schematic diagram of the fentanyl transdermal drug delivery system. Reprinted from Streisand et al. (3)

through the skin. Thus, the transdermal system, not the skin, dominates in controlling the rate of drug input to the skin surface and therefore to the systemic circulation. The fourth layer, a silicone skin adhesive, contains fentanyl. This allows the skin directly under the patch to rapidly absorb fentanyl just after the patch is attached. The rate of fentanyl delivered from the system is directly proportional to the size of the patch (Table 1) (4).

Table 1. Fentanyl transdermal drug delivery system: size, delivery rate, and plasma concentrations achieved.

Fentanyl size (cm^2)	**Content (mg)**	**Dose**		**Plasma concentration range (ng/ml)**
		(μg/h)	**(mg/24 hr)**	
10	2.5	25	0.6	0.3-0.6
20	5	50	1.2	0.5-2
30	7.5	75	1.8	0.8-3
40	10	100	2.4	1-4

Since substantial variation exists in intravenous fentanyl pharmacokinetics (5,6), it is not surprising that the same is true for transdermal fentanyl pharmacokinetics. Nevertheless, the goal of fentanyl transdermal delivery, to mimic a constant rate intravenous infusion and provide a stable plasma concentration of fentanyl over a 24- to 72-hour period, has been achieved with remarkably similar results from several independent investigators (7-9). The quantity of fentanyl released from each system (25 μg/hr per 10 cm^2), as well as the serum concentrations achieved, are directly proportional to the size of the patch (Table 1) (10).

When the system is first applied, fentanyl rapidly partitions from the drug-saturated adhesive layer of the patch into the skin. Nevertheless, absorption of fentanyl into the systemic circulation is quite slow during the first 4-8 hours after administration (Figure 2) (9). Serum

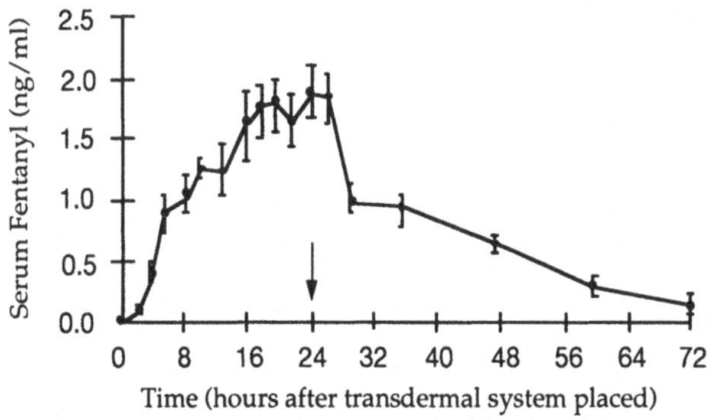

Figure 2. Fentanyl plasma concentrations following the placement of a 100 µg/hr transdermal drug delivery system; the patch was removed at 24 hr (shown by the arrow). Reprinted from Varvel et al. (9) .

concentrations reach steady state by 12-14 hours. These concentrations are maintained for as long as the system is in place. After the patch is removed, concentrations decrease slowly with detectable fentanyl still in the circulation for 36 hours. The terminal elimination half life after removal of the system is approximately 17 hours, 2-3 times that reported for intravenous fentanyl (9). Continuing absorption from the depot of fentanyl in the stratum corneum accounts for the prolonged elimination found after patch removal (9). The bioavailability of fentanyl after transdermal administration is 92% (compared to IV administration), therefore it is unlikely that transdermally administered fentanyl undergoes any cutaneous metabolism (9).

The above pharmacokinetic data for transdermal fentanyl delivery are derived from a single TTS fentanyl patch given to healthy surgical patients. Portenoy et al. (11) recently reported the repeated dose pharmacokinetics in opioid tolerant patients with cancer (Figure 3). Serum fentanyl concentrations reached steady state by 72 hours (beginning of second patch) and remained stable without a rise in serum fentanyl throughout the 15-day study (five 100 µg/hr patches were placed every 3 days). Remarkably, peak fentanyl concentrations and elimination half-lives were similar to values reported from healthy surgical patients. No data exists for patients with hepatic, renal, cardiac or other systemic impairment of physiologic function. In patients with a low clearance of

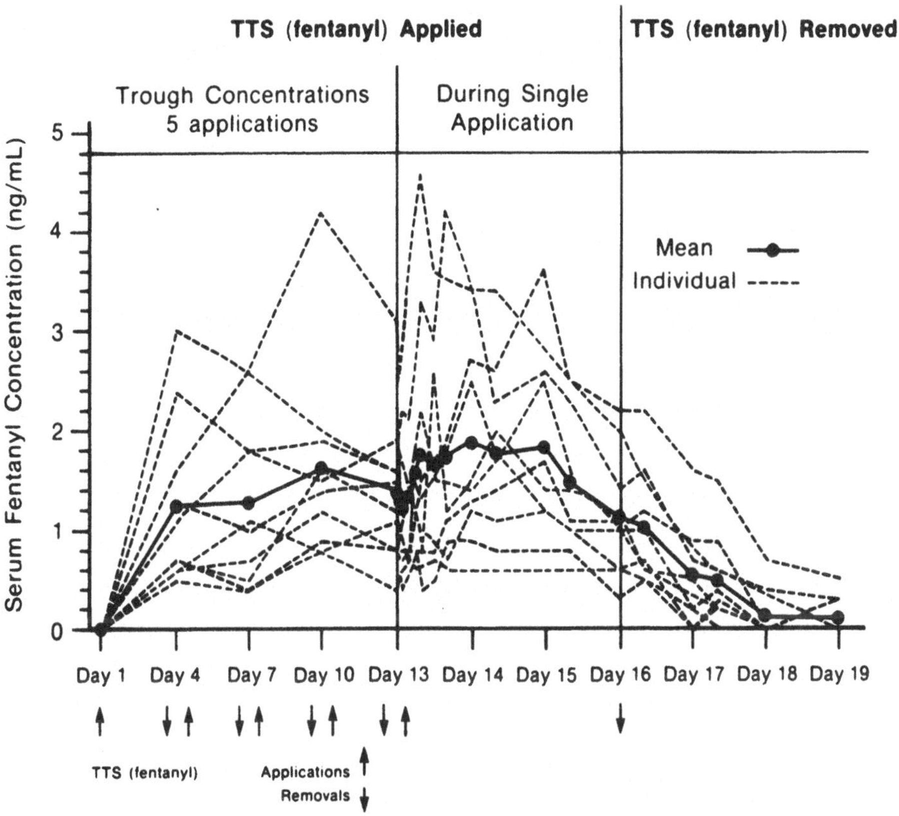

Figure 3. Fentanyl plasma concentrations measured from cancer patients over a 15-day period. The dashed lines are from individual patients while the bold lines and dots are the mean values. Reprinted from Portenoy et al. (11).

fentanyl, the kinetic profile of TTS-fentanyl would be expected to show a slower absorption and longer terminal elimination half-life. Finally, the system does not reliably reach a steady-state by 24 hours. Peak serum concentrations of fentanyl are greater when the patch is replaced every 24 hours for 3 days when compared to a single patch worn for 72 hours. This is why the manufacturer clearly states in the package insert that the system should not be changed more frequently than every 3 days (4).

TTS-fentanyl was first studied for treatment of acute postoperative pain. Well over three hundred patients were enrolled in a variety of open label and double blind placebo controlled studies in the United States, Europe, and Australia (8,12-17). TTS-fentanyl doses ranging from 25-100 μg/hr were utilized.

Caplan et al., Rowbotham et al., and McLesky found that patients receiving TTS-fentanyl had lower pain scores than placebo groups despite the availability of supplemental opioids (12,15,16). Patients from Caplan's study who wore the active patch expressed a significantly higher overall satisfaction rating of their pain control (16). In addition, Rowbotham et al. noted an improvement in the peak expiratory flow rate in patients receiving TTS-fentanyl, presumably from improved analgesia (12). Despite preoperative TTS-fentanyl placement and intraoperative fentanyl administration, the need for supplementary analgesics was greatest in the early postoperative period, reflecting the long lag time to attain effective fentanyl plasma concentrations (12-24 hr). The incidence of nausea and vomiting, the principle adverse effect observed with TTS-fentanyl, ranged from 30-70% but this incidence was no different from patients wearing placebo patches (12,15,16). Hypoventilation, defined as a respiratory rate <8 breaths/min or a $PaCO_2$ >55 mmHg was the most serious and clinically significant adverse effect observed in patients who were administered TTS-fentanyl. Six of the 177 (3.4%) patients receiving 75 μg/hr patches and 7 of the 105 (6.6%) receiving 100 μg/hr patches experienced one or more episodes of hypoventilation (17). There were no serious adverse outcomes in these patients, as they were closely monitored and treated rapidly with either naloxone or verbal prompting to breathe.

Thus, TTS-fentanyl is <u>not recommended nor approved</u> by the Food and Drug Administration in the United States for use in acute postoperative pain (4,17). Serum concentrations rise and fall too slowly to meet the rapidly changing states of acute postoperative pain. Patches should only be changed every 72 hours, and thus this system is not easily titrated for acute pain. Finally, there is a significant risk of hypoventilation in unmonitored, opioid naive patients.

Unlike acute postoperative pain, most cancer pain is constant, or nearly constant, and goes on for extended lengths of time. In addition, most patients with long-standing pain from cancer ultimately receive potent opioid analgesics. Therefore, part of an effective analgesic regimen for cancer pain aims at maintaining consistent concentrations of opioids in the blood. Continuous intravenous and subcutaneous infusions of opioids provide consistency, but their use requires a needle, catheter, and pump and experienced health-care workers to supervise administration. Transdermal fentanyl, on the other hand, is simple to administer, non-invasive, provides consistent serum concentrations, and, therefore, is ideally suited for cancer pain management.

Miser et al. were the first to report their findings in five patients with cancer pain treated with transdermal fentanyl (18). These patients were chosen because oral administration of opioids was either ineffective or not possible. The transdermal dose was selected by matching the μg/hr dose to an intravenous infusion of fentanyl that had been titrated to obtain satisfactory pain control. All five patients reported good to excellent pain control, using doses of TTS-fentanyl that ranged from 75-300 μg/hr for as long as 156 days. The major clinical difficulties were the delay in achieving steady state plasma concentrations, which led to minor overdosing in two patients and the prolonged effect of fentanyl after the system was removed. This became a significant clinical problem when new medical complications arose which required more rapid decline in opioid effect.

Over 150 patients with cancer pain have received TTS-fentanyl in a variety of clinical studies (13,17-21). The findings from these studies reinforce the concept that cancer pain is a dynamic process determined by multiple factors and make the effects of a single intervention difficult to analyze. Nevertheless, most of the patients who have received TTS-fentanyl prefer this treatment to other choices because of the achievement of satisfactory pain relief with a convenient, easy to use system.

To avoid the problems seen in opioid-naive patients (difficulty with titration, respiratory depression), TTS-fentanyl should not be used as a first line analgesic (4,22). After the patient has achieved adequate pain relief from conventional oral or parenteral opioids, the initial dose selection of TTS fentanyl is determined using the morphine equivalence chart found in the package insert and shown below (Table 2) (4). The conversion ratio is conservative, thus 50% of patients are likely to require an increase in fentanyl dose after initial application. Upward titration of

Table 2. Duragesic dose prescription based upon daily morphine equivalence dose.

Oral 24-hour Morphine (mg/day)	IM 24-hour Morphine (mg/day)	Duragesic Dose (μg/hr)
45-134	8-22	25
135-224	23-37	50
225-314	38-52	75
315-404	53-67	100
405-494	68-82	125
495-584	83-97	150
585-674	98-112	175
675-764	113-127	200
765-854	128-142	225
855-944	143-157	250
945-1034	158-172	275
1035-1124	173-187	300

Janssen Pharmaceutica. Duragesic Package Insert. Piscataway, New Jersey: 1991

the dose of TTS-fentanyl should occur no more frequently than every three days after the initial dose or every 6 days thereafter, as it may take that long to achieve equilibrium following a new dose. The majority of patients using TTS-fentanyl will require "rescue" dosing with rapidly acting, short duration oral or transmucosal opioids for treatment of breakthrough pain which may occur with routine daily activity. While dermatological reactions from TTS-fentanyl are mild and likely due to skin occlusion rather than contact dermatitis, it is advisable to rotate the sites of patched applications to minimize local irritation.

IONTOPHORESIS

Due to the limitations in passive transdermal drug delivery, physical and chemical methods of enhancing transdermal drug delivery are being developed. Iontophoresis is defined as the introduction of ions of soluble salts into the skin or mucosal surfaces of the body by means of an electrical current. Although interest in using this technique in medicine has waxed and waned during the past 50 years, advances in knowledge and equipment have expanded the capabilities of this simple technique.

An iontophoresis system consists of a power source that provides and controls an electrical current, a delivery electrode, and a current return electrode. When used on the skin, the delivery electrode contains an enclosed receptacle for the sterile placement of the drug. For iontophoresis in small or enclosed areas such as the tympanic membrane (23) or tip of the nose (24), the delivery electrode is brought in contact with a pledget or gauze (saturated with the drug solution) at the desired site. The current return electrode is placed on any convenient site, usually the skin near the delivery electrode. With activation of the current, electrons flow through the skin or mucosa beneath the electrode, through interstitial fluids, and back through the skin at the other electrode. An appropriately charged molecule will migrate along the same path. Positively charged drugs inserted into the reservoir at the anode are repelled toward the negative electrode. Conversely, negatively charged drugs placed at the cathode are repelled toward the positive electrode.

Local administration of dexamethasone sodium phosphate (DSP) by iontophoresis has been used for the treatment of acute and chronic musculoskeletal inflammatory conditions. Harris reported improvement (89% of patients treated) in pain scores, swelling, and range of motion after iontophoresis of DSP to patients with a localized inflammatory joint (lateral epicondylitis of the elbow, subacromial bursitis of shoulder, patellar tendonitis) (25). Most patients required three treatments over a one-week period with improvement of symptoms occurring 24 to 48 hours after a treatment. DSP iontophoretic treatment of an inflamed knee joint of a patient with rheumatoid arthritis improved muscle strength and joint range of motion, and decreased joint swelling (26). While clinical experience with DSP iontophoresis for acute localized inflammatory disease is limited, this technique has several advantages over the injection of steroids into inflamed joints: 1) the treatment is non-traumatic and painless; 2) tissue damage due to needle penetration and subcutaneous injection of a bolus of fluid is avoided; and 3) patients may be able to use this system at home.

Since new technologies in iontophoresis equipment and electrodes permit longer safe iontophoresis times, it is now possible to use iontophoresis for systemic drug administration. Morphine hydrochloride is a highly ionized molecule and, therefore, has the important physiochemical property necessary for its delivery through the skin by iontophoresis. Initial experience in human volunteers established analgesic morphine plasma concentrations after only 20 minutes of iontophoretic treatment (27). Plasma concentrations were proportional to the iontophoretic current. Subsequently, Ashburn and colleagues reported the use of morphine iontophoresis for acute postoperative pain in 38 patients undergoing total hip or knee arthroplasty (28).

Our lab has recently determined serum concentrations after two hours of fentanyl citrate iontophoresis in adult volunteers (Figure 4). While this data is preliminary (and to date unpublished), it is encouraging to note the rapid rise in serum fentanyl to concentrations associated with analgesia within an hour. Concentrations were directly proportional to the current administered. Finally, serum fentanyl concentrations decreased rapidly after the current was shut off. These preliminary

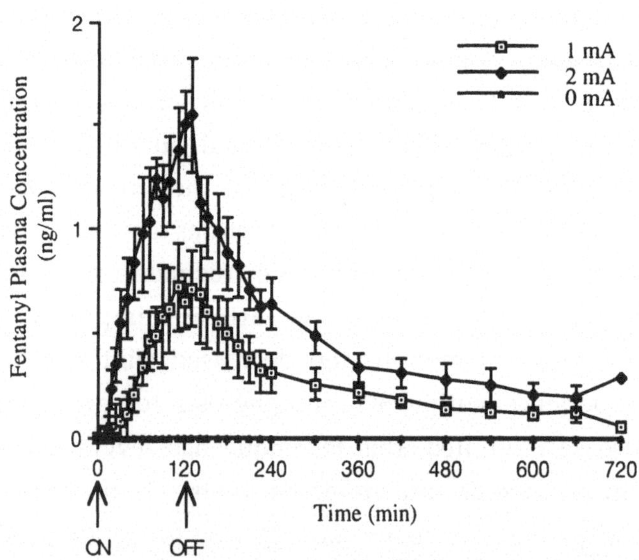

Figure 4. Serum fentanyl concentrations (mean ± SD) measured in volunteers during and after fentanyl iontophoresis. The arrows show the duration of patch placement.

results indicate a lack of depot, unlike passive transdermal delivery. Thus, it may be possible to rapidly change blood fentanyl with this delivery system.

While these initial reports demonstrate that systemic administration of morphine and fentanyl by iontophoresis is feasible, many questions remain concerning the utility of this system for acute pain management. The main advantages of iontophoresis over passive transdermal drug delivery (i.e., transdermal fentanyl) are: a) the ability to rapidly change the dose of opioid delivered by adjusting the iontophoretic current, and b) immediate discontinuation of drug delivery with removal of the delivery current (no "depot" effect is seen as occurs with transdermal fentanyl). Whether the advantage of rapid control of administered dose can be practically implemented for treating acute postoperative pain (i.e., patient controlled delivery) remains to be seen. In addition, the safety of prolonged (greater than 6 hours) iontophoresis times is unknown.

TRANSMUCOSAL DRUG ADMINISTRATION

In the past decade, a wide variety of drugs have been found to penetrate the oral and nasal mucosa to produce therapeutic plasma concentrations. Unfortunately, until recently, these anatomic sites have been overlooked as feasible routes for opioid administration. New vehicles and drug formulations (i.e., nasal sprays, buccal tablets, lozenges on a stick) are now being developed to enable efficacious transmucosal opioid delivery.

The advantages of transmucosal drug delivery over traditional routes of delivery are:

1. Rapid absorption. Since the drug does not have to pass through the long gastrointestinal tract, it can reach the systemic circulation within a short time. Also, the oral and nasal mucosa's high vascularity aids in rapid absorption.
2. No gastrointestinal or hepatic first-pass metabolism. Systemic absorption of drugs is greater (higher bioavail-

ability) and less erratic than oral administration. In addition, some drugs that are broken down in the acid milieu of the stomach or by gastrointestinal enzymes can be absorbed through the oral or nasal mucosa without metabolism or alteration.

3. Simple and noninvasive means of administration. Drugs can be easily applied to the mucosa without complicated delivery devices or painful injections.
4. Titratability. Medications can be easily removed from the oral mucosa when the desired effect is achieved.
5. Permeability Compared to the skin, the mucosa of the nose and mouth is much more permeable. Therefore, a greater variety of drugs can be administered through the oral and nasal mucosa than the skin. In addition, the skin's structure tends to form depots of drugs, unlike the oral or nasal mucosa. Continuous absorption of drug from a depot is undesirable when rapid discontinuation of drug effect is required.

Administration of morphine via the sublingual mucosa has been extensively practiced because of the need for nonparenteral methods of analgesic administration in patients with cancer pain (29-39). Sublingual morphine is useful when oral morphine is impractical (patient with nausea and vomiting, difficulty swallowing, or gastrointestinal problems) and parenteral injections are difficult and painful (patients with bleeding disorders, inaccessible veins, or muscle wasting).

Reports of systemic bioavailability of buccal and sublingual morphine have been quite variable. Reported relative bioavailabilities range from less than 9% (30,34) to 146% (39) of the bioavailability found after intramuscular morphine administration. This wide range in transmucosal morphine bioavailability may be attributable to several factors:

1. Adherence time (a longer contact of the dosage form with the mucosa seems to produce higher bioavailability) (30,32,39).
2. pH of the formulation (like with fentanyl, a higher pH results in better buccal absorption of morphine) (29). The

formulations (tablets, solutions) may have had quite different pH's.

3. The morphine assay utilized (some plasma morphine measurements may be subject to overestimation of plasma morphine concentrations due to poor resolution between morphine and its metabolites) (9).
4. Site of administration (in general, the sublingual mucosa is more permeable than the buccal mucosa).

The controversial results in buccal and sublingual morphine bioavailability and absorption kinetics indicate the lack of an optimized formulation. Morphine is probably a poor choice for transmucosal opioid administration due to its low lipid solubility and bitter taste.

In spite of this above problem, buccal and sublingual morphine have been used for preoperative sedation and anxiolysis (40), postoperative analgesia (15), and pain relief in patients with chronic cancer pain (37,38). Some reports find that buccal or sublingual morphine, produce similar or better analgesia, and cause less adverse effects than the same dose of intramuscular morphine (15,41). However, many patients complain of the bitter taste associated with most formulations of sublingual morphine. Finally, some clinicians administer a concentrated morphine solution (Roxanol™ UD, 20 mg/ml) sublingually with hope that onset of analgesia is faster than the oral route, However, there is no evidence of improved absorption or efficacy for this anecdotal practice.

Buprenorphine is a long-acting and highly potent mixed opioid agonist-antagonist. Due to its potency and high lipophilicity, buprenorphine is rapidly absorbed across mucosal membranes and is quite suitable for sublingual and nasal administration. The portion of the drug that is swallowed is almost completely metabolized by the liver and only a small fraction can reach the systemic circulation. The sublingual buprenorphine preparation is used as an analgesic for the control of moderate to severe pain, for premedication before surgery, and for detoxification of opioid addicts. Although parenteral buprenorphine is available for clinical use in the United States, the sublingual formulation has not met regulatory approval. Nevertheless, sublingual buprenorphine is utilized in 14 countries across Europe and Asia.

Clinical cross-over analgesic trials demonstrate that sublingual buprenorphine is 15 to 25 times more potent than intramuscular morphine 17,19). Buprenorphine is readily absorbed following sublingual administration, with a bioavailability of 55%, of which 30% is obtained in the first three hours (42). This is considerably higher than its oral bioavailability (15%) (42). However, sublingual absorption is slow. Following the administration of 0.8 mg, measurable plasma concentrations do not occur until after 30 minutes (Figure 5) (42). Peak concentrations are reached 200 minutes after administration, which is significantly slower than after intramuscular injection (25) or intranasal administration (43). The short presence of the tablet in the mouth (a few minutes) and the slow onset of plasma concentrations suggest the existence of a significant submucosal depot after sublingual buprenorphine administration. The analgesic effect following sublingual buprenorphine lasts 8 to 10 hours, much longer than buprenorphine's terminal elimination half-life (44). This unusual finding may be due to buprenorphine's high affinity and slow dissociation from the mu and kappa opioid receptors (45). This receptor interaction may also explain the inability of naloxone to easily reverse buprenorphine-induced respiratory depression (26).

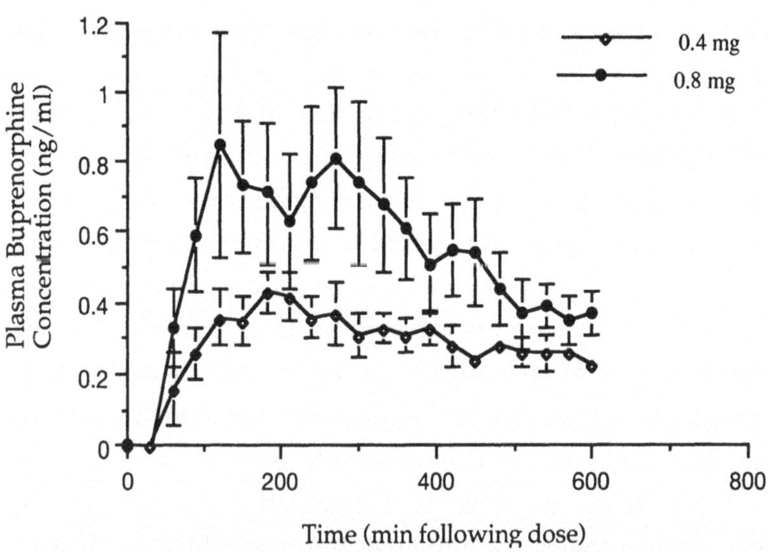

Figure 5. Buprenorphine plasma concentrations measured in healthy patients after a 0.4 mg or 0.8 mg sublingual tablet. Reprinted from Bullingham et al. (46).

Sublingual buprenorphine provides excellent , safe, and long lasting post-operative analgesia with less drowsiness and sedation than comparable doses of intramuscular morphine, (47) meperidine, (24,28) or buprenorphine (24). In addition, sublingual administration is more acceptable to children who dislike and sometimes refuse injections (48). Since buprenorphine is a partial opioid agonist and thus has a ceiling for analgesia, it may not be as efficacious as a pure mu agonist, such as morphine, in treating severe pain (19). Long-lasting respiratory depression, even after a single dose, is the most alarming side effect reported with sublingual buprenorphine (26,49). This is the primary reason for the unavailability of the sublingual dosage form in the U.S.

Oral transmucosal fentanyl citrate (OTFC) is a new formulation of fentanyl for transmucosal delivery. It consists of 100-800 μg of fentanyl in a sweetened lozenge on a stick. When placed in the mouth, fentanyl in the lozenge gradually dissolves into saliva and is rapidly absorbed by the oral mucosa. The fast onset of clinical effect allows the patient or clinician to regulate fentanyl delivery by stopping OTFC consumption when the desired effect is achieved. OTFC is currently undergoing clinical trials in the United States for premedication of children before surgery and painful procedures not requiring general anesthesia, for acute postoperative pain, and for break through pain in cancer patients.

Streisand et al. determined the pharmacokinetics of transmucosal, oral and IV fentanyl in healthy volunteers (50). Plasma concentrations peak at 3.0 ± 1.0 ng/ml (mean ± SEM) 23 minutes after OTFC administration, then decline to less than 1 ng/ml an hour later (Figure 6). Plasma concentrations rapidly (4-10 min) reach analgesic thresholds (0.63-1.0 ng/ml (51)) during OTFC consumption. This implies OTFC might be titratable for acute pain. The elimination half-life of OTFC is 7.7 hours which is similar to the intravenous route. Unlike transdermal fentanyl, OTFC leaves no significant depot in the mucosal tissues after it is remove (52). Some absorption of fentanyl continues after OTFC is removed from the patient's mouth due to absorption of swallowed fentanyl from the GI tract. The systemic bioavailability of OTFC, 50%, is therefore a combined effect of buccal and GI absorption. OTFC's bioavailability is similar to buprenorphine's (55%) (42) but much greater than buccal morphine and other less lipophilic opioids (Figure 7) (7,8).

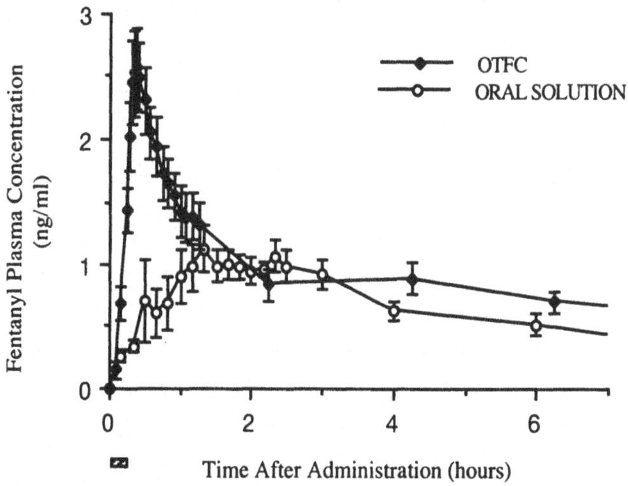

Figure 6. Plasma concentrations of fentanyl (mean = SEM) after 15 µg/kg of oral transmucosal fentanyl citrate or an oral fentanyl solution. The crosshatched bar represents the consumption time of OTFC (15 min).

Initial clinical trials with OTFC were performed in pediatric patients due to the need for less painful and less frightening methods of opioid administration in children. Over 800 doses of OTFC have been administered to children for premedication in 13 clinical trials at nine different hospitals in the United States (personal communication, William Moeller, Anesta Corporation, Salt Lake City, Utah). Children receiving OTFC before surgery are rapidly sedated and show reduced anxiety within 30 minutes of administration (53-57). OTFC produces only small, clinically insignificant decreases in respiratory rate and oxygen saturation. Yet close monitoring of respiration (pulse oximetry, respiratory rate) and the availability of supplemental oxygen is recommended when OTFC is used. In addition to being used as a premedication before surgery, OTFC is being used in children with leukemia to provide analgesia for lumbar punctures and bone marrow biopsies (general anesthesia is usually not given for these procedures (58). OTFC is not an ideal premedication for children undergoing ambulatory surgery due to the high incidence of postoperative nausea and vomiting which may delay discharge in this setting (59). While the risk of aspiration is a legitimate concern with OTFC premedication, Stanley et al. demonstrated the percentage of safe (gastric volume <0.4 ml/kg and pH>2.5) cases is no different whether children receive OTFC, a placebo lozenge, or no premedication (56). To date there are no reports of aspiration of stomach contents following OTFC administration.

In addition to the obvious advantages to pediatric patients, adults may also benefit from OTFC. Ashburn et. al. reported on a patient who self-administered OTFC, on an ambulatory basis, to provide analgesia for breakthrough cancer pain (12). Utilization of OTFC for breakthrough cancer pain may fill a niche because it provides rapid, analgesic blood levels of a potent opioid that can be used on an ambulatory basis without the use of expensive, invasive equipment such as pumps or catheters. Finally, OTFC has the potential to be used for sedation and analgesia in other areas outside of the operating room environment, such as the emergency room (60), dermatology clinic, and the surgeon's office for minor surgery.

Fentanyl's rapid absorption through the nasal mucosa suggest this route might be useful for managing acute pain. In fact, Striebel et al. recently reported on the intranasal administration of fentanyl (commercially available solution, 50 μg/ml) for acute postoperative pain

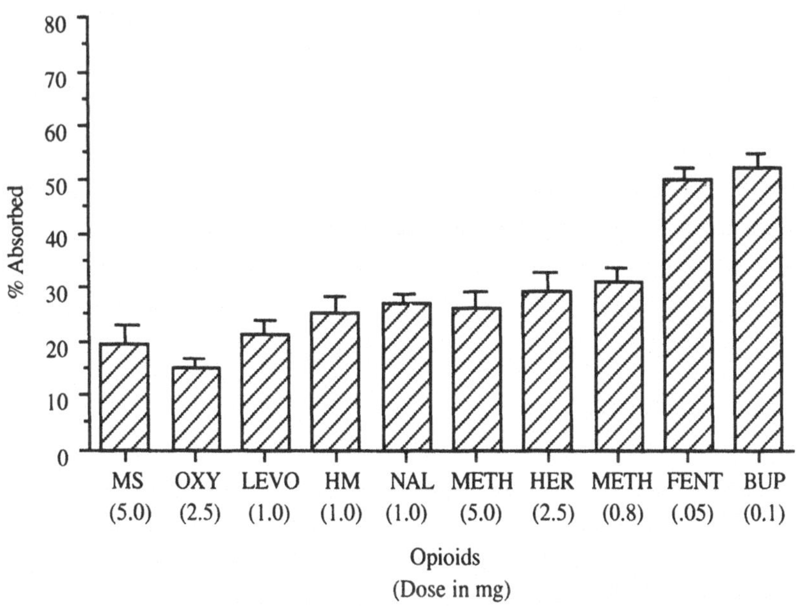

Figure 7. The sublingual absorption of various opioid agonists and antagonist solutions in volunteers. Reprinted from Weinberg et al. (30).

using 6 metered nasal sprays (0.09 ml/spray) per administration, such that each dose equaled 27 μg of fentanyl (61). Onset of analgesia occurred within 10 minutes, and was nearly as effective as the same dose of intravenous fentanyl. Interpatient variability was low which suggests a high bioavailability of fentanyl after intranasal delivery. No patients complained of pain or burning on administration. The authors suggest intranasal fentanyl administration might be particularly useful during the late postoperative period after intravenous access is removed or for patients suffering from breakthrough cancer pain. Further clinical investigation is necessary to examine the chronic effects of intranasal fentanyl administration on the nasal mucosa and to establish how upper respiratory viral infections effect absorption and bioavailability before this technique can be recommended for long term use.

Sufentanil's high potency and lipid solubility affirm its transnasal absorption. Nasal sufentanil has been investigated in children and adults as a premedication before surgery. There is no special formulation for nasal administration, therefore the commercially available parenteral solution is administered by nasal drops.

Helmers et al. determined plasma concentrations of sufentanil after a 15 μg intranasal or intravenous dose (62). The maximum plasma concentration, 0.08 ng/ml, occurred just 10 minutes after administration. The plasma concentration profiles of intranasal and intravenous sufentanil were virtually identical 30 minutes after administration. Nasal sufentanil provided the highest bioavailability, 78% of intravenous, of any transmucosally administered opioid studied to date.

While nasal sufentanil acts rapidly to sedate children within 10 minutes of administration, its routine use as a premedication is precluded by its side effects. In dose's of 2 μg/kg and above, it produces an unacceptable incidence of low oxygen saturation and chest wall rigidity (63,64). Furthermore, nasal midazolam provides more reliable sedation than nasal sufentanil without the respiratory side effects of sufentanil (63). Finally, most children are disturbed by this route of administration and complain of the bitter taste.

Vercauteren et al. and Helmers et al. both noted excellent sedation in adults with a low incidence of side effects with an intranasal sufentanil dose of 10-20 μg (33,34). Many of the problems with nasal sufentanil reported in children were not observed with adults, probably because a much lower dose was efficacious in adults.

The rapid absorption of nasally administered sufentanil suggest its use in acute pain management. However, to date no one has reported on its use in this arena.

REFERENCES

1. Elias PM: Protective role of the skin: The special role of the stratum corneum, Dermatology in Medicine. Vol 3. Edited by Fitzpatrick TB. New York, McGraw-Hill, 1987, pp. 213
2. Guy RH, Hadgraft J, Bucks DAW: Transdermal drug delivery and cutaneous metabolism. Xenobiotica 17:325-343, 1987
3. Streisand J, Stanley T: Opioids: new techniques in routes of administration. Current Opinion in Anesthesiology 2:456-462, 1989
4. Janssen Pharmaceutica: Duragesic Package Insert. 1991
5. Reilly CS, Wood AJJ, Wood M: Variability of fentanyl pharmacokinetics in man. Anaesth 40:837-843, 1984
6. McClain DA, Hug CC: Intravenous fentanyl kinetics. Clin Pharmacol Ther 28:106-114, 1980
7. Duthrie DJR, Rowbotham DJ, Wyld R, et al: Plasma fentanyl concentrations during transdermal delivery of fentanyl to surgical patients. Br J Anaesth 60:614-618, 1988
8. Holley FO, Van Steenis C: Postoperative analgesia with fentanyl: pharmacokinetics and pharmacodynamics of constant-rate iv and transdermal delivery. Br J Anaesth 60:608-613, 1988
9. Varvel JR, Shafer SL, Hwang SS, et al: Absorption characteristics of transdermally administered fentanyl. Anesthesiology 70:928-934, 1989
10. Lehmann KA, Zech D: Transdermal fentanyl: clinical pharmacology. J Pain Symptom Manage 7(Suppl. 3):S8-S16, 1992
11. Portenoy RK, Southam MA, Gupta SK, et al: Transdermal fentanyl for cancer pain: Repeated dose pharmacokinetics. Anesthesiology 78:36-43, 1993
12. Rowbotham DJ, Wyld R, Peacock JE, et al: Transdermal fentanyl for the relief of pain after upper abdominal surgery. Br J Anaesth 63:56-59, 1989
13. Zech D, Dauer HG, Stollenwerk B, Lehmann KA: PCA and TTS fentanyl in the treatment of cancer pain (abstract). Pain 5:S356, 1990
14. Gourlay GK, Kowalski SR, Plummer JL, et al: The transdermal administration of fentanyl in the treatment of postoperative pain: pharmacokinetics and pharmacodynamic effects. Pain 37:193-202, 1989
15. McLesky CH: Fentanyl TTS for postoperative analgesia. Eur J Pain 11:92-97, 1990

16. Caplan RA, Ready LB, Oden RV, et al: Transdermal fentanyl for postoperative pain management: a double blind placebo study. JAMA 261:1989
17. Wright C: Medical officer review, NDA #19813, Alza Corporation TTS Fentanyl, Pharmacokinetics and Pharmacodynamics. 2:1990
18. Miser AW, Narang PK, Dothage JA, et al: Transdermal fentanyl for pain control in patients with cancer. Pain 37:15-21, 1989
19. Simmonds MA, Payne R, Richenbacher J, et al: TTS (fentanyl) in the management of pain in patients with cancer (abstract). Proc Am Soc Clin Oncol 8:324, 1989
20. Levy MH, Rosen SM, Kedziera P: Transdermal fentanyl: seeding trial in patients with chronic cancer pain. J Pain Symptom Manage 7:48-50, 1992
21. Patt RB, Hogan LA: Transdermal fentanyl for chronic cancer pain: detailed case reports and the influence of confounding factors. J Pain Symptom Manage 7:51-53, 1992
22. Bailey PL, Stanley TH: Package inserts and other dosage guidelines are especially useful with new analgesics and new analgesic delivery systems. Anesth Analg 75:873-875, 1992
23. Comeau M, Brummett R: Anesthesia of the human tympanic membrane by iontophoresis of a local anesthetic. Laryngoscope 88:277-285, 1978
24. Maloney JM: Local anesthesia obtained via iontophoresis as an aid to shave biopsy. Arch Dermatol 128:331-332, 1992
25. Harris PR: Iontophoresis: Clinical research in musculoskeletal inflammatory conditions. JOSPT 4:109-112, 1982
26. Hasson SH, Henderson GH, Daniels JC, Schieb DA: Exercise training and dexamethasone iontophoresis in rheumatoid arthritis: A case study. Physiother Can 43:11-14,29, 1991
27. Petelenz TJ: Selected topics in iontophoresis. Ph.D. Thesis, University of Utah, Salt Lake City, Utah, U.S.A., 1989
28. Ashburn MA, Stephen RL, Ackerman E, et al: Iontophoretic delivery of morphine for postoperative analgesia. J Pain Symptom Manage 7:27-33, 1991
29. Al-Sayed Omar O, Johnston A, Turner P: Influence of pH on the buccal absorption of morphine sulphate and its major metabolite, morphine-3-glucuronide. J Pharm Pharmacol 39:934-935, 1987
30. Weinberg DS, Inturrisi CE, Reidenberg B, et al: Sublingual absorption of selected opioid analgesics. Clin Pharmacol Ther 44:335-342, 1988
31. Manara AR, Shelly MP, Quinn KG, Park GR: Pharmacokinetics of morphine following administration by the buccal route. Br J Anaesth 62:498-502, 1989
32. Bardgett D, Howard C, Murray GR, et al: Plasma concentration and bioavailability of a buccal preparation of morphine sulphate. Proceedings of the BPS 198P-199P, 1983

33. Fisher AP, Fung C, Hanna M: Absorption of buccal morphine. Anaesthesia 43:552-553, 1988
34. Fisher AP, Fung C, Hanna M: Serum morphine concentrations after buccal and intramuscular morphine administration. Br J Clin Pharmac 24:685-687, 1987
35. Hoskin PJ, Hanks GW, Aherne GW, et al: The bioavailability and pharmacokinetics of morphine after intravenous, oral and buccal administration in healthy volunteers. Br J Clin Pharmac 27:499-505, 1989
36. Pitorak EF: Pain control with sublingual or buccal morphine. ONF 18:941, 1991
37. Shepard KV, Bakst AW: Alternate delivery methods for morphine sulfate in cancer pain. Cleve Clin J Med 57:48-52, 1990
38. Pannuti F, Rossi AP, Iafelice G, et al: Control of chronic pain in very advanced cancer patients with morphine hydrochloride administered by oral, rectal and sublingual route. Clinical report and preliminary results on morphine pharmacokinetics. Pharmacol Res Commun 14:369-380, 1982
39. Bell MDD, Mishra P, Weldon BD, et al: Buccal morphine - A new route for analgesia? Lancet 1:71-73, 1985
40. Price NM, Schmitt LG, McGuire J, et al: Transdermal scopolamine in the prevention of motion sickness at sea. Clin Pharmacol Ther 29:414-419, 1981
41. Gourlay GK, Kowalski SR, Plummer JL, et al: Fentanyl blood concentration-analgesic response relationship in treatment of postoperative pain. Anesth Analg 67:329-337, 1988
42. Davis WT Jr: Use of iontophoresis for oral mucosal anesthesia. South Carolina Dent J 39:53-57, 1981
43. Kern DA, McQuade MJ, Scheidt MJ, et al: Effectiveness of sodium fluoride on tooth hypersensitivity with and without iontophoresis. J Periodontol 60:386-389, 1989
44. Sisler HA: Iontophoretic local anesthesia for conjunctival surgery. Ann Ophthalmol 10:597-598, 1978
45. Dundee JW, Samuel IO, Toner W, Howard PJ: Midazolam: a water-soluble benzodiazepine. Anaesthesia 35:454-458, 1980
46. Bullingham RES, McQuay HJ, Porter EJB, Allen MC: Sublingual buprenorphine used postoperatively: Ten hour plasma drug concentration analysis. Br J Clin Pharmac 13:665-673, 1982
47. Sloan JB, Soltani K: Iontophoresis in dermatology. J Am Acad Dermatol 15:671-684, 1986
48. Maunuksela E-L, Korpela R, Olkkola KT: Comparison of buprenorphine with morphine in the treatment of postoperative pain in children. Anesth Analg 67:233-239, 1988
49. Kennard CD, Whitaker DC: Iontophoresis of lidocaine for anesthesia during pulsed due laser treatment of port-wine stains. J Dermatol Surg Oncol 18:287-294, 1992

50. Bailey PL, Streisand JB, Pace NL, et al: Transdermal scopolamine reduces nausea and vomiting after outpatient laparoscopy. Anesthesiology 72:977-980, 1990
51. Eriksen J, Jensen N-H, Kamp-Jensen M, et al: The systemic availability of buprenorphine administered by nasal spray. J Pharm Pharmacol 41:803-805, 1989
52. Streisand J, Ashburn M, LeMaire L: Bioavailability and absorption of oral transmucosal fentanyl citrate. Anesthesiology 71:A230, 1989
53. Feld LH, Champeau MW, van Steennis CA, Scott JC: Pre-anesthetic medication in children: a comparison of oral transmucosal fentanyl citrate versus placebo. Anesthesiology 71:374-377, 1989
54. Friesen RH, Lockhart CH: Oral transmucosal fentanyl citrate for preanesthetic medication of pediatric day surgery patients with and without droperidol as a prophylactic anti-emetic. Anesthesiology 71:374-377, 1989
55. Nelson PS, Streisand JB, Mulder SM, et al: Comparison of oral transmucosal fentanyl citrate and an oral solution of meperidine, diazepam, and atropine for premedication in children. Anesthesiology 70:616-621, 1989
56. Stanley TH, Leiman BC, Rawal N, et al: The effects of oral transmucosal fentanyl citrate premedication on preoperative behavioral responses and gastric volume and acidity in children. Anesth Analg 69:328-335, 1989
57. Streisand JB, Stanley TH, Hague B, et al: Oral transmucosal fentanyl citrate premedication in children. Anesth Analg 69:28-34, 1989
58. Schechter NL, Weisman SJ, Rosenblum M, et al: Sedation for painful procedures in children with cancer using the fentanyl lollipop: A preliminary report, Advances in Pain Research Therapy. Vol 15. Edited by Tyler DC, Krane EJ. New York, Raven Press Ltd, 1990, pp. 209-213
59. Ashburn MA, Streisand JB, Tarver SD, et al: Oral transmucosal fentanyl citrate for premedication in paediatric outpatients. Can J Anaesth 37:857-66, 1990
60. Lind GH, Marcus MA, Ashburn MA, et al: Oral transmucosal fentanyl citrate for analgesia and anxiolysis in the emergency room. Anesth Analg 70:S241, 1990
61. Striebel H, Koenigs D, Kramer J: Postoperative pain management by intranasal demand-adapted fentanyl titration. Anesthesiology 77:281-285, 1992
62. Helmers JH, Noorduin H, Van Peer A, et al: Comparison of intravenous and intranasal sufentanil absorption and sedation. Can J Anaesth 36:494-497, 1989
63. Fisher A, Vine P, Whitlock J, Hanna M: Buccal morphine premedication. Anaesthesia 41:1104-1111, 1986
64. Evans WS, Borges JLC, Kaiser DL, et al: Intranasal administration of human pancreatic tumor GH-releasing factor-40 stimulates GH release in normal men. J Clin Endocrinol Metab 57:1081, 1983

PHYSICIAN-ASSISTED SUICIDE AND EUTHANASIA

K. M. Foley

The issues of euthanasia and physician-assisted suicide have emerged once again in the public and professional medical literature. Numerous factors contribute to this public debate, including the advancements in high technological medical support systems for patients with respiratory or cardiac failure, the AIDS epidemic, policy shifts to individual rights from societal rights, the increasing prevalence of cancer, the increasing aged population, and the limitation in health care resources, particularly, for the care of the dying. Coincident with this debate and in support of patient-centered care has been the wide expansion of the use of living wills, advanced directives and health care proxies to protect patients from the medical systems—physicians and hospitals—who care for them (1-3).

For purposes of this discussion, euthanasia is defined as the physician's intentionally administering a treatment (usually medication) to cause the patient's death with the patient's fully informed consent. Voluntary active euthanasia is another term used to describe this action. Involuntary active euthanasia is the act of a physician to intentionally administer a treatment (usually medication) to cause the patient's death without the patient's full consent. The patient may be either incompetent or never asked. Physician-assisted suicide is the provision of medication to a patient with the intent that the patient will use the drug to commit suicide. In contrast, physicians withdrawing or withholding treatment from a patient to let him or her die or, similarly, administering opioids or sedative drugs to relieve pain and suffering in the dying patient, with the incidental consequence of causing either respiratory depression and extreme sedation resulting in the patient's death, are not considered as either physician-assisted suicide or voluntary or involuntary euthanasia. It is critical to recognize that the last two approaches are considered to be

T. H. Stanley and M. A. Ashburn (eds.), Anesthesiology and Pain Management, 373–384.

both ethical and legal in some situations (4). At the present time, most states have developed a growing consensus supporting the ethics of withdrawing and withholding life-sustaining treatments (the "double effect" principle). As well, the Supreme Court allows such medical practices in certain conditions. In the management of the patient with severe pain and suffering, the ethical principle of "double effect" has long been accepted by both physicians and non-physicians (5); however, there is significant confusion among health care professionals about this very specific issue (6).

THE PUBLIC DEBATE

Several public events have fueled the debate. These include: 1) a series of acts by Dr. Jack Kevorkian of both physician-assisted suicide and euthanasia for patients with medical illness (7), 2) the publication by Derek Humphrey of his book *Final Exit*, which became a best seller on the *New York Times Book List* (8), 3) the experience of the Netherlands where euthanasia has been permitted, although not legalized (9), 4) the referendums in the states of Washington and California to legalize euthanasia (10), and a 5) a series of public surveys that have attempted to poll the public perspective on this topic (12).

Cases of Dr. Kevorkian

In the case of Dr. Jack Kevorkian, 19 patients have died using his suicide machine (physician-assisted suicide). At least 2 patients have died by direct acts of voluntary euthanasia. Although much has been published about Dr. Kevorkian, only some of the families of the dead patients have come forward in public support of his actions. Again the limited available data on those who have died has not clearly defined the medical problems of the individual patients, their prior care, their psychological state, or their options for alternative treatments. This lack of data has made it difficult to understand the decision making in this group of patients.

Publication of Final Exit

Derek Humphrey's successful book, *Final Exit,* describes various approaches patients may consider in killing themselves. These range from the use of large doses of barbiturates, to the use of carbon monoxide poisoning, to the use of large plastic bags appropriately tied to produce asphyxia. The success of the book suggests the public's fascination with the topic and further supports the broad public interest in having not only a good death but a controlled death.

Euthanasia in the Netherlands

Advocates for the legalization of euthanasia in the United States point to the Netherlands' experience where euthanasia is permitted, although it remains illegal. The Netherlands represents the only country in Western civilization where active voluntary euthanasia is permitted. Debate over euthanasia has a long history in the Netherlands beginning in the 1970's, in which a series of court cases, as well as a State Commission, began to investigate the legal aspects of euthanasia (13). The Royal Dutch Medical Association played an active role in these discussions, as did the Dutch Supreme Court, leading to the establishment of the Remmelink Commission. Although the Dutch Penal Code prohibits taking another person's life, even at his/her explicit and serious request, through the work of the Remmelink Commission and by the passage of a bill in 1993 by the Dutch Parliament, it explicitly grants physicians immunity from prosecution if they adhere to three conditions for a justifiable euthanasia They must notify the coroner about a euthanasia death.

Because of the overwhelming nature of the anecdotal data, the Remmelink Commission began an empirical study of euthanasia in the Netherlands (9). They also reviewed completed questionnaires from anonymous physicians on 5,197 deaths between August and December 1990. The study estimated that there were over 9,000 explicit requests for euthanasia in the Netherlands each year, with almost half including a written directive. Only 3,000 requests resulted in euthanasia—1.8% of all deaths were by euthanasia, 0.3% by physician-assisted suicide and 17.5% by the withdrawal or withholding of life sustaining technology. Of particular interest, oncology patients represented the majority of patients who died by euthanasia (68%) and 27% of all deaths in the Netherlands are from cancer. In attempting to define the most common reason to request euthanasia, loss of dignity (57%) followed by pain (46%), were the most common reasons. As part of this general survey, the Remmelink study found that 84% of Dutch physicians had discussed euthanasia with at least one patient at some time. Fifty-four percent had participated in euthanasia, and 25% had done so within the previous two years. Twelve-percent of Dutch physicians claimed that they would not commit euthanasia under any circumstances, and 35% claimed that they had never committed euthanasia, but might consider circumstances that might lead them to this act. Of interest, in 75% of cases, physicians listed the euthanasia death on the death certificate as a death from natural causes. Less than 20% of euthanasia cases are properly reported to the state prosecutor, and only 25% of Dutch physicians believe that euthanasia cases should be reported. Probably the greatest concern coming from the Remmelink report was that in 0.8% of all deaths, which represented over 40% of the euthanasia cases, drugs were administered with the explicit intention to shorten the patient's life without the strict criteria for euthanasia being fulfilled. In most of the cases, euthanasia had been discussed with the patient, but the patient was not fully competent. This extension of euthanasia to incompetent patients and to minors was further brought up by the Commission study. The lack of physician compliance with the existing guidelines for the administration of euthanasia, particularly with the extension to incompetent patients and to minors, portends the kind of abuse that may often occur when euthanasia legislation is introduced (14).

EUTHANASIA DEBATE IN THE UNITED STATES

In the United States, public attention on the euthanasia debate became quite focused in the referendums in the states of Washington and California (10,15). At the present time there are a series of states, at least six, whose efforts to legalize euthanasia or physician-assisted suicide are in development. Of particular interest, the initiatives both in the state of Washington and California were defeated by votes of 56% to 44%. Public surveys which attempt to define public attitudes on physician-assisted suicide and euthanasia are currently underway. In one collaborative study, between the *Boston Globe* and the Harvard School of Public Health, 1,004 people participated in the survey, with 64% believing that physicians should be legally permitted to give a terminally ill patient in pain a lethal injection to aid in dying (11). Seventy-five percent thought withdrawal of life-sustaining treatment should be permitted, 20% stated that they would ask their physician for euthanasia if they had a terminal illness causing great pain, and 19% would ask the physician to assist in suicide. Of particular interest, only 11% would consider asking their family or friends to help them die if they had a terminal illness, and only 14% would be willing to help a terminally ill relative or friend commit suicide to end their suffering.

In a survey of public attitudes about cancer and pain, 69% of those surveyed reported that they would consider suicide if their pain was not effectively treated (16). It is always difficult to interpret these polls because it is hard to know what the public knows about their options for care and the necessary decision making that might go into appropriate care, or of the fact that only 14% would be willing to help a terminally ill relative or friend commit suicide, suggests that their perceptions of transferring this responsibility to someone else heavily weighs on their decision making. What is apparent from these public polls is that the American public wants to have a say in their care at the end of life, and may see physician-assisted suicide and euthanasia as the only approach, the only option.

In summary, these series of public events have contributed to the controversy and helped to support a concept that improved education of healthcare professionals on the care of the dying, as well as the greater understanding of the public's perspective on it, might help to further effective care for patients with advanced disease.

HEALTH CARE PROFESSIONAL DEBATE

"It's Over Debbie"

There have been a series of recent medical articles in leading journals that have attempted to refocus the debate. These include the JAMA article entitled "It's Over Debbie" (17). In this short piece, a young woman with advanced cancer is given an intravenous dose of morphine by a physician whose intent it is to end her life, and, therefore, end her suffering. This published case led to a series of reviews and commentaries debating the well-known issues of physician-assisted suicide and euthanasia. The case report posed several problems. The physician was a resident who did not have a clear relationship with the patient. There was no discussion of the social, psychological and medical factors contributing to the patient's medical and psychological state. There were no descriptions of whether the patient's pain control was adequate or inadequately relieved, and what, if any, methods were used to achieve adequate analgesia. Only a small dose of morphine was administered but the report implied a negative connotation for the use of opioids in this population of patients, suggesting that opioids served as agents of death, rather than as effective means to control pain and other symptoms. The value of the case, however, was that it brought to the forefront a professional debate on the care of the dying patient in pain. Subsequent articles addressed the need to develop guidelines for appropriate care for patients who are hopelessly ill (18).

The Case of Diane

In an attempt to push this argument further from a discussion of euthanasia to that of a physician-assisted suicide, Dr. Timothy Quill published his famous case, "Diane" (19). In this case, Dr. Quill gave the patient an appropriate dose of medication that she could use at any time when she wished to commit suicide. Similarly, the Diane case is a complicated one. Subsequent to the publication of the case, Dr. Quill was investigated by a New York State Grand Jury and the body of Diane was exhumed. Following a series of hearings, he was not charged, and this was based upon the fact that he had not been present at the death of the patient. Dr. Quill has written a book, *Death and Dignity*, based on his experiences as a hospice medical director and as an internist (20). He proposes that physician-assisted suicide be available to competent patients and sets forth a series of guidelines, in both the text as well as in a published paper, to facilitate this clinical practice for physicians.

In this book Dr. Quill issues a series of directives to the public, physicians, medical institutions and governments to "take charge and make change" to improve the care of dying patients. This book capitalizes on the current doctor and hospital bashing mode to make its point. Using case discussions, Dr. Quill graphically demonstrates the frequent failure and rare successes of what he terms "comfort care" for dying patients. In his book, his language is inflammatory and the examples he uses are frightening, only furthering the distrust that currently exists for the medical profession in the care of the dying patient. This sensationalism is particularly dangerous, because what he suggests as the limits of comfort care are factually incorrect, without reference and outdated. His use of the term "comfort care" subtly trivializes the specialties of palliative care medicine or hospice care, which have emerged in the last 20 years as systems of medical care.

In his chapter on public policy, for example, he cites the case of a dying lung cancer patient with respiratory failure and symptoms of suffocation. He argues that no good "comfort care" is currently available to such a patient. This is simply not true. Opioids, and, if necessary, sedative drugs such as benzodiazepines and barbiturates, are used to control patients' physical and psychological distress even to the point of continuous sedation. Such procedures are now well-described in both the internal medicine and critical care literature, as well as in the palliative care literature. In a palliative care service or in a hospice, this would be considered the standard of care for the dying patient who had signed orders refusing resuscitation, or whose health care proxy had agreed to this approach. This is neither physician-assisted suicide nor euthanasia, but good medical care provided by a responsible physician to treat pain and suffering in the dying patient. Dr. Quill argues that such care is not available to patients, or when it is available it does not work efficiently, yet he provides no data to support this statement. Dr. Quill is correct in suggesting that there are limitations to comfort care. However, he fails to make distinctions among the populations of dying patients, patients with uncontrolled pain, those with uncontrolled symptoms, and those with intolerable psychological distress, with or without uncontrolled pain or excessive symptoms—that group of patients with significant existential suffering.

At the present time, current thinking in palliative care is that it is the responsibility of the physician to address the needs of all these patients and to define and carefully assess each component of these aspects of physical and psychological distress. As previously described, Dr. Quill cites as his most formative experience the case of Diane, for whom he provides adequate doses of barbiturates to allow her to kill herself on demand, alone at home at a point in time when she found her existence intolerable. It is this case that Dr. Quill uses to support his proposed guidelines to allow competent patients the opportunity to have available to them a death packet, that they may take at any point in time, should they view their suffering as intolerable (21). This proposal is narrow in its focus, denies a similar form of help to patients who are unable to administer drugs to themselves because of physical limitations and advocates physician assistance for a group of patients who may represent the highest percentage of patients with psychological factors contributing to their complaint, that is, the group of patients with existential suffering.

Although Diane's case is a formative experience for Dr. Quill, his discussions reflect his own concepts of medical care, and not the now broad existing literature on psycho-oncology and psychological complications of cancer. Diane had all the known risk factors for suicide. She had a family and a personal history of alcoholism. She had a past history of depression and a previous significant medical illness. Dr. Quill never suggests what might have happened if he had said no to Diane's request for barbiturates for sleep. In the case discussion, it was not clear to what extent Diane was either anxious or depressed, and what medications were tried to help control these symptoms. The fact that Dr. Quill, Diane's trusted physician, gave her the barbiturates, served as a signal to her that her greatest fears of any of the events surrounding her death were now being acknowledged as possible or real by her treating and trusted physician. This powerful acknowledgement of the truth of a patient's fears, whether real or unfounded, offers further credibility to the patient's belief that controlling their death is a necessity. In the case of Diane, the lack of detailed discussions of the psychological factors of the husband, son and patient and their family dynamics and Diane's need to control, and her degree of narcissism are not discussed. What of the role of the hospice nurse and hospice team caring for the patient? In short, this book *Death and Dignity* focuses on the need for humane and compassionate care of patients with terminal illness disregards and trivializes the recent developments in the entire field of pain management, palliative care and psycho-oncology, which offer better improved care for this population of patients.

SURVEYS OF PHYSICIAN ATTITUDES TOWARD PHYSICIAN-ASSISTED SUICIDE AND EUTHANASIA

As much as the cases of Debbie and Diane have served to charge the debate on this controversial issue, there have been a variety of professional surveys that have asked American physicians to comment on euthanasia. From these physician-based surveys, anywhere from 13% to 43% have been asked to commit euthanasia or physician-assisted suicide, and between 1% and 20% have committed some action that might be considered euthanasia. In addition, 28% to as many as 70% of physicians might consider euthanasia if it were legalized. There are numerous limitations to these surveys (10,22-26).

A recent survey was mailed to a total of 1137 professionals including internists, medical nurses and social workers at three institutions, a cancer research hospital, a university-based general hospital, and a hospital specializing in the care of the terminally ill (27). It was developed to measure the willingness to endorse assisted-suicide or euthanasia, and to evaluate demographics, professional status, perceived knowledge of symptom management approaches, religiosity, and "burnout." This survey, which had an overall response rate of 49.3%, included responses from 199 physicians, 276 nurses and 71 social workers. Initial analyses supported the validity and reliability of the derived scales, including a summary score for willingness to endorse assisted-suicide or euthanasia. This score was higher in social workers than physicians or nurses, and higher in physicians than nurses. Professionals at the hospital for the care of the terminally ill scored significantly lower than those at other sites. Scores were inversely correlated with religiosity, perceived knowledge of symptom control, and time spent in the management of cancer-related symptoms. Multiple regression analysis demonstrated that religiosity, professional discipline, institutional setting and the interaction between religiosity and perceived knowledge were all independent predictors of the willingness to endorse assisted-suicide or euthanasia, accounting for 43.8% of the variance. This particular survey points up the importance of several factors as determinants of professional attitudes toward physician-assisted suicide or euthanasia. Of interest from this study, the finding that professionals who perceive themselves to have relatively less knowledge or competence in symptom control, or who have less direct experience in the management of cancer related symptoms, are more likely to endorse the use of assisted suicide or euthanasia, raises substantial concerns about the implementation of these approaches should they become legal. Of particular interest, the study also addressed the issue of professional burnout. Although there was no significant correlation between the scores on the burnout scale and the willingness to endorse assisted suicide or euthanasia in the survey, further studies are clearly necessary to see to what degree this may play a role in the care of this population of patients.

A CALL TO ACTION: IMPROVED CARE FOR THE DYING PATIENT

In order to fully address this public and professional debate, there is an enormous need for better studies on the current status of the care of the dying. From available data, at least in cancer patients, evidence suggests that two-thirds of patients with advanced disease will have significant pain, and that currently available analgesic, drug and non-drug approaches will provide relief in 85% to 95% of patients. Yet several studies have pointed to the fact that upwards of 20% of patients may report moderate to severe pain in the last 4 weeks of life, and in a palliative care program upwards of 20% to 30% of patients may require sedation to control symptoms other than pain (29,30). To what extent patients dying in hospital settings have uncontrolled pain and uncontrolled symptoms remains unstudied. Similarly, the management of pain and other symptom control at home and in nursing homes has not been fully addressed. Moreover, there has clearly been a debate in the literature as to whether patients should "sleep before they die" (31). It is the physician's responsibility to control pain and suffering and to sedate patients, if necessary, to prevent undue suffering (32). To what extent and in what way should we care for those patients with profound existential distress? (33) Several authors have suggested that their dying patients can gain new growth and development and that it is the setting of care and the caregivers who can help support patients in these circumstances (34,35).

In short, we need to have a clear definition of the nature of suffering in this population of patients, develop a taxonomy, provide a system of care and study its outcome (36-38). Only in this way will we begin to really address the issues and needs of patient requests for physician-assisted suicide and euthanasia, and what should be the appropriate medical response.

REFERENCES

1. Reiser SJ: The era of the patient. JAMA 269:1012-1017, 1993
2. President's Commission for the Study of Ethical Problems in Medicine and Biomedical and Behavioral Research: Deciding to forego life-sustaining treatment. Washington D.C., U.S. Government Printing Office 1983
3. The Hastings Center: Guidelines on the termination of life-sustaining treatment and the care of the dying. Bloomington, IN, Indiana University Press, 1987
4. Emanuel EJ: A review of the ethical and legal aspects of terminating medical care. Am J Med 84:291-301, 1988
5. Ashley BM, O'Rourke KD: Healthcare ethics a theological analysis. Catholic Health Association, St. Louis, Mo., 1989
6. Coyle N, Adelhardt J, Foley KM, Portenoy RK: Character of terminal illness in the advanced cancer patient: pain and other symptoms during the last four weeks of life. J Pain Symptom Manage 5:83-93, 1990
7. Kevorkian placid under arrest, New York Times, Nov. 7, 1993
8. Humphrey D: Final Exit: The Practicalities of Self-Deliverance and Assisted Suicide for the Dying. Eugene, OR, Hemlock Society, 1991
9. The Remmelink Report. Health Policy. (Special Issue) 22:1-262, 1992
10. Initiative 119 WSMA membership survey. Seattle, Washington State Medical Association, March 1991
11. Knox RA: Poll: Americans favor mercy killing. Boston Globe, November 3, 1991:1,22
12. The Hemlock Society 1991 Roper Poll of the West Coast on Euthanasia. New York, Roper Organization, May 1991
13. de Wachter MAM: Active euthanasia in the Netherlands. JAMA 262:3316-3319, 1989
14. van der Maas PJ, van Delden JJM, Pinjnenborg L, Looman CWN. Euthanasia and other medical decisions concerning the end of life. The Lancet 338:669-674, 1991
15. Helig S: The San Francisco Medical Society Euthanasia Survey: Results and Analysis. San Francisco, CA, San Francisco Medicine 61:24-34, 1988
16. Cleeland CS, Cleeland LM, Dar R, Rinehardt LC: Factors influencing physician management of cancer pain. Cancer 58:796-800, 1986
17. Anonymous: It's Over Debbie. JAMA 259:272, 1988

18. Wanzer SH, Federman DD, Adelstein J, et al: The Physician's responsibility toward hopelessly ill patients. N Engl J Med 320:844-849, 1989
19. Quill T: Diane. New Engl J Med 324:691-694, 1991
20. Quill T: Death & Dignity. WW Norton & Co, New York, 1993
21. Quill TE, Cassel CK, Meier DE: Care of the hopelessly ill: Proposed clinical criteria for physician-assisted suicide. N Engl J Med 327:1280-1384, 1992
22. Overmyer M: National survey: physicians' views on the right to die. Physician's Management 31:40-60, 1991
23. Crosby C: Internists grapple with how they should respond to requests for aid in dying. The Internist 33:10, 1992
24. Caralis PV, Hammond JS: Attitudes of medical students, housestaff, and faculty physicians toward euthanasia and termination of life-sustaining treatment. Crit Care Med 20:683-690, 1992
25. Fried TR, Stein MD, O'Sullivan PS, Brock DW, Novack DH: The limits of patient autonomy: physician attitudes and practices regarding life-sustaining treatments and euthanasia. Arch Intern Med (in press)
26. Heilig S: The SFMS euthanasia survey: results and analysis. SF Medicine 61(5):24-26,34, 1989
27. Portenoy RK, Coyle N, Kash K, et al: Determinants of the willingness to endorse assisted suicide: a survey of physicians, nurses and social workers. Manuscript in preparation, 1993
28. Foley KM: The treatment of cancer pain. NEJM, 313:84-95, 1985
29. Coyle N: The euthanasia and physician-assisted suicide debate: Issues for nursing. Oncol Nurs Forum 19:41-46, 1992
30. Ventafridda V, Ripamonti C, DeConno F, Tamburini M, Casseleth BR: Symptom prevalence and control during cancer patients' last days of life. J Palliative Care 6:7-11, 1990
31. Roy D: Need they sleep before they die. J Palliative Care 6:3-4, 1991
32. Foley KM: The relationship of pain and symptom management to patient requests for physician-assisted suicide. J Pain Symptom Manage 6:289-297, 1991
33. Callahan D: The Troubled Dreams of Life. Simon and Schuster, New York, 1993
34. Byock I: The euthanasia/assisted suicide debate matures. Amer J Hospice and Palliative Care, March/April, 1993
35. Mount B: A final crescendo of pain. J Palliative Care 6:3-4, 1991
36. Cassell E: The nature of suffering and the goals of medicine. NEngl J Med 306:639-645, 1982
37. Cherny NI, Coyle NM, Foley KM: Aggressive treatment of suffering. Manuscript in preparation, 1993

DEVELOPMENTS IN CRITICAL CARE MEDICINE AND ANESTHESIOLOGY

1. O. Prakash (ed.): *Applied Physiology in Clinical Respiratory Care*. 1982 ISBN 90-247-2662-X
2. M. G. McGeown: *Clinical Management of Electrolyte Disorders*. 1983 ISBN 0-89838-559-8
3. T. H. Stanley and W. C. Petty (eds.): *New Anesthetic Agents, Devices and Monitoring Techniques*. Annual Utah Postgraduate Course in Anesthesiology. 1983 ISBN 0-89838-566-0
4. P. A. Scheck, U. H. Sjöstrand and R. B. Smith (eds.): *Perspectives in High Frequency Ventilation*. 1983 ISBN 0-89838-571-7
5. O. Prakash (ed.): *Computing in Anesthesia and Intensive Care*. 1983 ISBN 0-89838-602-0
6. T. H. Stanley and W. C. Petty (eds.): *Anesthesia and the Cardiovascular System*. Annual Utah Postgraduate Course in Anesthesiology. 1984 ISBN 0-89838-626-8
7. J. W. van Kleef, A. G. L. Burm and J. Spierdijk (eds.): *Current Concepts in Regional Anaesthesia*. 1984 ISBN 0-89838-644-6
8. O. Prakash (ed.): *Critical Care of the Child*. 1984 ISBN 0-89838-661-6
9. T. H. Stanley and W. C. Petty (eds.): *Anesthesiology: Today and Tomorrow*. Annual Utah Postgraduate Course in Anesthesiology. 1985 ISBN 0-89838-705-1
10. H. Rahn and O. Prakash (eds.): *Acid-base Regulation and Body Temperature*. 1985 ISBN 0-89838-708-6
11. T. H. Stanley and W. C. Petty (eds.): *Anesthesiology 1986*. Annual Utah Postgraduate Course in Anesthesiology. 1986 ISBN 0-89838-779-5
12. S. de Lange, P. J. Hennis and D. Kettler (eds.): *Cardiac Anaesthesia*. Problems and Innovations. 1986 ISBN 0-89838-794-9
13. N. P. de Bruijn and F. M. Clements: *Transesophageal Echocardiography*. With a contribution by R. Hill. 1987 ISBN 0-89838-821-X
14. G. B. Graybar and L. L. Bready (eds.): *Anesthesia for Renal Transplantation*. 1987 ISBN 0-89838-837-6
15. T. H. Stanley and W. C. Petty (eds.): *Anesthesia, the Heart and the Vascular System*. Annual Utah Postgraduate Course in Anesthesiology. 1987 ISBN 0-89838-851-1
16. D. Reis Miranda, A. Williams and Ph. Loirat (eds.): *Management of Intensive Care*. Guidelines for Better Use of Resources. 1990 ISBN 0-7923-0754-2
17. T. H. Stanley (ed.): *What's New in Anesthesiology*. Annual Utah Postgraduate Course in Anesthesiology. 1988 ISBN 0-89838-367-6
18. G. M. Woerlee: *Common Perioperative Problems and the Anaesthetist*. 1988 ISBN 0-89838-402-8
19. T. H. Stanley and R. J. Sperry (eds.): *Anesthesia and the Lung*. Annual Utah Postgraduate Course in Anesthesiology. 1989 ISBN 0-7923-0075-0
20. J. De Castro, J. Meynadier and M. Zenz: *Regional Opioid Analgesia*. Physiopharmacological Basis, Drugs, Equipment and Clinical Application. 1990 ISBN 0-7923-0162-5
21. J. F. Crul (ed.): *Legal Aspects of Anaesthesia*. 1989 ISBN 0-7923-0393-8

DEVELOPMENTS IN CRITICAL CARE MEDICINE AND ANESTHESIOLOGY

22. E. Freye: *Cerebral Monitoring in the Operating Room and the Intensive Care Unit.* 1990 ISBN 0-7923-0349-X
23. T. H. Stanley and R. J. Sperry (eds.): *Anesthesiology and the Heart.* Annual Utah Postgraduate Course in Anesthesiology. 1990 ISBN 0-7923-0634-1
24. T. H. Stanley, M. A. Ashburn, P. G. Fine (eds.): *Anesthesiology and Pain Management.* 1990 ISBN 0-7923-1073-X
25. T. H. Stanley and R. J. Sperry (eds.): *Anesthesia and the Lung 1992.* Annual Utah Postgraduate Course in Anesthesiology. 1992 ISBN 0-7923-1563-4
26. G. M. Woerlee: *Kinetics and Dynamics of Intravenous Anesthetics.* 1992 ISBN 0-7923-1506-5
27. A. Willner (ed.): *Cerebral Damage before and after Cardiac Surgery.* 1993 ISBN 0-7923-1928-1
28. R. J. Sperry, J. O. Johnson and T. H. Stanley (eds.): *Anesthesia and the Central Nervous System.* Annual Utah Postgraduate Course in Anesthesiology. 1993 ISBN 0-7923-2083-2
29. T. H. Stanley and M. A. Ashburn (eds.): *Anesthesiology and Pain Management.* 1994 ISBN 0-7923-2662-8

KLUWER ACADEMIC PUBLISHERS – DORDRECHT / BOSTON / LONDON

The manufacturer's authorised representative in the EU is Springer Nature Customer Service Centre GmbH, Europaplatz 3, 69115 Heidelberg, Germany. If you have any concerns regarding our products, please contact ProductSafety@springernature.com

Printed and bound by CPI Group (UK) Ltd, Croydon, CR0 4YY
27/07/2026
02177365-0004